AF361680

Emergencies and Public Health Crisis Management-Current Perspectives on Risks and Multiagency Collaboration

Emergencies and Public Health Crisis Management-Current Perspectives on Risks and Multiagency Collaboration

Editors

Amir Khorram-Manesh
Frederick M Burkle

MDPI • Basel • Beijing • Wuhan • Barcelona • Belgrade • Manchester • Tokyo • Cluj • Tianjin

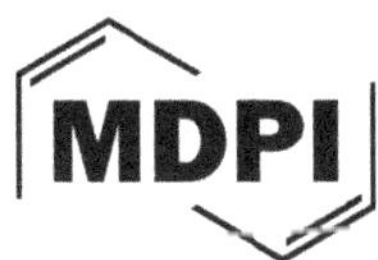

Editors
Amir Khorram-Manesh
Institute of Clinical Sciences,
Department of Surgery,
Gothenburg University
Sweden

Frederick M Burkle
Harvard Humanitarian Initiative,
Harvard University & T.H. Chan
School of Public Health
USA

Editorial Office
MDPI
St. Alban-Anlage 66
4052 Basel, Switzerland

This is a reprint of articles from the Special Issue published online in the open access journal *Sustainability* (ISSN 2071-1050) (available at: https://www.mdpi.com/journal/sustainability/special_issues/emergencies_crisis_management).

For citation purposes, cite each article independently as indicated on the article page online and as indicated below:

LastName, A.A.; LastName, B.B.; LastName, C.C. Article Title. *Journal Name* **Year**, *Article Number*, Page Range.

ISBN 978-3-03943-681-1 (Hbk)
ISBN 978-3-03943-682-8 (PDF)

Contents

About the Editors

Amir Khorram-Manesh currently works as a senior lecturer in surgery and disaster medicine, trauma, and public health. He has international engagement as a visiting professor in various countries, such as at Mahidol University in Bangkok, Thailand, and Shiraz University of Medical Sciences in Shiraz, Iran. He is research advisor and executive member of the Gothenburg Emergency Medicine Research Group (GEMREG) and at the Center for Disaster Medicine in Gothenburg, Sweden. He conducts research in disaster and emergency medicine, trauma, and public health.

Frederick M Burkle currently works as a senior fellow and scientist at the Harvard Humanitarian Initiative, Harvard University, and T.H. Chan School of Public Health. He is also a senior international public policy scholar at Woodrow Wilson International Center for Scholars, Washington, DC, U.S.A. Frederick conducts research in international and humanitarian medicine, emergency medicine, and disaster medicine. He is trained in emergency medicine, pediatrics, psychiatry, public health, and tropical medicine. His major interest is in global public health advancement.

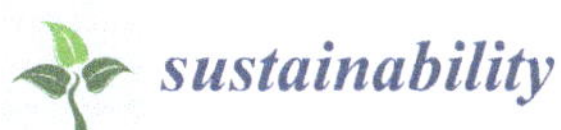 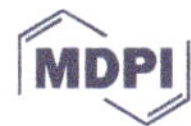

Editorial

Disasters and Public Health Emergencies—Current Perspectives in Preparedness and Response

Amir Khorram-Manesh [1,2,*] and Frederick M. Burkle Jr. [3]

[1] Institute of Clinical Sciences, Department of Surgery, Sahlgrenska Academy, University of Gothenburg, 405 30 Göteborg, Sweden
[2] Department of Research and Development, Swedish Armed Forces Centre for Defense Medicine, 426 76 Göteborg, Sweden
[3] Harvard Humanitarian Initiative, T.H. Chan School of Public Health, Harvard University, Boston, MA 02115, USA; skipmd77@aol.com
[*] Correspondence: amir.khorram.manesh@gmail.com or amir.khorram-manesh@surgery.gu.se; Tel.: +46-707-722-741

Received: 7 October 2020; Accepted: 15 October 2020; Published: 16 October 2020

Disasters and public health emergencies are inevitable and can happen anywhere and anytime. However, they can be mitigated and their impacts can be minimized by utilizing appropriate measures in all four different phases of disaster management, i.e., mitigation and prevention, preparedness, response, and recovery. Several factors are crucial for achieving successful disaster management. In the mitigation and preparation phase, all risks should be reviewed and new ones should be added and analyzed carefully to propose proper solutions and plans. In the preparedness phase, the ability and knowledge of each organization and all individuals in the management system should be tested and evaluated to ensure good readiness in responding to an emergency. Furthermore, plans should be available at all levels of the emergency chain of action to cope with all issues in the response and recovery phases [1,2]. This Issue of *Sustainability* aimed to cover emergency and public health crisis management from a multiagency perspective, by discussing lessons learned, introducing new ideas about flexible surge capacity, and showing the way it can practice multiagency collaboration.

One important part of mitigation and prevention is to analyze the potential risks in society. Risks are dynamic and may change due to social and political changes. In her paper, Posluszna reports the prognostic view on the ideological determinants of violence in the radical ecological movement [3]. She argues that ecologically motivated violence that manifests itself in animal and environmental rights has been increasing. Along with the multiplicity of the methods used (arson, food poisoning in supermarkets, destruction of equipment, and attacks with the use of incentivized devices), this type of violence should be considered as a dynamic and difficult-to-grasp phenomenon (eco-terrorism) that can endanger our society and its inhabitants and has the potential to create new public health emergencies and disasters. Starting with the ecosystem, there are other important natural resources and environmental factors, such as water, that are essential for the management of disasters and public health emergencies. In their report, Bross et al. discuss emergency preparedness planning in the water supply [4] and emphasize that various scenarios such as floods, power failures, or even a pandemic can influence the supply and provision of water. They present a newly developed composite indicator system to assess the status of emergency preparedness planning and compare two weighting methods. The results show that there is a need for action in emergency preparedness planning at several levels, especially in the area of risk analysis and the evaluation of measures.

Preparedness enables staff to act confidently, but do they act efficiently? Goniewicz et al. try to answer this question by using a questionnaire to assess the relationship between hospital and staff preparedness and disaster response efficiency among healthcare providers in Poland. They reported that the evaluation of the preparedness and effectiveness of disaster response is essential for finding and removing possible gaps and weaknesses in the functioning and effective management of a hospital during mass-casualty incidents [5]. Thus, preparedness is crucial, but how prepared are we? From this perspective, the emergency staff's "perception of preparedness is particularly important, since they influence risk assessment and risk communication to the public, policy agendas, and implementation of policies and initiatives [6–8]".

In their report, Sultan et al. assessed the perceived disaster readiness of emergency nurses in the southern part of Saudi Arabia by using a self-assessment questionnaire. The participating nurses reported good perceived knowledge in almost all investigated aspects of the theoretical dimensions, but perceived weaknesses in practical dimensions of emergency management and difficulties in assessing their own efforts. Simulation exercises, including theoretical and practical aspects of emergency management, were suggested to continuously examine and strengthen nurses' knowledge, skills, and abilities [9]. These results are concordant with those reported by Diakakis et al., who also found a correlation between knowledge and perception of risks and readiness with personal characteristics of participants, such as education level, qualification, age, years in service, etc., whereas, handling the everyday issues, practices and processes was correlated with their positions in the hierarchical chain [10]. Although prepared and knowledgeable, are healthcare providers really willing to risk their lives to work during disasters and public health emergencies? The willingness of healthcare providers to stay and fight in an emergency and the impact of social support on job engagement and retention intention was examined by Kim et al., among nurses struggling in the continuing scenes of the current pandemic (COVID-19). Data collected in this study showed that nurses' job engagement and job retention intention were high, depending on their age and work experience. However, in terms of factors related to the Covid-19 pandemic, the group with experience in nursing patients infected with COVID-19 and nurses working in COVID-19 divisions had low job-retention intentions. They could also identify possible differences in job engagement and job-retention intention due to the category and type of social support. These results suggest that social support should be provided strategically to ensure nurses' job retention [11].

Preparedness should be enhanced by multiagency exercises and training, and in all environments, i.e., water, air, and land. Carlström et al. [12] investigated differences between on-shore and off-shore exercises and aimed to compare findings from trained emergency staffs' perceptions of the impact of exercises. Data collected from surveys showed that collaboration is a predictor for some of the items in learning, and learning was a predictor for some of the items in utility. There was, however, a stronger covariation between collaboration, learning, and utility in the off-shore exercises than in the on-shore. This result is interesting, as it points out the potential of cultural differences in different organizations as well as professional attitudes and legal restrictions in the outcome of training and exercises. Karlsson et al. [13] aimed to explore the collaborative learning process of exercise organizers from the rescue service, mining companies, the emergency medical service, a training company, and academia. They used the theory cycle of expansive learning to the material consisting of documents from collaboration meetings and full-scale exercises to make tools in collaboration with the participants. These tools were further examined and tested during collaboration meetings and were implemented during full-scale exercises. The exercise organizers believed that this process led to organizational development and a better understanding of the other organizations' perspectives. Consequently, a tentative model for developing the learning process of exercise organizers was developed. Dealing with collaboration as an important factor in the teamwork, Sørensen et al. [14] conducted a study to test whether there is a relationship between exercise participation and perceived levels of learning and utility by using an online survey. Data were collected from participants in a two-day, full-scale, wildland-fire collaboration exercise in southeastern Norway, using an already existed instrument, the collaboration, learning, and utility (CLU) scale. According to their findings, joint evaluations, improvising, and testing of new and alternative strategies across sectors are important when exercises are constructed. Finally, Steiro et al. [15] presented lessons learned from a case study in the Norwegian armed forces to exemplify the importance of preparedness and multiagency collaboration. The paper aimed to investigate the structure for learning and the learning outcomes from a paper exercise based on multiagency collaboration and point to potential benefits for crisis leadership and management in civil organizations by using the participant observation model in one exercise and a questionnaire in the following exercise to measure outcomes. They identified five management principles for interaction under unforeseen conditions: (1) develop a pedagogical view for the organization, (2) facilitate and train using processes for complementary process development, (3) develop a precise and common language, (4) train the organization in concurrent learning, and (5) develop tolerance and mutual respect. These reports all indicate the need for collaboration and coordination, not only among various agencies but also among different states and nations. Current pandemic shows that all nations and states can be influenced, and indicates a need for a collaborative and coordinated approach to healthcare, and economic and social issues resulting from a disaster [16,17].

Besides preventive measures and proper preparedness, the response to the disaster and public health emergency management requires both structural and non-structural resources. Glantz et al. emphasize the concept of flexible surge capacity and the need for extra resources in an expanding emergency to increase local and regional surge capacity in a flexible manner [18]. They investigated the use of alternative care facilities within a community and found interest and ability in the primary healthcare centers; veterinary and dental clinics; and schools, sports, and hotel facilities, to participate in such a system, either by receiving resources and/or drills and exercises. Limiting factors for potential participation in this response system consisted of a varying lack of devices, healthcare materials, competences, clear organizational structure, legal support, medical responsibility, and sufficient funding. Raidla et al. [19] argue that an alternative care facility can also be organized within or near to a hospital to improve the flexibility needed in peacetime as well as during disasters. They investigated this concept by examining how the establishment of an urgent care center (UCC), i.e., a secondary emergency department (ED), co-located and in close collaboration with an ED, can influence the outcome of treatment in terms of length of stay, time to a physician, and use of medical services. The results showed reduced waiting times at the UCC, both in terms of length of stay, and time to a physician. They concluded that creating a primary care-like facility in close proximity to the hospitals may not only relieve overcrowding of the hospital's EDs in peacetime but may also provide an opportunity to create a flexible resource to be used during disasters and public health emergencies. A flexible surge capacity needs trained leadership and other personal resources. Phattharapornjaroen et al. [20] searched for alternative leadership among emergency physicians (EP) in Thailand [17]. Using an established method for training collaboration, two training courses were arranged for over 50 Thai EPs, who were divided into three teams of prehospital, hospital, and incident command groups. Three scenarios of a terror attack, along with a bomb explosion, riot, and shooting, and high building fire, were presented, and the participants' performance was evaluated regarding their preparedness, response, and knowledge gained. The results obtained in this study showed that Thai EPs' perceived ability in command and control, communication, collaboration, coordination, and situation assessment improved in all groups systematically. New perspectives and innovative measures were presented by participants, which improved the overall management on the final day. They conclude that tabletop simulation exercises can be used to increase the perceived ability, knowledge, and attitude of Thai EPs in managing major incidents and disasters, providing alternative leadership as part of the concept of a flexible surge capacity response system.

Finally, the current Covid-19 pandemic has shown the importance of the public-private partnership (PPP) during both the response and the recovery phases of disasters and public health emergencies. In these phases, there is the possibility of widespread project failures and constrained budgets, which makes governments search for ways to prioritize projects in the need of relief and bolster post-pandemic recovery plans. To meet this need, Baxter et al. conceptualized a triage system for PPP programs based on five categories: (1) projects without a need for economic stimulus (blue); (2) projects experiencing minor economic/financial losses (green); (3) projects needing temporary/stop-gap support or restructuring (yellow); (4) projects unable to survive without significant economic relief (red); and

(5) projects that cannot survive, even with government intervention (black) [21]. They also stress the importance of launching and sustaining a central crisis command to support PPP triage decisions and encourage PPP stakeholders to collectively craft win–win solutions for post-pandemic recovery efforts.

Altogether, this Issue offers new insights into emergency and public health crisis management from a multiagency perspective and allows discussion about new potential risks; lessons learned; and the introduction of new concepts such as flexible surge capacity, and shows some new aspects of practicing multiagency collaboration before, during, and after disasters and public health emergencies.

Funding: The research received no external funding.

Conflicts of Interest: The authors declare no conflict of interest.

References

1. Burkle, F.M., Jr. Disaster management, disaster medicine and emergency medicine. *Emerg. Med. Aust.* **2001**, *13*, 143–144. [CrossRef] [PubMed]
2. Khorram-Manesh, A. Flexible Surge Capacity—Public heaklth, public education, and disaster management. *Health Promot. Prespect.* **2020**, *10*, 175–179. [CrossRef] [PubMed]
3. Posluszna, E. A prognostic view on the ideological determinants of violence in the radical ecological movement. *Sustainability* **2020**, *12*, 6536. [CrossRef]
4. Bross, L.; Wienand, I.; Krause, S. Batten Down the Hatches—Assessing the status of emergency preparedness planning in the German water supply sector with statistical and expert-based weightng. *Sustainability* **2020**, *12*, 7177. [CrossRef]
5. Goniewicz, K.; Goniewicz, M. Disaster preparedness and professional competence among healthcare providers: Pilot study results. *Sustainability* **2020**, *12*, 4931. [CrossRef]
6. Donovan, A.; Eiser, J.R.; Sparks, R.S.J. Scientists' views about lay perceptions of volcanic hazard and risk. *J. Appl. Volcanol.* **2014**, *3*, 1–14. [CrossRef]
7. Boholm, Å.; Prutzer, M. Experts' understandings of drinking water risk management in a climate change scenario. *Clim. Risk Manag.* **2017**, *16*, 133–144. [CrossRef]
8. Beck, U. *Risk Society: Towards a New Modernity*; Sage: Newcastle upon Tyne, UK, 1992.
9. Sultan, M.H.S.; Khorram-Manesh, A.; Carlström, E.; Sørensen, J.L.; Al Sulayyim, H.J.; Taube, F. Nurses' readiness for emergency and public health challenges—The case of Saudi Arabia. *Sustainability* **2020**, *12*, 7874. [CrossRef]
10. Diakakis, M.; Damigos, D.G.; Kallioras, A. Identification of Patterns and Influential Factors on Civil Protection Personnel Opinions and Views on Different Aspects of Flood Risk Management: The Case of Greece. *Sustainability* **2020**, *12*, 5585. [CrossRef]
11. Kim, Y.J.; Lee, S.Y.; Cho, J.H. A study on the job retention intention of nurses based on social support in the Covid-19 situation. *Sustainability* **2020**, *12*, 7276. [CrossRef]
12. Carlström, E.; Magnussen, L.I.; Kristiansen, E.; Berlin, J.; Sørensen, J.L. Inter-Organizational exercises in dry and wet context-Why do maritime response organizations gain more knowledge from exercises at sea than those on shore. *Sustainability* **2020**, *12*, 5604. [CrossRef]
13. Karlsson, S.; Saveman, B.I.; Hultin, M.; Eklund, A.; Gyllencreutz, L. Expansive learning process of exercise organizers: The case of major fire incident exercises in underground mines. *Sustainability* **2020**, *12*, 5790. [CrossRef]
14. Sørensen, J.L.; Halvorsen, C.; Aas, J.P.W.; Carlström, E. "Share Your Tools"—A utility study of a Norwegian Wildland-Fire collaboration exercise. *Sustainability* **2020**, *12*, 6512. [CrossRef]
15. Steiro, T.J.; Torgersen, G.E. Preparedness and multiagency collaboration—Lessons learned from a case study in the Norwegian Armed Forces. *Sustainability* **2020**, *12*, 7240. [CrossRef]
16. Khorram-Manesh, A.; Carlström, E.; Hetelendy, A.J.; Goniewicz, K.; Carter, B.C.; Burkle, F.M. Does the prosperity of a country play a role in COVID-19 outcomes? *Disaster Med. Public Health Prep.* **2020**, 1–10. [CrossRef] [PubMed]
17. Goniewicz, K.; Khorram-Manesh, A.; Hetelendy, A.J.; Goniewicz, M.; Naylor, K.; Burkle, F.M. Current response and management decisions of the European Union to the COVID-19 outbreak: A review. *Sustainability* **2020**, *12*, 3838. [CrossRef]

18. Glantz, V.; Phattharapornjaroen, P.; Carlström, E.; Khorram-Manesh, A. Regional Flexible Surge Capacity—A flexible response system. *Sustainability* **2020**, *12*, 5984. [CrossRef]

19. Reidla, A.; Darro, K.; Carlson, T.; Khorram-Manesh, A.; Berlin, J.; Carlström, E. The outcomes of establishing an Urgent Care Centre in the same location as an emergency department. *Sustainability* **2020**, *12*, 8190. [CrossRef]

20. Phattharapornjaroen, P.; Glantz, V.; Carlström, E.; Dahlén Holmqvist, L.; Khorram-Manesh, A. Alternative leadership in Flexible Surge Capacity—The perceived impact of tabletop simulation exercises on Thai emergency physicians' capability to manage a major incident. *Sustainability* **2020**, *12*, 6216. [CrossRef]

21. Baxter, D.; Casady, C.B. A Coronavirus (COVID-19) Triage framework for (Sub) National Public-Private Partnership (PPP) Programs. *Sustainability* **2020**, *12*, 5253. [CrossRef]

Publisher's Note: MDPI stays neutral with regard to jurisdictional claims in published maps and institutional affiliations.

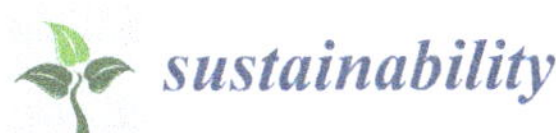 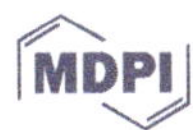

Article

A Prognostic View on the Ideological Determinants of Violence in the Radical Ecological Movement

Elżbieta Posłuszna

Faculty of Aviation Safety, Military University of Aviation, 08-521 Dęblin, Poland; e.posluszna@law.mil.pl

Received: 2 July 2020; Accepted: 9 August 2020; Published: 13 August 2020

Abstract: Ecologically motivated violence that manifests itself in the animal-rights and environmental forms is not a declining phenomenon. The fluctuating increase of the number of ecologically motivated crimes during the last 50 years, the multiplicity of the methods used (arson, food poisoning in supermarkets, destruction of equipment, attacks with the use of incentivized devices) should make us look at eco-extremism as a dynamic and difficult to grasp phenomenon. The paper is of both explanatory and prognostic nature; its goal is to present the genesis and essence of ecological radicalism, as well as to formulate the predictions for the future. In these forecasts, I wish to depart from the frequent, albeit somewhat simplistic, argument that, since the environmental extremist groups have not yet resorted to direct violence (targeting humans), and the animal-rights groups have reached for it very rarely, this state of affairs will continue in the future. This claim does not necessarily have to be true. I argue that some aspects of ideology can induce, in certain circumstances (a growing ecological catastrophe, further departure from the anthropocentric perspective), a change of the potential of radicalism within the environmental and animal-rights movements. In the case of animal-rights groups, the principle of not causing harm to people may be openly rejected, and in the case of environmental groups, the actions aimed at the annihilation of the whole human species may be undertaken.

Keywords: ecoterrorism; environmental extremism; animal-rights extremism; deep ecology; ecologically motivated violence

---

1. Introduction

We live in the shadow of the coming crisis. However, this crisis will be different from all the previous ones, for it will cover all spheres of life and will be total in its nature. It is a crisis of paradigms; the paradigms, like anthropocentrism or dichotomism, that for centuries, brought forth achievements of our civilization. These paradigms, however, have eventually led to the threat of self-destruction.

In 1962, Rachel Carson emphasized the need for attention to the emerging ecological crisis, by describing the impact of insecticides (such as DDT or aldrin) on the natural environment and the life support system over the longer term [1]. According to Carson, the greed and egoism of the lethal pesticide industry cannot be easily stopped, just as it is the case with the pursuit of technological progress that has become a permanent element of the post-war world. Therefore, the natural world, and consequently, human beings, are in mortal danger, and this cannot be easily reversed. Many ecological thinkers, such as Clarence Morris, Lynna White, and Christopher Stone followed this way of thinking, as well as numerous radical environmental and animal-rights organizations (Earth First!, Earth Liberation Front, and Animal Liberation Front).

British scientist James Lovelock presented a slightly different vision of the catastrophe (disaster) in his Gaia hypothesis in the early 1970s [2]. According to this hypothesis, the Earth is not merely a collection of living and inanimate entities, but a living superorganism that manipulates the Earth's atmosphere for its benefit, and strives for optimal harmony that promotes the development of life [2].

It is in Gaia's interest to keep all life on Earth in the state of dynamic balance (homeostasis). When this balance is disturbed, e.g., due to pollution or collision with a meteorite, it usually leads to the extinction of species, but not necessarily to the disappearance of life on Earth. The reason might be the fact that the earth will be able to adapt to new conditions and will survive; however, this adaptability may not necessarily be applied to its individual parts that have not developed such capabilities.

Although both concepts differ in the way that they see the future of the ecological system (according to the first, it will degrade, while the second states that it will cope), there is something that undoubtedly links them together, namely the belief that a catastrophe caused by humanity will destroy the foundations of its existence, and thus the whole species. Indeed, the changes that have been taking place in the world do not engender optimism. The surface temperature of our planet has risen by 1 °C over the past 150 years [3]. The effects of global warming include climatic anomalies such as floods, drought, desertification, cyclones, and hurricanes. In many regions of the world, progressive soil degradation occurs, which is manifested by erosion, loss of organic components, desertification, acidification, salinity or alkalization (excessive accumulation of sodium compounds). The increased emission of sulfur oxide (SO_2) contributes to the formation of acid rain, which then cause the degradation of forests, vegetation, and diseases of animals and people [4]. As many as 50% of the animals that once shared the Earth with us have already disappeared. A significant population decrease has been observed in another 30% of species. In recent years, most of them have lost over 40% of their natural habitat area, and almost half of them have lost more than 80% of their areas of occurrence in 1900–2015 [3]. Modern meat production, mass-scale fishing, and modern chemistry-based agriculture destroy the natural environment, and in moral terms, they bring forth the death and suffering of millions of animals. All these changes are brought forth because of human activity. Unfortunately, that is not all. Mass deforestation and the destruction of meadows destroy habitats of wild animals that massively move near human homes. This, in turn, results in the occurrence of numerous zoonoses, such as Spanish flu, AIDS, measles, Nipah disease, Ebola hemorrhagic fever, swine flu, SARS, MERS or COVID-19 [5].

Radical ecologists believe that humans are destructive beings, who use and misuse nature in the process of satisfying their non-vital needs. Being part of nature, they, of course, are entitled to protection, but as misusers, they deserve condemnation, and perhaps even exclusion from the biological community. The aim of this paper is to discuss the risks posed by eco-terrorism, and to investigate which branch of the ecological movement will radicalize and hence create new threats.

It should be noted that many researchers have doubts regarding the usage of the term "terrorism" concerning radical animal rights and environmental groups. Among such scholars, there is, for example, Christopher C. Harmon, according to whom activists whose actions are motivated by the will to protect animals and natural environment do not usually have an inclination towards acts that could be described as "terrorist." This means that they do not seek to destroy the social order, and are usually opposed to all forms of bodily integrity violations. Their goal is not to generate a sense of threat, but to stop the activities of certain classes of people (vivisectors, entrepreneurs, foresters). It is in this narrow-range mode of operation that they try to influence the policy of a given country or region [6]. A similar opinion is expressed by Leonard Weinberg and Paul Davis [7] or Bron Taylor, according to whom "despite the frequent use of revolutionary and martial rhetoric by participants in these movements, they have not, as yet, intended to inflict great bodily harm or death" [8].

Of course, environmental activists, who construct their conceptual framework on a different philosophical basis than their opponents, do not accept the term "terrorism" to be used to describe their actions. They argue, taking a completely "non-anthropocentric" position (egalitarian in relation to sentient beings or holistic in relation to the natural world), that the use of the term "terrorism" to denote activities that do not target natural (the environmentalist perspective) or sentient beings (the animal-rights perspective) is an abuse originating from the traditional (anthropocentric) moral perspective. This perspective leads to the erroneous perception of violence and terrorism as something that can occur only in relation to human beings and their property, and not in relation to other non-human beings. If we abandon this erroneous factor, which is based on our harmful habits of thought and perspective, we will have to recognize that the "real terrorists" are not those who fight for "oppressed beings" (animal and natural), but rather those "that promote or defend the exploitation of the natural world" [9].

The term "terrorism" is not neutral. This word has strong negative connotations and is associated with the need to take decisive defense measures to combat it. Therefore, even if we do not revise our conceptual framework and do not take the non-anthropocentric position, we will have to recognize that using this term to refer to groups that operate according to the non-violence principle must give rise to a feeling of inadequacy, or even injustice. It is especially so when we compare their "violent" actions with the activities of such groups as the Islamist Al-Qaeda or the anti-abortion Army of God, which are undoubtedly much more brutal. Moreover, the radicalism of the animal-rights and natural environment defenders is not particularly "impressive" when compared to other types of radicalism born in Western civilization (e.g., religious, nationalist, single issue, far right, and far left), both in terms of the numbers and violent nature of attacks [10].

At this point, it should be noted that the environmental activists are often the target of "terrorist" attacks. According to David Helvarg, the author of *The War Against the Greens*, some of these attacks in the US are organized by the robust Wise Use movement, that gathers farmers, property developers, hunters, SUV users, miners, free-market advocates, and religious fundamentalists. This movement, in Helvarg's opinion, is, in fact, not a grassroots campaign, but a kind of "astroturf", behind which big business hides [11], as well as those who are responsible for a series of acts of violence, such as intimidation, arson, assault, rape, and even murder towards people involved in the environmental movement [11]. Carl Deal, in his book *The Greenpeace Guide to Anti-Environmental Organizations*, expresses a similar opinion [12]. Public Employees for Environmental Responsibility (PEER) that studies and analyzes the actions of Wise Use, lists on its websites a number of acts of violence perpetrated by supporters of the Wise Use ideology, among which there are shooting at buildings, beating and intimidating, and planting bombs [13–15].

2. Methodology

The goal of the paper is to provide a narrative, based on interdisciplinary research, review on the topic of eco-terrorism. The study was carried out on the philosophical, political, sociological, and historical level. The basis of the entire research process was, of course, analysis and synthesis. The analytical method was deployed to examine original source texts, and all types of other studies (scientific and non-scientific). The purpose of the analysis of the source texts was to extract the truth about a given document, and to ascertain on its basis, as well as on the previously acquired knowledge, what the actual facts were. The goal of the analysis of the secondary literature was to, apart from expanding knowledge about the phenomenon, extract "alternative truths" and confront them with the author's own research intuitions. With the use of synthesis in the research process, the author intends to go beyond the mere merging of reconstructed fragments of the studied phenomenon, and to create a complete, and most importantly, meaningful and rich picture of the whole.

The paper is based on many sources that can be classified into a few groups. The first one are scientific works. Some concern the phenomenon of eco-extremism, others broadly understood security. The second group of sources includes reports of analytical centers and statistical materials. Some reports come from government agencies, some from private agencies. The third group of sources consists of propaganda materials of the discussed groups and the so-called narrative sources, namely "testimonies" (i.e., confessions of environmental radicals). These materials are posted on websites or published in a traditional form. The fourth group consists of documentary sources (official documents, court records, trial transcripts, official letters). The fifth group of sources includes press releases and news agencies reports. There are difficulties related to all those sources because, as it happens, various sources often give contradictory information (sometimes it is due to the imperfection of human memory, and sometimes it stems from a deliberate bending of facts in the sake of one's own, usually ideological, interests). It also happens that the authors are not neutral in their approach, which often leads to a distortion of the image of a given phenomenon. Therefore, in my research, I had to place great emphasis on identifying the most reliable data and distinguishing between facts and ideological propaganda, which I did by relying on my knowledge about the authors, the source of materials, and socio-political context.

3. Results

3.1. The Characteristics of Ecoterrorism

The belief of human superiority over all other beings [16] was rarely negated within the European culture. However, everything changed in the 1970s, when, within the framework of the culture, an extremist trend appeared that changed gentle activism into unprecedented committed radicalism. Today, ecologically motivated violence is no longer a marginal phenomenon. The data published by the FBI shows that among 112 attacks carried out between 1986 and 2005 in the United States, classified as terrorism, 57 were organized by groups or individuals motivated by environmental or animal-rights ideologies, such as Animal Liberation Front, Earth Liberation Front, Stop Huntingdon Animal Cruelty, Arissa, Animal Rights Militia, Band of Mercy, Justice Department, Animal Liberation Brigade, Vegan Dumpster Militia, Sea Shepherd Conservation Society, Direct Action Front.

Although, in the United States, there were only nine attacks in 1986–1997, the number grew to 48 in 1998–2005 [17]. The total number of incidents in the USA between 1979 and 2008 committed by ecological extremists was around 2000, and their total cost was estimated at $110 million [18]. These statistics do not include minor vandalism attacks, or small acts of violence against people, or, finally, botnet swarm attacks [19]. R. L. Young's doctoral dissertation examined the period, 1993–2003, and identified over 1400 incidents of terrorism committed by environmental and animal rights extremists [20], while Varriale-Carson, LaFree, and Dugan documented 1069 criminal incidents committed by these groups between 1970 and 2007 [21].

According to the data of the Foundation for Biomedical Research, in 1981–2005, there were 529 ecology-related crimes committed in the United States, including 53 arson attacks, 123 thefts, 36 bombings, 238 acts of vandalism, and 79 cases of harassment. A particular increase in crimes occurred after 1999. In 1998, there were only seven registered incidents of that kind, but in 1999, the number grew to 27, and the trend continued—in 2000 there were 28 of them, in 2001—42, 2002—17, 2003—101, 2004—99, 2005—82, and so on [22]. According to the data presented by the National Consortium for the Study of Terrorism and Responses to Terrorism, in the United States alone, there were 239 attacks between 1995 and 2010—arson (38%) and bombing attacks (62%), perpetrated by environmental (54.8%) and animal-rights extremists (45.2%)—mainly the ALF (Animal Liberation Front) and the ELF (Earth Liberation Front). More than 42% of these attacks resulted in severe financial losses [23,24]. These data indicate an increase in the number of incidents in 1995 through 2001, a variation in the number of incidents until 2010, and a relatively stable level after 2010 [24].

According to the data gathered by AnimalRighstsExtremism.info, there were 27 serious incidents worldwide between April 2012 and 5 September 2016 [25]. In 2010–2019, animal rights organizations carried out approximately 2521 prohibited acts, including sabotage, arson, "liberation" actions (in 2019—264, in 2018—306, in 2017—225, in 2016—124, in 2015—139, in 2014—214, in 2013—241, in 2012—251, in 2011—387, in 2010—370) [26]. The Global Terrorism Index states that attacks on facilities and infrastructure were the most common form of terrorist attacks in the US between 2002 and 2018, with a total number of 239 attacks. The majority of attacks were carried out by animal rights and environmentalist groups. It should be stressed, however, that these types of attacks result in very low casualties and rarely have loss of life as the main goal [27]. According to William Braniff, the Director of National Consortium for the Study of Terrorism and Responses to Terrorism, between 2000–2009, animal rights and environmentally motivated terrorist attacks were carried out by Animal Liberation Front (Coalition to Save the Preserves, Earth Liberation Front, Environmentalists, Revenge of the Threes,

Revolutionary Cells, Animal Liberation Brigade). In 2010—2019, in the US, there were six terrorist attacks that can be attributed to Animal Liberation Front, one attributed to the Justice Department, and three to environmentalist groups. One deadly attack was carried out by an anonymous person driven by broadly conceived ecological ideology [10]. Of course, these statistics are highly selective and do not take into account the attacks carried out in Europe and other various parts of the world.

3.2. Reasons for the Emergence of Ecological Extremism

The reasons for the emergence of environmental and animal-rights extremisms seem to be different. The sources of the former could be found in the early 1960s, when the correlation between the increase of exploitation of natural resources and the growth of prosperity started to be questioned for the very first time. Moreover, more and more people (mainly in the U.S.) began to realize that the possibility of an ecological crisis is real, and when it occurs, it will threaten all the species living on the earth. This emerging environmental awareness quickly resulted in protective activities. As early as in the second half of the 1960s, the consumer movements in the United States started to demand the right for "the natural environment that would correspond to the needs of the human body and high quality of life." More and more organizations were established to lobby for the natural environment. Despite the high activity of these movements, their actions did not bring forth expected results, or the results did not satisfy all of the members, who increasingly demanded more radical forms of fighting for the conservation of the natural environment. The 1979 decision of the U.S. Forest Service to use 36 million acres of forest areas for commercial purposes; the so-called RARE II ("Roadless Area Review and Evaluation II") was, as it seems, a turning point in the formation of green extremism. The decision was a great shock for some environmental activists. It not only showed the lack of ecological awareness of the agency, but also demonstrated the weakness of the traditional environmental organizations that were not able to oppose it, or did not want to, due to e.g., their relationship with large corporations and government agencies, as well as large internal bureaucracy. Because of general dissatisfaction caused by this decision and the unfavorable climate around the "legal environmental organizations", several groups were established, the sole purpose of which was to decisively (and not necessarily lawfully) combat the growing indifference towards the natural environment [28].

The emergence of the animal rights extremism is more difficult to picture, since it is problematic to point out a turning point that could be considered to be an "ideological trigger" of the animal-rights radicalism. It is so probably because the process of becoming radical was evolutionary, not revolutionary; it was a consequence of ever stronger and courageous demands regarding broadening moral horizons, so they included all previously discriminated groups of beings, including those who are unable to articulate the liberation postulates themselves. The animal rights movement was born in the 19th century in England, and although initially, the source of its motivation were not animals but human beings, more precisely, their spiritual and moral development; the movement relatively quickly tried to reject this "narrow anthropocentric perspective" in order to entirely equalize the respect of the interests of all sentient beings. This was the path that facilitated a formulation; in the 1970s, the most radical (and yet very catchy) claim of the modern "liberation movement" so far, namely that the discrimination of a creature only because of its belonging to a particular species is a superstition as immoral as racism or sexism. In contrast to the environmental extremism, which constituted to the influence of an eco-systemic threat, the radical movement of animal protection came into being, because of an altruistic development of moral awareness.

In the second half of the 20th century, this development brought about a real abundance of radical animal-rights groups fighting for a total ban on exploitation and killing of animals. The activities of radical groups defending the rights of animals, as well as those fighting for protection and conservation of the natural environment, are often analyzed together under the umbrella terms "ecological terrorism" or [29–31]. Such an approach is justified by the fact that many organizations belonging to the two movements closely cooperate, because their objectives, in many respects, confluence. Despite the convergence of the goals and quite similar intra-organizational structure (leaderless resistance model), there are some ideological differences between the radical environment activists and animal rights defenders that prevent them from a complete organizational convergence. Such differences also mean that some researchers (such as Wayman Mullins, Kenneth Dudonis, David Schulz, Sean Eagan) distinguish between ecoterrorism or environmental terrorism, understood as violence in defense of nature, and animal rights terrorism, understood as violence in the defense of animals [32–34]. The Earth Liberation Front and the Animal Liberation Front are, respectively, the most prominent representatives of those two types.

The Earth Liberation Front (ELF) was founded in England in 1992, by former members of Earth First!. The group's aim is to restore the original ecosystems, which in the opinion of the group's members, have been destroyed as a result of immoral and selfish human activities. According to Earth First!, adopting an uncompromising view, based on the philosophy of deep ecology attitude towards the natural environment, is a necessary condition to achieve this goal. Moreover, such an attitude should be expressed by direct actions. The ELF's attacks are aimed primarily at timber companies, institutions promoting genetic engineering, construction companies, car sellers, and power generating and distribution businesses, as well as, it is worth emphasizing, all structures that embody the "greed and injustice of the capitalist state" [35]. This last point requires a short elucidation, for the ELF does not only want to destroy the capitalist system, but also to remove profit as a motive for action from all spheres of social life [36].

The Animal Liberation Front (ALF), the largest extremist animal-rights group, was founded in 1976 by Ronnie Lee. The main goal of the group is to fight all forms of human exploitation of animals. Their attacks are aimed primarily at the meat production, food, pharmaceutical, fur, zoological industries, as well as research institutions. In the first period of its activity, the most frequent method used by the group was sabotage: freeing animals, inserting sticky substances into holes in locks, destroying equipment, painting on windows or breaking them. This relatively mild period of the ALF's activity ended in the 1980s, when the group began to organize acts of economic sabotage, like arson, planting explosive and incendiary devices, devastating laboratory equipment, or bricking up windows in butcher shops. The radicalism of the ALF grew in the mid-1980s, when the group started attacking people. The attacks most often consisted of threats, intimidation, and relatively minor cases of assault and battery, although sometimes, more drastic acts of violence also occurred (planting explosive devices in the homes of people working in companies exploiting animals) [37].

3.3. Ideological Basis as a Source of Radicalism

The ideological foundation of the radical environmental and animal rights movements is undoubtedly anti-anthropocentrism that manifests itself in the belief that the human being is not a unique and superior element of the world. Human beings, therefore, should not occupy a privileged place among other beings. However, the category of "other beings" is not shared by the two ecological radical movements. According to the animal rights activists, it is limited to sentient beings (who possess the so-called interests), and according to environmentalists, it includes all-natural creatures (including those inanimate as well).

Another difference is the placement of moral value. In the case of environmental radicals, this placement is of holistic nature, i.e., it is based on the belief that nature is not a mere collection of living and inanimate beings, but a biogenic whole that is infinitely more perfect than its individual human or non-human forms of existence [38]. This whole is not an aggregate—it possesses peculiar characteristics that cannot be reduced to the characteristics of its constituents (i.e., it is not merely a sum of the properties of its individual parts). Analyzing this claim from an ethical perspective, may lead to the conclusion that nature as a whole has a higher moral value than the individuals that constitute it. It is well reflected by the words of Aldo Leopold from his *A Sand County Almanac*: "A thing is right when it tends to preserve the integrity, stability, and beauty of the biotic community. It is wrong when it tends otherwise" [39]. Hence, nature is, primarily, entitled to respect and protection, and its less perfect parts should be considered in the second place. The practical dimension of this claim refers to the threat posed by environmental extremists, which may be the gradation of beings (certain parts of the whole that belong to the lower levels of the food chain have higher moral value than the ones that are on the top, e.g., the existence of oceanic plankton or soil bacteria is essential for the functioning of the ecosystem, while the existence of humans or tigers is not necessary). Secondly, due to the integrity of the ecosystem, the life of the representative of the endangered species should be given a higher value than the life of the human being, whose species is not threatened with extinction. Thirdly, since the human being threatens the entire ecosystem and does not seem to be necessary for its functioning, it can be stated that it would be better for the ecosystem if the human species disappeared entirely from the surface of the planet.

From the perspective of prognostic considerations, it should be acknowledged that the above claim may also lead to a hypothesis that, as long as human activities do not directly threaten nature as a whole, but merely harm certain parts of it that do not possess a full autonomous moral value, it can be expected that the environmental organizations will use non-threatening forms of persuasion. It is especially so because of their strong conviction of the sanctity of all life, including human life precluding such attacks. Still, for many radical environmentalists, the human beings are "problematic"—they are, indeed, a part of nature, but, at the same time, go beyond it through their hostile actions towards nature. As part of nature, they are obviously entitled to protection; as the beings that destroy nature—condemnation, or perhaps even exclusion from the biological community. These two perspectives of looking at the human being overlap and intersect. However, this standoff does not have to be permanent. It may change as soon as a severe ecological crisis occurs; one that will not pose a threat to some parts of the ecosystem, but to nature as a whole, which is given almost divine status by environmentalists. Then, one can expect a significant radicalization of their actions, that might target not only individual people, but all humankind.

Of course, the belief that human activity threatens the ecosystem as a whole is always a subjective, to a certain degree, conviction. Moreover, apparently, such a subjective conviction guided the actions of the R.I.S.E group [40], which, in 1972, hoping for the annihilation of the human species [32], decided to reach for, in their opinion the most reliable remedy—pathogens (corynebacterium diphtheria, neisseria meningitides, salmonella typhi, shigella sonnei) [40]. The pathogens were to be sprayed in supermarkets and large buildings using special aerosols, and for contamination of the water supply system of Chicago. It was not the only case of using a biological weapon by an environmental group. In 1981, a not well-known group called Dark Harvest Commando in protest against anthrax contamination, during World War II, of a small Gruinard Island located close to the Scottish mainland, placed a package containing the soil taken from the island in front of the Chemical Defense Establishment in Porton Down in Wiltshire. A few days later, a similar package was dropped off at the conference of the ruling Conservative Party in Blackpool [41].

The animal rights movements place moral value in individuals. A distinctive feature of their ideology is what could be called an "individual approach", which is manifested in the belief that the life and well-being of the individual has the priority. A person has the right to defend them even if, in consequence, it will necessarily lead to an infringement of the well-being of the ecological community they are a part of. Moral value is attributed here, above all, to individuals [42]. The latter category, according to the defenders of animal rights, includes all living beings capable of feeling pleasure and suffering, and thus has interests [43]. Among such beings, there are, of course, human beings and animals. Killing morally significant individuals (the one possessing moral value) is treated as the greatest crime that has to be firmly fought against. The consequences stemming from the adopted by the animal activists' assumptions are unequivocal. If we accept that animals, as well as people, have the same capacity for suffering and the right to equal treatment, then we must also recognize that their often cruel exploitation is evil and comparable to what slaves experienced at plantations or prisoners in concentration camps [44]. If it is additionally accepted that this evil must be necessarily opposed with the use of all possible and adequate means, then using violence against humans begins to appear as the supreme moral obligation [37].

Still, the evil that the animal rights activists fight against is rather individual, not collective in nature. In their writings, there are not many references to the collective responsibility or catastrophic visions of the end of the world. "Animal executioners" have names and addresses; they are concrete people who must be stopped or even "neutralized" at any cost. There have been several attempts of such "neutralization." One dramatic attempt of resorting to violence in the United States was an incident involving an activist, who in November 1988, was apprehended at the premises of the United States Surgical Corporation (a company that used dogs for testing surgical staples), while she was planting a high-class explosive device equipped with a radio igniter at the parking spot of the head of the facility. In February 1990, the Dean of the Veterinary School of the University of Tennessee was shot to death on his private farm. A month earlier, local police received a warning from the FBI National Crime Information Center that animal rights extremists threatened to murder the Dean in the next 12 months. On 6 May 2002, another activist committed a murder, which was intended to protect the "weakest part of society", in which, as it seems, he included animals [45]. In spite of the attacks of that type, humanity, according to animal-rights extremists, is not an impediment to the liberation of animals. People and animals can live in peace and harmony. Therefore, it seems impossible that the radical animal-rights activists would be willing to target humans. On the other hand, it is plausible and should be assumed that violence against individuals blamed for the oppression of animals is unlikely to diminish. On the contrary, it can even, given the growing willingness to challenge anthropocentrism, significantly escalate and radicalize.

4. Tactics

However, the differences between the two types of groups are not limited merely to ideology. They also manifest themselves in relation to violence and the tactics derived from it. In its struggle for "restoring ecological balance", the environmental movement employs, almost exclusively, indirect violence that is based on acts of ecological sabotage, whereas animal-rights groups, apart from indirect violence, use also, although in a limited scope, direct violence targeting human beings.

a. **Sabotage:** Sabotage, also known as ecotage (ecological sabotage) or "monkeywrenching" (from a monkey wrench, the most popular tool of saboteurs), is a common tactic to both types of groups, and involves a variety of methods, among which the most commonly used are: setting fire to tourist centers in construction, "tree spiking" (inserting long metal rods into the trunks of trees that are to be cut down. When the saw chain hits such a spike, it is torn, and its pieces often hurt the loggers). Destruction of machines and equipment, knocking down billboards, removing signs from the ski trails, dismantling power lines (environmental groups), releasing animals, destruction and setting fire to laboratories, walling up windows in butcher stores, destroying equipment used for transport or the slaughter of animals (animal-rights groups). "Monkeywrenching is believed to be more than just sabotage. It is revolutionary, Jihad, which even affects innocent bystanders, because in these desperate hours, bystanders are not innocent" [8].

b. **Arson:** The most spectacular method of ecotage has always been arson. This method was used in a famous attack on the Vail Ski Resort in Colorado on 19 October 1998. Its purpose was to protect the land inhabited by lynxes, and resulted in the destruction of the restaurant, four hotel buildings, and three chairlifts. Monkeywrenchers caused damage assessed at $12 million. Burning down the Vail Ski Resort is no longer the most costly act of environmental sabotage. Another arson attack that caused a total burn down of a residential complex and a crane in San Diego on 1 August 2003, resulted in losses at around $50 million. The most costly case of sabotage motivated by animal-rights ideology in the United States was undoubtedly the arson attack on the University of California Veterinary Diagnostic Center in Davis on 16 April 1987, in which several buildings and 18 vehicles were destroyed, with a cost of about $3.5 million [46]. This attack was the first classified as "domestic terrorism" by the FBI [47]. In June 2006, ALF members claimed responsibility for a firebomb attack on a UCLA researcher. A firebomb was planted on the doorstep of a house occupied by a 70-year-old tenant. However, it failed to ignite. The attack was used by the acting Chancellor of UCLA, to constitute the Animal Enterprise Terrorism Act. In December 2015, the ALF admitted that they had organized an arson attack on a clubhouse operated by the Fox Terrier Association in Germany, in consequence of which, the building burned down. This attack came after an incident in June of the same year, when the ALF released several foxes from an enclosure on the club's plot [48]. In June 2015, another arson attack took place—fire was set to two trucks belonging to Harlan Laboratory in Mississauga, Canada. The activists accused Harlan of supplying research animals and animal feed for vivisectionists [49].

c. **Direct attacks on humans**: Sabotage actions are not the only ones that radical environmentalists carry out. Some of them who belong to a not a very numerous group fighting for animal rights reach for more violent forms of persuasion, namely, the attacks directly targeting humans. There are two groups that should be mentioned here—the Animal Rights Militia (ARM) and the Justice Department (JD). The ARM's actions have always been organized as single, isolated attacks, and their primal aim was to intimidate "animal enemies." The first action carried out by the ARM probably took place in England on 30 November 1982. Explosives were sent to the offices of the leaders of four major political parties. Three of them were disabled, but the fourth one exploded in the hands of an official, and caused minor injuries [50]. Another ARM's action consisted of poisoning of Mars candy bars on 18 November 1984, which forced the company to withdraw the "suspicious" batch of products from the stores, and a loss of £3 million. A similar action was carried out by the Canadian ARM in 1992 [51]. At the beginning of the 1990s, the ARM's attacks became more violent. The most common practice was planting incendiary bombs in stores. Other attacks reported are; threats to kill (1998), poisoning (2006), contamination (2007) [48,52]. The ARM also took responsibility for attacks in Sweden, mainly against vivisection personnel and fur farm owners. The actions involved planting firebombs at a McDonald's restaurant in Gothenburg in 2011, bomb threats, letter bombs, and vandalism, targeting fur companies and vivisection personnel. According to the Animal Liberation Press Office, in 2011–2012, there was a wave of ARM-claimed attacks in Sweden, which occurred after the arrest of a young animal rights activist, who was sentenced to prison in 2011 [48].

d. **Other methods**: The methods used by the animal-rights group Justice Department were in many respects similar to those employed by the ARM, i.e., beatings, blackmail, and relatively harmless bomb attacks. The first action of the JD consisted of sending several package bombs to people who practiced "bloody" off-road sports, such as hunting or fishing. The packages did not reach the recipients—the explosion occurred at the sorting office in Watford. In 1996, the JD attacked representatives of the leather industry with the allegedly soaked in HIV infected blood razor blades. In 1999, yet again, the Justice Department Anti-Fur Task Force sent a letter containing razor blades to the representatives of the American fur industry. In February 2009, two scientists from Wake Forest University in North Carolina experimenting on animals received letters with razor blades covered in rat poison [53]. A similar action took place on 22 November 2010, when the Justice Department at UCLA sent bloody AIDS tainted razor blades to a neuroscientist and animal researcher. The North American Animal Liberation Press Office posted an anonymous communiqué from the group, who claimed that they had carried out the action because the scientist used primates for government-funded testing of drug addiction [54].

5. Discussion

It is undoubtedly the fact that the sensitivity of society to environmental problems has considerably increased over the past few decades. Nobody now negates the need to care for the welfare of our planet and its inhabitants. Despite sustained development and the increasing popularity of the environmentalist movement, as well as eco-friendly legislation adopted by many governments, the destruction of the natural environment progresses rapidly. Oil stains, clusters of trash in the oceans, the mass felling of Siberian and Amazon forests, air pollution, water poisoning, soil degradation, not to mention the greenhouse effect, are the facts to which, despite the declared indignation, one gets no real widespread and spirited reaction. Environmental and animal-rights activists often see this incapacity for self-restraint as a manifestation of destructive property intrinsic to human nature, which leads to a global ecological disaster/catastrophe. The catastrophe could be avoided not only by rejecting the anthropocentric culture, but also everything that it has created (modern medicine and agriculture, technology, industrialism). There is much skepticism regarding human nature and the possibility of the voluntary abandonment of anthropocentrism, which could foster the occurrence of a hostile attitude towards the human species and the readiness to eliminate it, at least partially [55].

Moreover, the times when animals were considered to be only tools whose sole purpose was to serve humans have already happened. More and more people are willing to see in animals the beings that, due to their ability to experience suffering, must be respected and protected, and even have the right to life and unfettered development. Ninety years ago, when industrial production changed farming into agribusiness, the living conditions of breeding animals have dramatically deteriorated. In those who are sensitive to the suffering of animals, such a state of affairs must necessarily cause frustration and outrage, which can easily lead to a desire to punish those who are responsible for that suffering. Here, as well, it is anthropocentrism (speciesism) that is blamed for that situation, but because of a strong individualistic attitude and a lack of a holistic approach, this "placing blame" is never of a total nature, i.e., it does not encompass the whole species. This is why the response to the evil that is experienced by sentient beings (animals) has to be individual (attacks on particular human individuals).

Can ecological radicalism change its nature or intensity? As it seems, the number of sabotage actions have not significantly changed. Due to a slow overcoming of anthropocentrism, one should instead expect the opposite trend. However, one thing should be noticed—over the past twenty years, radical ecological organizations have constantly broadened the scope of their goals. Nowadays, these organizations do not limit themselves to attacking forest-felling companies, ski resorts, high-voltage power lines, or laboratories where experiments on animals are carried out. More and more often, large corporations, private houses, SUVs, as well as various symbols of capitalism, become the subject of attacks [46]. The anti-capitalist attitude is obviously nothing new among the radical environmentalists and animal-rights activists. It was there before, but open criticism of capitalism and globalization occurred in the late 1990s, especially after the protests in Seattle in the fall of 1999, when people closely associated with anarchism and alter globalism started to have more influence on these movements. For them, the liberation of the earth has become closely linked to the abolition of capitalism and social liberation. The way to achieve that was not a slow reform, but a revolutionary spurt, preceded by mass attacks on the elements of the capitalist system [56]. The actions of the ELF can be comprehended as acts of revolution, not reform. The liberation of the Earth equals the liberation of every one of us [28,57]. Paradoxically, the broadening of the scope of objectives by incorporating the social ones that are specifically human (and hence pro-anthropocentric) can in fact, lead to the intensification of actions, but rather not to their brutalization. Such a situation in the case of environmental groups can even become an ideological safeguard against anti-human activities, which, in the era of the ecological catastrophe and relatively easy access to means of mass destruction, will become more than probable.

The word "jihad" used by many activists should be understood as the "jihad of the sword" but also, and perhaps even above all, as the "jihad of the heart", which is a profound transformation in the way of thinking and feeling, and which must arise in the minds of all monkeywrenchers. It seems that although many interpretations of Islam propagate the intrinsic value of animals [58] and there are even calls for Islamic eco-jihad [59], the above mentioned activists had in mind rather a common perception of the word as a wide-raging fight against the enemy. The actions of destroying machinery and objects that pose a threat to nature are such a fight. It is, however, not only a strategy, but an attempt to reorganize the world; an attempt of introducing an order that initially existed in the world, and which was lost by the people at some moment in time. The destruction of machinery is not violence but the only appropriate and necessary way of restoring these machines to their original form, their true unadulterated nature, which has been brutally taken away from them. Animal-rights radicals speak in a similar vein. In April 1989, the Animal Liberation Front organized a raid on the University of Arizona in Tucson, in the result of which, 1200 animals were liberated, and material losses stemming from the destruction of several buildings that were set on fire amounted to $250,000. After the action, the activists released a statement in which they claimed that the Arizona raid was conducted as "an act of mercy and compassion for the individual animal victims and also as part of a larger international campaign against the scientific/medical industry's misguided, anti-human, anti-earth, profit-oriented practices of vivisection, bio-technology, and synthetic pharmaceutical research" [60]. It is worth noting that the ALF always considered its sabotage activities to be completely violence-free [61]; violence can occur only in actions involving attacks on living beings capable of feeling joy and sadness. Military-type actions targeting objects used for inflicting suffering to animals are, in their opinion, purely defensive, and cannot be compared to bloody acts of terror.

As we observe emerging risk factors that may affect the future occurrence of public health emergencies, we may not forget the impact of eco-terrorism on the future development of the world. The actions conducted by eco-activists may be isolated but may also extend to a larger magnitude than we may be able to handle, resulting in major incidents and disasters. These actions should be taken into serious considerations, and contingency plans should also include suggestions to mitigate the impact of these actions. Whatever the causes, sabotage, arsons, direct violence, threats, bombs, etc. are all methods used in eco-terrorism. As we label these acts as instruments for terrorists, we may also consider that eco-terrorism might be easier to perform and the enemy may not be as visible as we believe.

6. Limitation

There are a few limitations to this study. This narrative review is an evidence-round up, on eco-terrorism, and not a systematic evidence-based investigation. Although this review may not have the same value as a systematic review, given the fact that the topic is seldom discussed, it still gathers enough information for further studies or a systematic review. Having this in mind, the selection of the literature used might be biased and based on the author's preferences.

7. Conclusions

Although the environmental extremist groups have not yet resorted to direct violence (targeting humans), and the animal rights groups have reached for it very rarely, the phenomenon itself and some aspects of ideology can induce, in certain circumstances, such as a growing ecological catastrophe, further departure from the anthropocentric perspective, a change of the potential of radicalism within the environmental and animal-rights movements. In the case of animal-rights groups, the principle of not causing harm to people may be openly rejected, and in the case of environmental groups, the actions aimed at the annihilation of the whole human species may be undertaken. This change may result in more extensive actions, and eventually major incidents and disasters. The will and threats from all radical organizations should be taken into serious considerations, and preventive measures should be established to prevent a future catastrophe.

Funding: This research received no external funding.

Conflicts of Interest: The author declares no conflict of interest.

References

1. Macnagten, P.; Urry, J. *Alternatywne Przyrody. Nowe Myślenie o Przyrodzie i Społeczeństwie*; Scholar: Warszawa, Poland, 2005; p. 67.
2. Lovelock, J. *Gaia: A New Look at Life on Earth*; Oxford University Press: Oxford, UK, 2000; p. 9.
3. Globalne i Regionalne Problemy Środowiskowe. Available online: https://geografia.na6.pl/globalne-i-regionalne-problemy-srodowiskowe (accessed on 1 July 2020).
4. Sustainable Development Goals "UN Report: Nature's Dangerous Decline 'Unprecedented'; Species Extinction Rates 'Accelerating'". Available online: https://www.un.org/sustainabledevelopment/blog/2019/05/nature-decline-unprecedented-report/ (accessed on 1 July 2020).
5. The Environmental Justice Foundation. Lynn Dicks, "Viral Diseases from Wildlife in China. Could SARS Happen Again?". 2020. Available online: https://ejfoundation.org/resources/downloads/EJF_Viral-diseases-from-wildife-in-China-2003-final.pdf (accessed on 1 July 2020).
6. Harmon, C.C. *Terrorism Today*; Frank Cass Publishers: London, UK, 2000; p. 8.
7. Weinberg, L.B.; Davis, P.B. *Introduction to Political Terrorism*; McGraw-Hill: New York, NY, USA, 1989; p. 7.
8. Taylor, B. Religion, violence and radical environmentalism: From earth first! to the Unabomber to the Earth Liberation Front. *Terror. Political Violence* **1998**, *10*, 1. [CrossRef]
9. Best, S. Behind the Mask: Uncovering the Animal Liberation Front. In *Terrorist or Freedom Fighters? Reflections on the Liberation of Animals*; Best, S., Nocella, A.J., II, Eds.; Lantern Books: New York, NY, USA, 2004; p. 31.
10. National Consortium for the Study of Terrorism and Responses to Terrorism (START); Homeland Security and Governmental Affairs Committee. Countering Domestic Terrorism: Examining the Evolving Threat. *Testimony of William Branif*, 25 September 2019, pp. 31–32. Available online: https://www.start.umd.edu/sites/default/files/publications/local_attachments/START_HSGACTestimony_CounteringDomesticTerrorism_Braniff_09252019.pdf (accessed on 14 March 2020).
11. Helvarg, D. *The War Against the Green. The 'Wise Use' Movement, the New Right, and Anti-Environmental Violence*; Sierra Club Books: San Francisco, CA, USA, 1994; pp. 120–122, 374–375, 385–389.
12. Deal, C. *The Greenpeace Guide to Anti-Environmental Organization*; Odonian Press: Berkley, CA, USA, 1993; p. 1.
13. Profile in Courage. Available online: http://www.peer.org/watch/wiseuse/profileincourage.php (accessed on 13 December 2008).
14. Employee Violence Report Covering 2004 Incidents. Available online: http://www.peer.org/watch/wiseuse/employee_violence_report_upto2004.pdf (accessed on 13 December 2008).
15. Vohryzek-Bolden, M.; Olson-Raymer, G.; Whamond, J.O. *Domestic Terrorism and Incident Management. Issue and Tactics*; Charles C Thomas Publisher: Springfield, IL, USA, 2001; p. 151.
16. Gen. 1:26. In *The Holy Bible: New Revised Standard Version*; Cambridge University Press: Cambridge, UK, 2005; p. 1.
17. U.S. Department of Justice, Federal Bureau of Investigation, "Terrorism 2002–2005". Available online: https://www.fbi.gov/stats-services/publications/terrorism-2002--2005 (accessed on 1 September 2019).
18. FBI. Putting Intel to Work: Against ELF and ALF Terrorists. 30 June 2008. Available online: https://archives.fbi.gov/archives/news/stories/2008/june/ecoterror_063008 (accessed on 1 September 2019).
19. Arquilla, J.; Ronfeld, D. Networks and Netwar. Available online: http://radio-weblogs.com/0107127/stories/2002/09/10/networksAndNetwar.html (accessed on 2 September 2019).
20. Young, R.L. A Time Series Analysis of ECO Terrorist Violence in the United States: 1993–2003. Ph.D. Thesis, Sam Houston State University, Huntsville, TX, USA, 2004.
21. Varriale-Carson, J.; LaFree, G.; Dugan, L. Terrorist and non-terrorist criminal attacks by radical environmental and animal rights groups in the United States, 1970–2007. *Terror. Political Violence* **2012**, *24*, 298–319.
22. *Illegal Incidents Report: A 25 Year History of Illegal Activities by Eco and Animal Extremists*; Foundation for Biomedical Research: Washington, DC, USA, 2006.
23. U.S. Department of Homeland Security. An Overview of Bombing and Arson Attacks by Environmental and Animal Rights Extremists in the United States, 1995–2010: Final Report to the Resilient Systems Division, Science and Technology Directorate. May 2013. National Consortium for the Study of Terrorism and Responses to Terrorism A Department of Homeland Security Science and Technology Center of Excellence. Available online: https://www.dhs.gov/sites/default/files/publications/OPSR_TP_TEVUS_Bombing-Arson-Attacks_Environmental-Animal%20Rights-Extremists_1309-508.pdf (accessed on 23 July 2019).

24. START, National Consortium for the Study of Terrorism and Responses to Terrorism. Ideological Motivations of Terrorism in the United States, 1970–2016. Available online: https://www.start.umd.edu/pubs/START_IdeologicalMotivationsOfTerrorismInUS_Nov2017.pdf (accessed on 23 July 2019).

25. AnimalRighstsExtremism.info, ARE INCIDENT MAP. Available online: http://www.animalrightsextremism.info/are-incident-map/ (accessed on 14 March 2020).

26. Bite Back Direct Action Info. Available online: http://www.directaction.info/news.htm (accessed on 14 March 2020).

27. Institute for Economics and Peace. Global Terrorism Index 2019. Measuring the Impact of Terrorism, Sydney, November 2019. Available online: http://visionofhumanity.org/app/uploads/2019/11/GTI-2019web.pdf (accessed on 14 March 2020).

28. Posłuszna, E. *Environmental and Animal Rights: Extremism, Terrorism, And National Security*; Elsevier: Amsterdam, The Netherlands, 2015.

29. Statement of James, F.; Jarboe, Domestic Terrorism Section Chief. Counterterrorism Division Federal Bureau of Investigation Before the House Resources Committee. Subcommittee on Forest and Forest Health. 12 February 2002. Available online: http://www.cdfearchives.org/jarboe.htm (accessed on 1 February 2009).

30. Laqueur, W. *The New Terrorism. Fanaticism and the Arms of Mass Destruction*; Oxford University Press: Oxford, UK; New York, NY, USA, 1999; pp. 199–204.

31. Liddick, D.R. *Eco-Terrorism. Radical Environmental and Animal Liberation Movement*; Praeger, Westport: London, UK, 2006.

32. Mullins, W.C. *A Sourcebook on Domestic and International Terrorism. An Analysis of Issues, Organizations, Tactics and Responses*; Charles C. Thomas Publisher: Springfield, IL, USA, 1997; pp. 229, 232.

33. Kushner, H.W. *Encyclopedia of Terrorism*; Sage Publications: Thousand Oaks, CA, USA; London, UK; New Delhi, India, 2003; pp. 32–35, 116–118.

34. Bolz, F.; Dudonis, K.J.; Schulz, D.P. *The Counterterrorism Handbook. Tactics, Procedures, and Techniques*; Taylor & Francis: Boca Raton, FL, USA; London, UK; New York, NY, USA; Singapore, 2005; pp. 157, 164.

35. U.S. Department of Justice. Federal Bureau of Investigation. Terrorism 2002/2003. Available online: http://www.fbi.gov/publications/terror/terrorism2002_2005.htm#page_21a (accessed on 8 October 2008).

36. Pickering, L.J. *The Earth Liberation Front 1997–2002*; Arissa Media Group: Portland, OR, USA, 2007; p. 47.

37. Henshaw, D. *Animal Warfare, The Story of the Animal Liberation Front*; Fontana Press: London, UK, 1989.

38. Callicott, J.B. Elements of an Environmental Ethics: Moral Considerability and the Biothic Community. *Environ. Ethics* **1979**, *1*, 71–81. [CrossRef]

39. Leopold, A. *A Sand County Almanac*; Oxford University Press: New York, NY, USA, 1991; p. 262.

40. Carus, S. R.I.S.E. In *Toxic Terror*; Tucker, J.B., Ed.; MIT Press: Cambridge, CA, USA; London, UK, 2001.

41. Eagan, S.P. From Spikes to Bombs: The Rise of Eco-Terrorism. *Stud. Confl. Terror.* **1996**, *19*, 7–8. [CrossRef]

42. Singer, P. *Animal Liberation*; Thorsons: New York, NY, USA, 1991.

43. Regan, T. *All that Dwell Therein. Animal Rights and Environmental Ethics*; University of California Press: Berkeley, CA, USA; Los Angeles, CA, USA; London, UK, 1982.

44. Jensen, D.; Opening the cages with the ALF. An Interview with David Barbarash. DerricJensen.org (17 December 2001). Available online: https://www.derrickjensen.org/2001/12/opening-the-cages-with-the-theALF/ (accessed on 1 September 2019).

45. Carnell, B. Volkert van der Graaf in Court, Brian.Carnell.Com. 14 April 2003. Available online: https://brian.carnell.com/articles/2003/volkert-van-der-graaf-in-court/ (accessed on 30 September 2019).

46. ADL. Ecoterrorism: Extremism in the Animal Rights and Environmentalist Movements. Available online: https://www.adl.org/education/resources/reports/ecoterrorism (accessed on 12 September 2019).

47. U.S. Department of Justice, U.S. Department of Agriculture, Report to Congress on the Extent and Effects of Domestic and International Terrorism on Animal Enterprises. 2 September 1993. Available online: http://www.rpoatexasoutreach.org/Brochurs_Flyers/Flyer%20-%20FBI_Report.pdf (accessed on 12 September 2019).

48. START—National Consortium for the Study of Terrorism and Responses to Terrorism. Available online: https://www.start.umd.edu/gtd/search/IncidentSummary.aspx?gtdid=201512020058 (accessed on 15 March 2020).

49. UPDATED: Animal Rights Group Claims Responsibility for Blaze that Destroyed Two Trucks in West Mississauga. Mississauga News. 8 June 2015. Available online: https://www.mississauga.com/news-story/5666768-updated-animal-rights-group-claims-responsibility-for-blaze-that-destroyed-two-trucks-in-west-mississauga/ (accessed on 16 March 2020).

50. Ezard, J. Animal Group says it sent bomb to PM. Guardian.co.uk, 1 December 1982. Available online: http://www.guardian.co.uk/fromthearchive/story/0,,1362801,00.html (accessed on 22 June 2019).
51. Smith, G.D. (Tim), Commentary No. 21: Militant Activism and the Issue of Animal Rights. April 1992. A Canadian Security Intelligence Service Publication. Available online: http://www.datapacrat.com/True/INTEL/CSIS/COM21E.HTM (accessed on 27 June 2019).
52. Facebook. Animal Liberation Press Office. 7 May 2019. Available online: https://www.facebook.com/AnimalLiberationPressOffic/posts/animal-rights-militiathe-animal-rights-militia-arm-is-a-banner-used-by-animal-ri/2278788152207848/ (accessed on 16 March 2020).
53. Bite Back Direct-Action Info. News from the Frontlines. Available online: http://www.directaction.info/news_aug28_07.htm (accessed on 16 March 2020).
54. North American Animal Liberation Press Office. Justice Department at UCLA sent bloody AIDS tainted razor blades to David Jentsch. Available online: https://animalliberationpressoffice.org/NAALPO/2010/11/22/justice-department-at-ucla-sent-bloody-aids-tainted-razor-blades-to-david-jentsch/ (accessed on 17 March 2020).
55. Aiken, W. Ethical Issues in Agriculture. In *Earthbound. New Introductory Essays in Environmental Ethics*; Tom, R., Ed.; Random House: New York, NY, USA, 1984; p. 269.
56. Leslie, J.P. ELF Communique. In *The Earth Liberation Front 1997–2002*; Arissa Media Group: Portland, OR, USA, 2007; p. 29.
57. Pickering, L.J. Final Statement of Leslie James Pickering as Spokesperson of the North American Earth Liberation Front Press Office. In *The Earth Liberation Front 1997–2002*; Arissa Media Group: Portland, OR, USA, 2007; p. 234.
58. Bernat, P. Sustainable development and the values we share—Sustainability as the confluence if islamic and western frameworks. *Probl. Sustain. Dev.* **2012**, *7*, 33–41.
59. Zbidi, M. The Call to Eco-Jihad, Environment and Ecology. 2013. Available online: http://environment-ecology.com/religion-and-ecology/738-the-call-to-eco-jihad.html (accessed on 28 July 2020).
60. Strand, R.; Strand, P. *The Hijacking of the Humane Movement*; Doral Publishing: Wilsonville, OR, USA, 1993; p. 121.
61. Stallwood, K. A Personal Overview of Direct Action in the United Kingdom and the United States. In *Terrorist or Freedom Fighters? Reflections on the Liberation of Animals*; Best, S., Nocella, A., II, Eds.; Lantern Books: New York, NY, USA, 2004; p. 83.

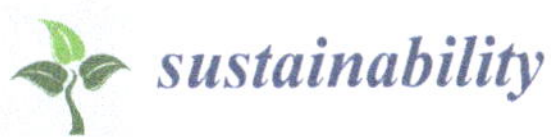 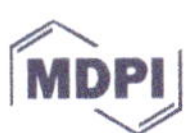

Article

Batten Down the Hatches—Assessing the Status of Emergency Preparedness Planning in the German Water Supply Sector with Statistical and Expert-Based Weighting

Lisa Bross [1,*], **Ina Wienand** [2] **and Steffen Krause** [1]

[1]   Research Center RISK, Bundeswehr University Munich, Werner-Heisenberg-Weg 39, 85577 Neubiberg, Germany; steffen.krause@unibw.de
[2]   Federal Office of Civil Protection and Disaster Assistance, Provinzialstrasse 93, 53127 Bonn, Germany; ina.wienand@bbk.bund.de
*   Correspondence: lisa.bross@unibw.de

Received: 31 July 2020; Accepted: 26 August 2020; Published: 2 September 2020

Abstract: Emergency preparedness planning in the water supply sector includes preventive measures to minimize risks as well as aspects of crisis management. Various scenarios such as floods, power failures or even a pandemic should be considered. This article presents a newly developed composite indicator system to assess the status of emergency preparedness planning in the German water supply. Two weighting methods of the indicators are compared: the indicator system was applied to a case study and a Germany-representative data set. The results show that there is a need for action in emergency preparedness planning in the German water supply. This is in particular due to a lack of risk analyses and insufficient crisis management. Numerous water supply companies and municipalities are already well-prepared, however, there is a need for action at several levels, especially in the area of risk analysis and evaluation of measures. In Germany, responsibility for this lies primarily with the municipalities.

Keywords: crisis; critical infrastructure; disaster; drinking water; risk management; risk reduction

---

1. Introduction

The corona pandemic in 2020 affects society, as well as essential services such as the water utilities, in a new and profound way [1]. Critical infrastructures like water utilities and the provision of their vital services in such a scenario have an outstanding importance to a nation's society. Their failure or degradation could result in sustained supply shortages, which affect public health, economy and national security. Quarantined personnel, working from home to distance employees and unpredictable supply chains for consumables are new and unfamiliar conditions that make the operation of water supply companies more difficult and potentially endangers overall water supply [2].

A resilient drinking water supply is consequently one of the basic requirements for a stable social and economic system. However, impairments cannot be completely avoided, so that water supply companies have to deviate from normal operation, e.g., in the event of pipe bursts. Such minor disturbances occur comparatively frequently and have only minor effects [3]. They can usually be quickly identified and repaired. As a consequence they usually remain unnoticed to the consumers [4]. On the contrary, failures or more extensive impairments of the water supply systems can have serious impacts on the affected population and the economy [3,5–7]. Causes can be serious natural events, man-made accidents or intentional attacks [8,9], whose probability of occurrence is constantly increasing [10].

The corona pandemic puts the importance of critical infrastructures, and the need for proactive emergency preparedness planning to increase their resilience, at the forefront of civil protection and disaster management [1]. The understanding, analysis and quantification of resilience by water utilities, authorities, decision-makers and other stakeholders is a prerequisite for this.

The resilience of water supply systems can be increased by appropriate emergency preparedness planning instead of ad hoc coping responses. This includes the conceptual, organisational and technical preconditions for risk reduction and prepares structures for response in the event of a crisis [11]. Emergency preparedness planning in the water supply sector thus comprises, in addition to measures to avoid damaging events, especially preventive, safeguarding, reactive and restorative aspects of risk and crisis management.

Effective emergency preparedness planning is characterised, among other things, by the fact that the planning is carried out as preventive measures and the measures can be implemented in emergency situations. Beyond preventive measures to minimise risks, emergency preparedness planning in the water supply sector includes in particular aspects of crisis management [12]. Such emergency preparedness planning takes into account different scenarios and their possible effects on the water supply. In addition to preventive measures, the numerous aspects of crisis management also lead to risk minimization by limiting the extent of damage. Figure 1 shows the five steps of risk and crisis management according to the German Federal Ministry of the Interior [13] and the Federal Office of Civil Protection and Disaster Assistance [12,14].

Thorough preliminary planning forms as the first process step the basis for the successful establishment of risk and crisis management [13]. Basic specifications should be made in advance of the establishment or expansion of a risk and crisis management system. These include the promotion of risk awareness and the definition of key players as well as responsibilities in the course of the emergency preparedness planning process [14].

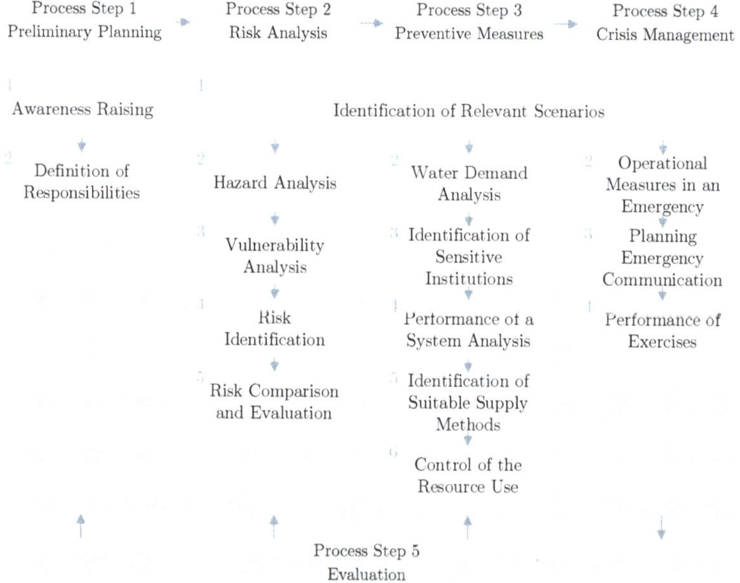

Figure 1. Structuring of the procedure for emergency preparedness planning in water supply based on [12,13,15].

A risk analysis structures and objectifies the collection of information on existing and potential risks to the water supply [14]. The analysis considers the reasons and causes of risks, examines the possible effects and determines the framework within which these consequences can occur [16]. In addition, risk analysis provides the basis for effective and efficient use of limited resources by comparing the various identified risks of processes and components of water supply.

Preventive measures contribute to the reduction of risks for critical processes. They also contribute to achieve operational protection goals and thus raise the barrier for events with crisis potential in the facility [12]. In this way, the number of crisis-prone events can be minimized or the intensity of the events can be reduced.

The processes of crisis management help to protect facilities and thus critical infrastructures and the population. Interactions exist with risk management, since not all risks can be reduced by risk-minimizing measures and a residual risk always remains [12]. Crisis management therefore offers a structure for coping with crises that cannot be prevented [13,17].

The evaluation refers to all phases, i.e., both the examination of points defined in the preliminary planning, the examination of the topicality of the information on existing risks, the examination of the effectiveness of the implemented preventive measures and the examination of the crisis management [14]. It should be repeated regularly.

2. Materials and Methods

The emergency preparedness planning indicator (EPP) developed in this study is based on a number of main, partial and individual indicators. These indicators cover organisational as well as technical aspects of emergency preparedness planning. The contents of the indicator correspond to the processes and components of effective emergency preparedness planning in water supply. For the development and calculation of the EPP, a multi-stage and iterative process according to [18] was carried out (Figure 2).

1   Description of approach for the development of composite indicators

2   Data acquisition and selection

3   Imputation of missing data

4   Normalisation of data

5   Weighting and aggregation

     5a Statistical   5b Expert-Based

6   Visualisation

Figure 2. Procedure for the compilation of a composite indicator based on [18].

2.1. Description of Approach for the Development of Composite Indicators

The theoretical framework of the EPP is the systematic procedure of risk and crisis management according to [13,14], the necessary scope of which is described by five process steps. The EPP therefore consists of the five main indicators of preliminary planning, risk analysis, preventive measures, crisis management and evaluation. The Table 1 shows the subdivision of the five main indicators and the 19 sub-indicators in total. Appendix A Tables A1–7 show all individual indicators. In addition to a literature study and existing theoretical models, the individual indicators representative for emergency preparedness planning were developed on the basis of expert and stakeholder knowledge in different workshops, thus applying a stakeholder-oriented methodology. This methodology is usually used in the development of composite indicators (e.g., [19,20]), if, as in the present case, their use is intended as a self-assessment tool for municipalities or authorities.

Table 1. Composition and hierarchy of the emergency preparedness planning indicator through five main indicators as well as their sub and individual indicators.

	Main Indicator		Sub Indicator	Individual Indicator	Source	In NoWa I Dataset
PP	Preliminary Planning	PP_1	awareness raising	$PP_{1,1}$ to $PP_{1,9}$	[12,14,21,22]	Yes
		PP_2	definition of responsibilities	$PP_{2,1}$ to $PP_{2,3}$	[14,21,23]	No
RA	Risk Analysis	RA_1	hazard analysis	$RA_{1,1}$ to $RA_{1,8}$	[14,17,24]	Yes
		RA_2	vulnerability analysis	$RA_{2,1}$ to $RA_{2,8}$	[14,17]	No
		RA_3	risk identification	$RA_{3,1}$ to $RA_{3,7}$	[14,16,17,25]	Yes
		RA_4	risk comparison and assessment	$RA_{4,1}$ to $RA_{4,2}$	[14]	No
PM	Preventive Measures	PM_1	structural redundancies	$PM_{1,1}$ to $PM_{1,2}$	[14,17]	Yes
		PM_2	interrelation of supply	$PM_{2,1}$	[14,17,26]	Yes
		PM_3	grid construction	$PM_{3,1}$ to $PM_{3,2}$	[17,27,28]	No
		PM_4	remote monitoring, control systems	$PM_{4,1}$ to $PM_{4,2}$	[14,17,29.30]	No
		PM_5	general measures	$PM_{5,1}$ to $PM_{5,3}$	[17,31,32]	Yes
CM	Crisis Management	CM_1	organisation and coordination	$CM_{1,1}$ to $CM_{1,7}$	[12,14,17.23,33–35]	Yes
		CM_2	provision of resources	$CM_{2,1}$ to $CM_{2,2}$	[12,14]	Yes
		CM_3	exercises	$CM_{3,1}$ to $CM_{3,2}$	[12,14,17.23]	Yes
		CM_4	communication	$CM_{4,1}$	[14,17,36.37]	Yes
E	Evaluation	E_1	evaluation preliminary planning	$E_{1,1}$ to $E_{1,2}$	[14,17]	No
		E_2	evaluation risk analysis	$E_{2,1}$ to $E_{2,4}$	[14,17,38]	Yes
		E_3	evaluation preventive measures	$E_{3,1}$ to $E_{3,5}$	[14]	No
		E_4	evaluation crisis management	$E_{4,1}$ to $E_{4,4}$	[14,17,23.36]	Yes

2.2. Data Acquisition and Selection

The indicators shown in Table 1 are necessary for the quantitative assessment of the status of implementation of emergency preparedness planning. Thus, data are required that allow both a review of the applicability and significance of the EPP and the determination of the status quo in Germany. However, the required information cannot be determined from publicly available data, as this is utility-specific and relevant to the security of the water utility and its services. A targeted assessment is therefore necessary.

2.2.1. Case Study for Verification of Indicator

To check the applicability and significance of the EPP, all indicators were collected on the basis of a questionnaire for a water supply company as a case study. The case study shows a real water supply utility which supplies a total of 230,000 inhabitants in 120 municipalities and districts. In total, the water supply company delivers about 10 million cubic meters of water annually.

2.2.2. Germany-Representative Dataset

In order to assess the status quo of emergency preparedness planning in Germany, an existing dataset of a nationwide survey on emergency preparedness planning in water supply was analysed. The data set was collected in 2015 by means of a partially standardised questionnaire within the framework of the NoWa I research project with the assistance of the federal level in order to obtain a general, supra-regional overview of the current status of emergency planning in the districts and municipalities. As the responsible bodies, the districts and municipalities had to ask for input from the water supply companies to fill out the data collection form, if the information was not already available. In total, a completed survey questionnaire was returned by 194 districts and 166 municipalities. The data thus consists of 360 individual data sets, which contain data from nationwide distributed municipalities and districts with a population of around 39 million inhabitants.

Each dataset contains information on 37 questions concerning different aspects of emergency preparedness planning and existing water supply systems. To determine the status quo, 21 relevant individual indicators from the data entry form with 37 questions were identified and considered in the EPP. In total, the data sets are assigned to twelve of the 19 sub-indicators (Table 1).

A subsequent data collection or data supplement could not be implemented, since the data collection within the framework of the NoWa I project and an additional collection of a representative data set could not be repeated. Thus, the determination of the status quo does not include all identified indicators.

2.3. Imputation of Missing Data

Missing data impairs the development and evaluation of composite indicators and can lead to a distortion of the results [18]. In the present study, a case-by-case elimination of data sets is only applied if the data that are absolutely necessary for the situation analysis (e.g., allocation of the data set to the municipality) are not available.

The analysed data of the NoWa I project were collected before the methodology of the emergency preparedness planning indicator was developed. They do not include all indicators relevant to the EPP. Since it was not possible to collect such a data set subsequently, the NoWa I data sets were used to determine the indicator, although they did not include complete indicator data sets (as shown in Table 1). The missing individual indicators are therefore not included in the evaluation.

2.4. Normalisation of Data

In order to be able to compare the indicators of different municipalities or the individual sub-indicators with each other, a normalisation process is necessary. This is especially true if the data sets differ in their units of measurement [18].

The questions with "yes-no" or "yes-partial-no" possible answers are converted into a [0,1] scale. Likert scales with a given answer scale were also transformed into a [0,1] scale. The answer option "not known" was equated to the answer option "no", since this is equivalent in terms of content for the evaluation of the indicator. This was necessary because the originally planned survey in the NoWa I project had a different assignment of the questions.

2.5. Weigthing and Aggregation

The individual indicators are integrated into the composite indicator with different weightings (see Equation (1)). This is because the composite indicator is calculated by the weighted sum of its main indicators (see Equation (2)). For the contingency planning indicator, the weighted sum of the five main indicators is determined. As described in [39], there are several ways to determine the weighting of composite indicators.

$$CI = \sum_{j=1}^{m} x_j X_j \tag{1}$$

$$EPP = x_{PP} \cdot PP + x_{RA} \cdot RA + x_{PM} \cdot PM + x_{CM} \cdot CM + x_E \cdot E \tag{2}$$

CI Composite indicator
m Number of main indicators
x_j weight of main indicator j
X_j normalized value of the main indicator (PP, RA, PM, CM and E)

For the EPP this paper compares the results of a statistical and an expert-based weighting approach. The main difference between the two approaches is how the indicator weights are derived. Since the weighting of the main and sub-indicators significantly influences the result of the EPP, the composite indicator is determined with identical main and sub-indicators for both weighting approaches.

If the main indicators are equally weighted, they are equally included in the composite indicator. Due to the different weighting of the individual summands (main indicators or sub-indicators), they are assigned a differentiated significance for the composite indicator.

To determine the expert-based weighting, the weights were derived from expert opinions. Using a budget allocation approach, fourteen experts with different specialist backgrounds were asked to assess the main and sub-indicators in a questionnaire using a Likert scale according to their relevance for target-oriented emergency preparedness planning. The weightings of the main indicators derived from the equal distribution and from the expert opinions are presented in Section 3.1.

2.6. Visualisation

The results of the composite and main indicators are visualized in an anonymized representation using treemap diagrams. This type of presentation was chosen because the data set depicts a large number of municipalities and water supply utilities, but the number of inhabitants varies greatly. The hierarchical structure of the treemap diagrams makes the proportions of the municipalities and water supply companies under consideration clear. At the same time all results are visible. Rectangles of different sizes are used to display the number of inhabitants of the district or the district-free city or municipalities (E_i) in relation to the inhabitants of the entire data set (E_{ges}) (see Figure 3). Thus, each rectangle corresponds to a municipality, which is always at the same position in the respective diagrams. The color of the rectangles represents the value of the indicator. The evaluation of the data sets is carried out anonymously. In addition, the possibilities of drawing conclusions about individual municipalities are minimized by the following selected representation.

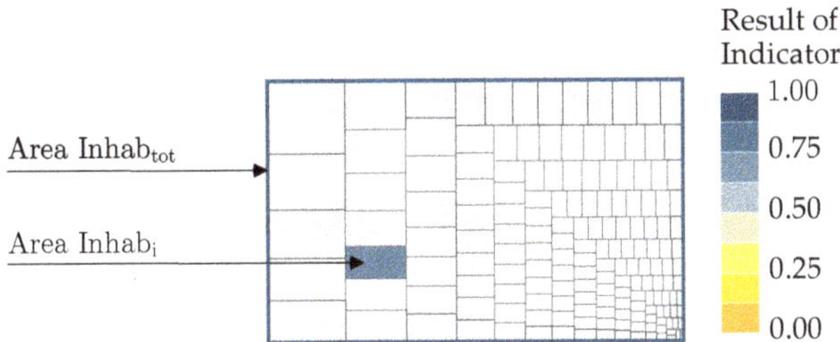

Figure 3. Explanation of the visualization of the analysis of the status of emergency preparedness planning through treemap diagrams.

3. Results

3.1. Determination of the Weighting of the Indicators

Emergency preparedness planning comprises the five process steps preliminary planning (1), risk analysis (2), preventive measures (3), crisis management (4) and evaluation (5). In case of equal distribution, the weighting of the five process steps corresponds to 20% or $x_j = 0,2$ each. The expert-based weights are between 17 and 22% (Figure 4). The mean value of the expert-based weight of the process step Preliminary Planning (1) is 0.22, the highest value, and the mean value of the expert-based weight of the process step Evaluation (5) is 0.17, the lowest value of the five weight. The expert opinion regarding the weight of the process step Evaluation (5) varies the strongest. The difference in the mean values of the expert-based weightings is statistically significant ($p < 0.05$).

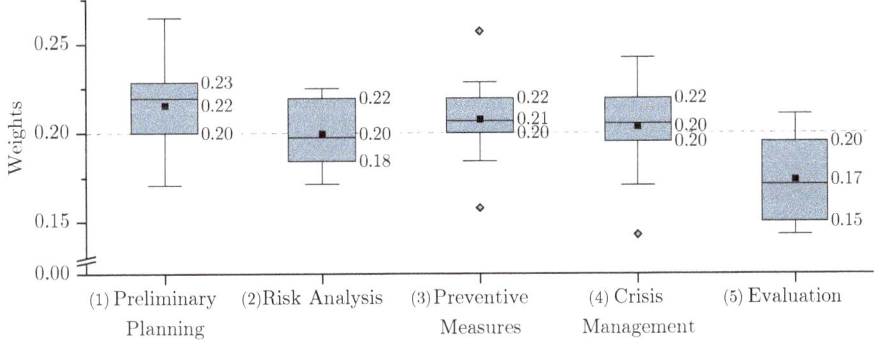

Figure 4. Expert-based weighting of the five process steps of emergency preparedness planning ($n = 14$).

3.2. Assessment of the Applicability and Significance of the Emergency Preparedness Planning Indicator Based on the Case Study

In order to determine the status quo of emergency preparedness planning, a data collection form was compiled from the indicators listed. This was answered by the water supply company and the responsible disaster control authority from the case study and the data was evaluated.

For the case study, this results in an EPP$_S$ of 0.66 and an EPP$_E$ of 0.67 (Figure 5). The main indicator PP with a value of 0.96 corresponds to the highest result of the five main indicators. The lowest value is obtained for the main indicator CM with 0.43 and 0.44. This means that in the area of preliminary planning almost all aspects have been implemented in the company and district, but in the area of preventive crisis management aspects are not yet sufficiently practiced.

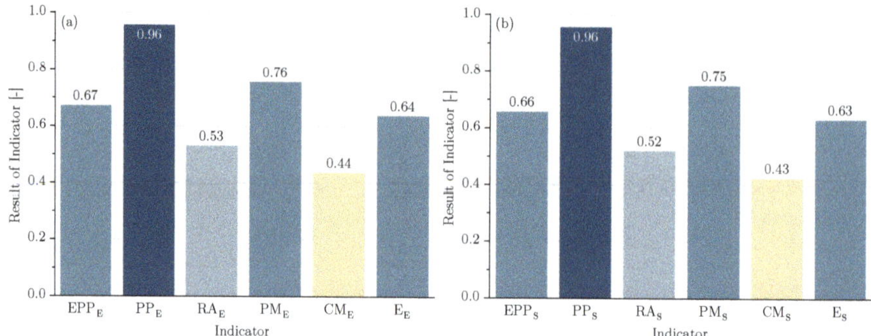

Figure 5. Results of the EPP and the main indicators for the case study based on the different weightings (**a**) Expert-based Weights (**b**) Equal Weights.

The methodology developed in this study to assess the status of emergency preparedness planning is applicable in practice. The applied questionnaire captures the relevant aspects for assessing the status quo and deriving the need for action. The quantitative results also enable a comparison between municipalities and the prioritisation of planned measures to address the need for action.

3.3. Status of Emergency Preparedness Planning in Germany

3.3.1. Data Basis for the Analysis of the Status Quo of Emergency Preparedness Planning

In order to determine the status of emergency preparedness planning in the water supply sector, a total of 360 data sets were analysed and evaluated. These comprise 194 data sets from districts and 166 data sets at the municipal level. Due to the different responsibilities in Germany, the data sets of the districts and municipalities are evaluated separately from the data sets at the municipal level (Table 2). The data sets are each divided into four groups of approximately equal size according to the number of inhabitants covered. In addition, a distinction was made between the areas of responsibility of the senders of the data collection forms. It is therefore necessary to examine, whether differences can be identified with regard to the level of preparation of the different senders and the size of the municipality.

Table 2. Size of the municipalities and districts as well as the field of activity of the senders of the survey forms.

Inhabitants	Proportion of Survey Forms					
	Water Utility	Administration	Civil Protection	Health Department	Multiple Senders	Line Sum
Municipalities (*n* = 166)						
to 3.000	7%	20%	0%	0%	0%	27%
3.001 to 5.000	4%	16%	0%	0%	0%	20%
5.001 to 10.000	11%	14%	0%	0%	0%	25%
more than 10.000	19%	3%	0%	3%	3%	28%
Column Sum	41%	53%	3%	0%	3%	100%

Table 2. *Cont.*

Inhabitants	Proportion of Survey Forms					
	Water Utility	Administration	Civil Protection	Health Department	Multiple Senders	Line Sum
Districs (n = 194)						
to 100.000	0%	6%	10%	3%	4%	23%
100.001 to 150.000	0%	7%	12%	4%	2%	25%
150.001 to 250.000	2%	5%	18%	1%	4%	30%
more than 250.000	2%	1%	11%	6%	2%	22%
Column Sum	4%	19%	51%	14%	12%	100%

3.4. Assessment of the Status of Emergency Preparedness Planning in Germany

In order to assess the status of the emergency preparedness planning of the districts as well as the municipalities, the composite indicator EPP and the main indicators PP, RA, PM, CM and E were determined on the basis of the data sets presented. For this purpose, the results of the emergency preparedness planning indicators with weighting according to expert opinion (EPP_E) and with equally distributed weighting (EPP_S) are presented below.

The results of the EPP_E and EPP_S vary for the districts in a few cases (Figure 6) The mean value of the EPP_E as well as the EPP_S is equal to 0.42 (Table 3). The small differences in the weighting show only a little effect in the result. Moreover, these differences are not statistically significant ($p > 0.05$).

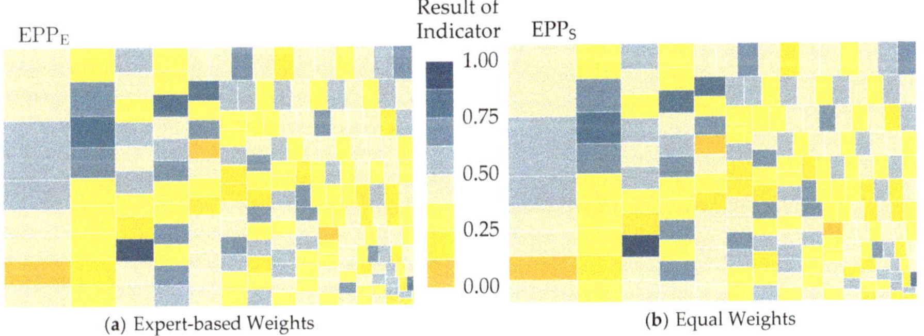

Figure 6. Emergency preparedness planning indicator according to the size of the districts.

Table 3. Results of the emergency preparedness planning indicator with expert based and equally distributed weighting and the main indicators.

	Indicator	Mean Value of Indicator (Standard Derivation)	
		Districs and Municipalities	
EPP	EPP_E	0.42 (SD = 0.17)	0.32 (SD = 0.18)
	EPP_S	0.42 (SD = 0.16)	0.32 (SD = 0.18)
Main Indicator	PP	0.43 (SD = 0.25)	0.30 (SD = 0.27)
	RA	0.16 (SD = 0.32)	0.14 (SD = 0.29)
	PM	0.57 (SD = 0.31)	0.39 (SD = 0.38)
	CM	0.55 (SD = 0.32)	0.43 (SD = 0.22)
	E	0.38 (SD = 0.22)	0.31 (SD = 0.25)

The participating districts show a different level of preparation. Districts with more inhabitants achieve a higher EPP (Figure 7). The range of EPP increases with the number of inhabitants, so that the largest districts show the greatest difference in the level of emergency preparedness within a size group. The differences in the mean values by size of the districts are significant in both cases ($p < 0.05$).

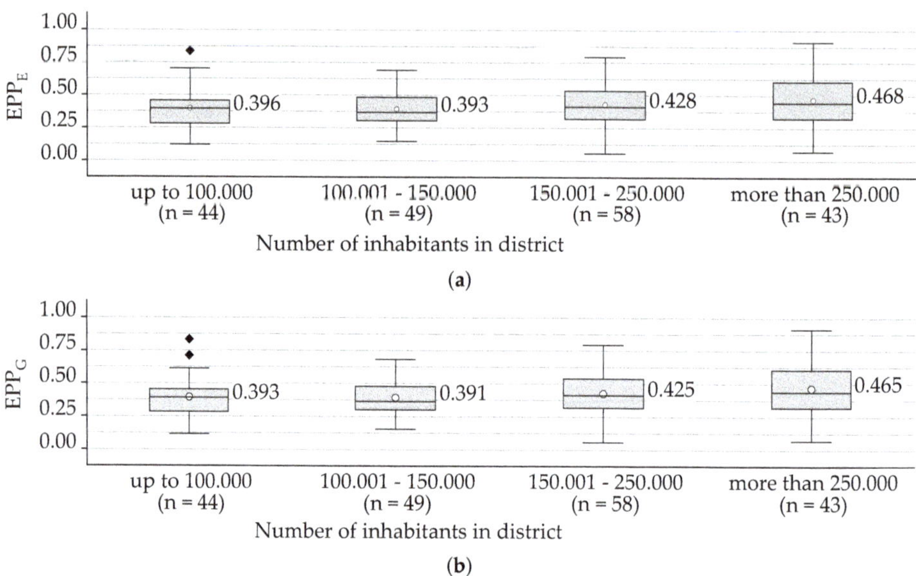

(a)

(b)

Figure 7. EPP according to the size of the districts. (**a**) Expert-based weighting of the main and sub-indicators; (**b**) Equally distributed weighting of the main and sub-indicators.

The mean values of the EPP_E and EPP_S for municipalities are 0.32. Some municipalities have thus already implemented certain aspects of emergency preparedness planning. However, these implementations are still in their beginnings. Differences between the EPP_E and EPP_S are only evident in a few cases (Figure 8), but do not show statistical significance ($p > 0.05$).

Municipalities with an increasing number of inhabitants achieve higher results in the EPP_E as well as in the EPP_S. The differences in the mean values between the size of the municipalities are significant ($p < 0.05$). However, the range of the EPP_E does not increase with a growing number of inhabitants in the municipality, which can be seen at the level of districts.

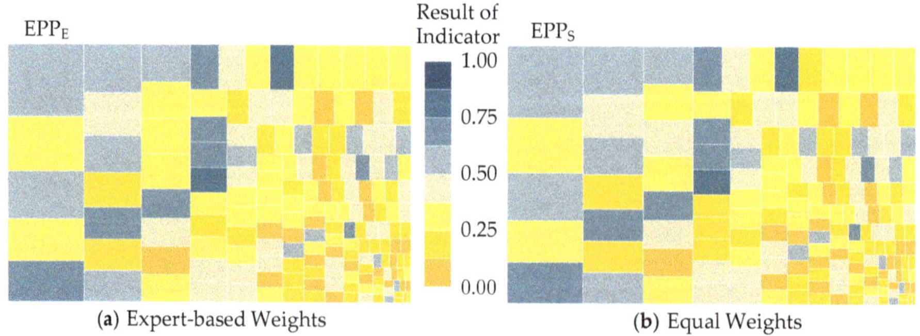

Figure 8. Emergency preparedness planning indicator by size of municipalities.

The Figure 9 shows the differences of the EPP_E and EPP_S between expert-based and equally distributed weighting. The colored variance of the rectangles shows that the different weightings affect the results of the EPP_E and EPP_S. In addition, the figure shows that the difference between EPP_E and EPP_S is in the range of ± 0.018 and is therefore only noticeable in a few cases when the result is rounded to the second decimal place.

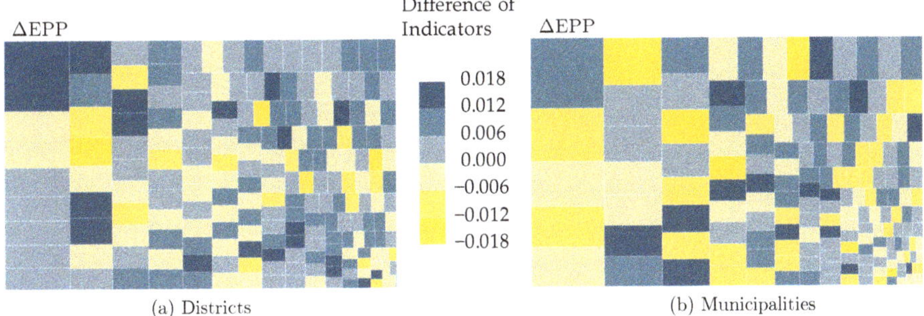

Figure 9. Difference between the emergency preparedness planning indicators EPP_E and EPP_S according to the size of the data sets taken into account.

4. Discussion

4.1. Discussion of the Applied Methods

For effective planning and implementing of measures to increase the resilience of water supply systems, it is necessary to assess the status of emergency preparedness. The Emergency Preparedness Planning Indicator was developed to increase transparency by quantifying this assessment. The EPP was tested on the basis of the case study for its applicability and significance. The determination of the status of emergency preparedness planning was implemented by means of a data set of the research project NoWa I which is representative for Germany.

The composite indicator developed in this study enables a measurable assessment of the status of emergency preparedness planning. The main and sub indicators included are based on scientific publications (e.g., [12,14,17,23]), so that they reflect the current state of research on emergency preparedness planning. The development and application of the composite indicator is based on two main motivations. Firstly, the indicator can serve as a tool for self-assessment of emergency preparedness planning by asking specific questions. The self-assessment can be used by water utilities, regional or national authorities and municipalities to improve the prevention measures. The result of the indicator can also raise awareness of the relevance of emergency preparedness planning and show the need for action.

Secondly, the indicator supports local and regional authorities as well as national and international organisations in the assessment process, by comparing different municipalities, e.g., in the context of benchmarking processes of water supply systems. The results should support these institutions in decision-making, e.g., on the allocation of resources, and make them more transparent and consistent.

Two weighting methods were used to determine the emergency preparedness planning indicator. An equally distributed weighting of indicators is the standard assumption in the literature (e.g., [40,41]). If equal weightings are used, the indicators are either constructed in such a way that each variable or branch of a hierarchy level is equally weighted. To determine the EPP, equal weighting was applied to each hierarchical level. Furthermore, a weighting of the main and sub-indicators was applied based on expert knowledge. However, no strict participatory method has been applied here, where all weightings included are based on expert opinion [39]. This was only used for the weighting of the main and sub-indicators, but not for the individual indicators. For the individual indicators, aggregation at each level by arithmetic means was applied. Due to the different number of partial and individual indicators, they have a different weight despite their apparent equal weighting [42]. This also applies to the evaluated data set of the NoWa I project and must be taken into account when deriving the need for action.

The results show only minor differences with the two different weighting methods, both for the data set of the NoWa I project and the case study. Consequently the experts' opinions confirm the relevance of all five process steps of risk and crisis management according to [13,14]. In order to increase the acceptance of the indicator and to simplify the calculation, it is therefore recommended that the weighting be applied by using statistically equally distributed weights.

4.2. Discussion of the Indicator and Assessment Results

The results of the status of emergency preparedness planning for the case study show that some measures have already been implemented. An advanced state of implementation can be seen, particularly in the preliminary planning (1) and preventive measures (3). However, since the status of the risk analysis (2) still needs to be improved, the appropriate identification and implementation of preventive measures cannot be in a targeted manner. For this reason, the evaluation of the preventive measures (3) is necessary following the complete implementation of the risk analysis (2). Further action is needed in the area of crisis management (4). The sub-indicator results of this process step refer to the lowest level of implementation in the case study. However, since the crisis management (4) measures are based on the risk analysis (2) and the preventive measures (3), the implementation of a systematic approach step-by-step is an important prerequisite. Nevertheless, the individual process steps must still be evaluated and updated regularly.

The results of the composite indicator show a very heterogeneous picture with regard to the implementation status of emergency preparedness planning in the German water supply sector. The heterogeneity of the emergency preparedness planning indicator exists both in the districts and at the municipal level. Furthermore, the results of the respective five process steps are very diverse. Thus, some aspects of emergency preparedness planning have already been implemented. Nevertheless, implementation is still insufficient in some districts and municipalities.

The differentiation of districts or municipalities according to their number of inhabitants indicates that in both cases, larger municipalities have on average better emergency preparedness planning than smaller ones. Nevertheless, both groups contain outliers in both directions. Reasons for a more sophisticated emergency preparedness planning in larger municipalities may be, on the one hand, an extensive staffing or optimized structural conditions. On the other hand, the water supply in larger municipalities in Germany often lies in the responsibility of larger supply utilities, which often devote themselves more intensively to this task due to their corporate structure.

Indicator methods can reduce their usefulness for policy-makers or even lead to disadvantageous decision-making due to over-simplification of complex concepts and the use of aggregation procedures that are difficult to understand [43]. Although the answers to the questions used to determine the EPP are checklist-based self-assessments, the scope of the questions could lead to little attention being paid to the individual answers. The result of the case study shows that the procedure is applicable and the self-assessment questionnaire with 74 questions is appropriate. A shorter list of questions would lead to a less meaningful result.

The emergency preparedness planning indicator enables a quantitative comparison between municipalities or water supply utilities as well as the five process steps and the identification of the need for action. In the German water supply sector, the implementation of risk analysis should be emphasized. Preventive measures that have already been taken have to be checked for their appropriateness following the successful implementation of a risk analysis. Threshold values for sufficient or improvable emergency preparedness planning have to be defined. However, this cannot be achieved by science alone. This requires in particular a discourse between scientists, technical experts and political decision-makers.

5. Conclusions

Effective emergency preparedness planning is characterised, among other things, by the fact that its process steps can be carried out with foresight and the defined measures can be effectively put into practice in emergency situations. The five process steps of risk and crisis management have to be systematically taken into account.

The status of emergency preparedness planning in Germany was determined using a composite indicator. The data basis of the indicator system is formed by the case study of a water supply company and a survey of the NoWa I research project, which is representative for Germany. The results indicate a need for action in the different processes of emergency preparedness planning, because the process steps (1–5), especially risk analysis (2) are carried out rarely or insufficiently. However in the area of preliminary planning (1), numerous water supply companies and municipalities are already well positioned, and several preventive measures (3) are also being implemented. The regular evaluation (5) of these measures could be improved.

A need for action is especially identified in the development of practicable tools for implementation of an integrated risk and crisis management process in order to intensify the exchange of the relevant actors. Furthermore training in the area of risk and crisis management with the emphasis on extraordinary or extreme events should be conducted by water utilities and local authorities.

Author Contributions: Conceptualization: L.B., S.K., and I.W.; methodology: L.B. validation: S.K. and I.W.; formal analysis: S.K. and I.W.; investigation: L.B., I.W., and S.K.; resources: S.K. and I.W.; data curation: L.B.; writing—original draft preparation: L.B.; writing—review and editing: L.B., S.K., I.W.; visualization: L.B.; supervision: S.K. and I.W.; project administration: S.K. and I.W.; funding acquisition: S.K. All authors have read and agreed to the published version of the manuscript.

Funding: This research received no external funding.

Acknowledgments: The authors would like to thank all those involved in the survey for their commitment and support. Furthermore, the authors would like to thank Salomé Parra and Christian Platschek, who laid the foundation for further work through their preliminary work within the framework of the NoWa I project, as well as Renate Solmsdorf, Sybille Rupertseder and Karolina Eggersdorfer, who helped to digitise the data sets. This study was supported by the Research Center RISK and the Bundeswehr University Munich.

Conflicts of Interest: The authors declare no conflict of interest.

Abbreviations

The following abbreviations are used in this manuscript:

CM	Crisis Management
E	Evaluation
EPP	Emergency Preparedness Planning Indicator
EPP_S	Emergency Preparedness Planning Indicator with statistical weights of main indicators
EPP_E	Emergency Preparedness Planning Indicator with weights based on expert knowledge
PM	Preventive Measures
PP	Preliminary Planning
RA	Risk Analysis
E	Evaluation

Appendix A

Table A1. Survey sheet to assess the Emergency Preparedness Planning Indicator—Part 1.

ID	Question	Reply Options	Source	Individual Indicator
	Main Indicator PP—Preliminary Planning			
	Sub Indicator PP_1—Awareness Raising			
1	Is it known how the supply zone is divided into municipalities or neighbourhoods?	Yes, partially, no	[14]	$VP_{1,1}$
2	Does the possible amount of water discharge correspond to the defined protection goals?	Yes, partially, no	[14]	$VP_{1,2}$
3	Is the technically maximum possible discharge quantity from the own extraction plant known?	Yes, partially, no	[14]	$VP_{1,3}$
4	Is the technically maximum possible water supply from other water utilities known?	Yes, partially, no	[14]	$VP_{1,4}$
5	Is the capacity of your own extraction plants known?	Yes, partially, no	[14]	$VP_{1,5}$
6	Is it known which part of the supply zone is supplied by which water extraction plant?	Yes, partially, no	[14]	$VP_{1,6}$
7	Is the following known for the individual tanks for water storage?			$VP_{1,7}$
7.1	Origin of water	Yes, partially, no	[14]	$VP_{1,7,1}$
7.2	Capacity of the storage tanks	Yes, partially, no	[14]	$VP_{1,7,2}$
7.3	max. possible feed-in quantity from the storage tanks into the grid	Yes, partially, no	[14]	$VP_{1,7,3}$
8	Is there an awareness in your community that there may be a quantitative impairment of the water supply?	Yes, partially, no	[14,21]	$VP_{1,8}$
9	Is there an awareness in your community that there may be a qualitative impairment of the water supply?	Yes, partially, no	[14,21]	$VP_{1,9}$
	Sub Indicator PP_2—Definition of Responsibilities			
10	Is it known who is the contact person for emergency situations in the water supply utility/ies?	Yes, partially, no	[12,14]	$VP_{2,1}$
11	Has a crisis task force been set up?	Yes, partially, no	[12,14]	$VP_{2,2}$
12	Is the organizational and operational structure defined?	Yes, partially, no	[12,14, 44]	$VP_{2,3}$

Table 2. Survey sheet to assess the Emergency Preparedness Planning Indicator—Part 2.

ID	Question	Reply Options	Source	Individual Indicator
	Main Indicator RA—Risk Analysis			
	Sub Indicator RA_1—Hazard Analysis			
13	Has a risk analysis been carried out?	Yes, partially, no	[14,17]	$RA_{1,1}$
14	Is there a list of which hazards have already been considered and which are not yet part of the risk analysis?	Yes, partially, no	[14]	$RA_{1,1}$
15	From the point of view of the water supply utility, do the following exceptional events represent relevant hazards for the water supply?		[14,24]	$RA_{1,2}$
15.1	Natural hazards	Yes, partially, no	[14,24]	$RA_{1,2,1}$
15.2	Accidents (human failures)	Yes, partially, no	[14,24]	$RA_{1,2,2}$
15.3	Accidents (technical failures)	Yes, partially, no	[14,24]	$RA_{1,2,3}$
15.4	Terrorism	Yes, partially, no	[14,24]	$RA_{1,2,4}$
16	Does the hazard analysis include experiences from past events?	Yes, partially, no	[14]	$RA_{1,3}$
17	Have qualitative impairments of the water supply occurred in the past so that substitute supply measures were necessary?	Yes, partially, no	[12,22]	$RA_{1,4}$
18	Have quantitative impairments of the water supply occurred in the past so that substitute supply measures were necessary?	Yes, partially, no	[12,22]	$RA_{1,5}$
19	Does the hazard analysis include other potential hazards that have not yet occurred?	Yes, partially, no	[14,17]	$RA_{1,6}$
20	Have hazards been identified that need to be prioritised?	Yes, partially, no	[14,17]	$RA_{1,7}$
	Sub Indicator RA_2—Vulnerability Analysis			
21	Has a vulnerability analysis been conducted?	Yes, partially, no	[14,17]	$RA_{2,1}$
22	Was the vulnerability analysis carried out in cooperation with water supply utilities and disaster management?	Yes, partially, no	[12,14]	$RA_{2,2}$
23	Have scenarios been identified for the vulnerability analysis?	Yes, partially, no	[12,14]	$RA_{2,3}$
24	Are the components to be analysed specified?	Yes, partially, no	[14]	$RA_{2,4}$
25	Have you checked which components would be exposed to which hazards (exposure)?	Yes, partially, no	[14]	$RA_{2,5}$
26	Has the functionality of the components been checked?	Yes, partially, no	[14]	$RA_{2,6}$
27	Has the technical replaceability of the components been checked?	Yes, partially, no	[14]	$RA_{2,7}$
28	Has the organizational replaceability of the components been checked?	Yes, partially, no	[14]	$RA_{2,8}$

Table 3. Survey sheet to assess the Emergency Preparedness Planning Indicator—Part 3.

ID	Question	Reply Options	Source	Individual Indicator
	Main Indicator RA—Risk Analysis			
	Sub Indicator RA_3—Risk Identification			
29	Was the risk assessment carried out with the involvement of specialist authorities or research institutions?	Yes, partially, no	[14]	$RA_{3,1}$
30	Has the extent of damage in the scenarios considered been determined?	Yes, partially, no	[14]	$RA_{3,2}$
31	Was the assessment of the extent of damage carried out with the involvement of those responsible for civil protection in the county/city?	Yes, partially, no	[14]	$RA_{3,3}$
32	Was the probability of occurrence determined in the scenarios considered?	Yes, partially, no	[14,21,45]	$RA_{3,4}$
33	Was the probability of occurrence carried out with the involvement of specialist authorities or research institutions?	Yes, partially, no	[16]	$RA_{3,5}$
34	Was the number of inhabitants affected in the scenarios considered determined?	Yes, partially, no	[14]	$RA_{3,6}$
35	Has the probability of occurrence and the extent of damage been classified on a scale (e.g., according to [14])?	Yes, partially, no	[14]	$RA_{3,7}$
	Sub Indicator RA_4—Risk Comparison and Evaluation			
36	Were the scenarios compared using a risk matrix?	Yes, partially, no	[14]	$RA_{4,1}$
37	Were the scenarios prioritized using a risk matrix?	Yes, partially, no	[14]	$RA_{4,2}$

Table 4. Survey sheet to assess the Emergency Preparedness Planning Indicator—Part 4.

ID	Question	Reply Options	Source	Individual Indicator
	Main Indicator PM—Preventive Measures			
	Sub Indicator PM_1—Structural Redundancies			
38	Are the extraction plants designed redundantly?	Yes, partially, no	[14]	$PM_{1,1}$
39	Are the storage tanks designed redundantly?	Yes, partially, no	[17]	$PM_{1,2}$
39 1	quantitatively redundant?	Yes, partially, no	[14]	$PM_{1,2,1}$
39 2	structurally redundant?	Yes, partially, no	[14]	$PM_{1,2,2}$
	Sub Indicator PM_2—Interrelation of Supply			
40	Are there supply links with other water utilities?	Yes, partially, no	[14,26]	$PM_{2,1}$
	Sub Indicator PM_3—Grid Construction			
41	Are there supply links with other water utilities?	Yes, partially, no	[17,28]	$PM_{3,1}$
42	Have grid development measures, which are necessary to ensure security of supply, been implemented?	Yes, partially, no	[27]	$PM_{3,2}$
	Sub Indicator PM_4—Remote Monitoring, Control Systems			
43	Is the supply system connected to a remote monitoring system?	Yes, partially, no	[17,29,30]	$PM_{4,1}$
44	Is the supply system equipped with a state-of-the-art control system?	Yes, partially, no	[14]	$PM_{4,2}$
	Sub Indicator PM_5—General Measures			
45	Have renewal measures necessary to ensure security of supply been implemented?	Yes, partially, no	[17,32]	$PM_{5,1}$
46	Have maintenance measures necessary to ensure security of supply been implemented?	Yes, partially, no	[17,32]	$PM_{5,2}$
47	Have physical protection measures, which are necessary to ensure security of supply, been implemented?	Yes, partially, no	[14,31]	$PM_{5,3}$

Table 5. Survey sheet to assess the Emergency Preparedness Planning Indicator—Part 5.

ID	Question	Reply Options	Source	Individual Indicator
	Main Indicator CM—Crisis Management			
	Sub Indicator CM_1—Organisation and Coordination			
48	Does the water utility develop contingency plans in addition to the action plans according to the Drinking Water Ordinance?	Yes, partially, no	[14,35]	$CM_{1,1}$
49	Are contingency plans for emergency situations in the water supply developed by the civil protection authority?	Yes, partially, no	[14,35]	$CM_{1,2}$
50	Are you familiar with the content of these plans?	Yes, partially, no	[14,34]	$CM_{1,2}$
51	Are the contact details of the following contact persons known?	Yes, partially, no		$CM_{1,3}$
51.1	Water utility	Yes, no	[17,23]	$CM_{1,3,1}$
51.2	Emergency management / civil protection	Yes, no	[17,23]	$CM_{1,3,2}$
51.3	Principal administrator	Yes, no	[14]	$CM_{1,3,3}$
51.4	Fire department	Yes, no	[12]	$CM_{1,3,4}$
51.5	Federal Agency for Technical Relief	Yes, no	[12]	$CM_{1,3,5}$
51.6	Red Cross	Yes, no	[12]	$CM_{1,3,6}$
51.7	Civil-Military Cooperation	Yes, no	[12]	$CM_{1,3,7}$
51.8	National Command	Yes, no	[12]	$CM_{1,3,8}$
51.9	Other authorities (e.g., health, environment, police)	Yes, no	[12]	$CM_{1,3,9}$
51.10	Press	Yes, no	[12]	$CM_{1,3,10}$
52	Are sensitive facilities available in the supply area?		[14]	$CM_{1,4}$
52.1	Hospital	Yes, no		$CM_{1,4,1}$
52.2	Nursing home	Yes, no		$CM_{1,4,2}$
52.3	Kindergarten/School	Yes, no		$CM_{1,4,3}$
52.4	Dialysis centers	Yes, no		$CM_{1,4,4}$
53	Are sensitive facilities in the supply area included?		[14]	$CM_{1,5}$
53.1	Hospital	Yes, partially, no		$CM_{1,5,1}$
53.2	Nursing home	Yes, partially, no		$CM_{1,5,2}$
53.3	Kindergarten/School	Yes, partially, no		$CM_{1,5,3}$
53.4	Dialysis centers	Yes, partially, no		$CM_{1,5,4}$
54	Are the telephone number, location and capacity of the following facilities in the district/district free city recorded?		[12]	$CM_{1,6}$
54.1	Brewery/beverage manufacturer	Yes, partially, no		$CM_{1,6,1}$
54.1.1	telephone number	Yes, partially, no		$CM_{1,6,1,1}$
54.1.2	location	Yes, partially, no		$CM_{1,6,1,2}$
54.1.3	capacity	Yes, partially, no		$CM_{1,6,1,3}$
54.2	Beverage suppliers (beverage market)			$CM_{1,6,2}$
54.2.1	telephone number	Yes, partially, no		$CM_{1,6,2,1}$
54.2.2	location	Yes, partially, no		$CM_{1,6,2,2}$
54.2.3	capacity	Yes, partially, no		$CM_{1,6,2,3}$
54.3	Carriers			$CM_{1,6,3}$
54.3.1	telephone number	Yes, partially, no		$CM_{1,6,3,1}$
54.3.2	location	Yes, partially, no		$CM_{1,6,3,2}$
54.3.3	capacity	Yes, partially, no		$CM_{1,6,3,3}$
54.4	Neighbouring Utilities			$CM_{1,6,4}$
54.4.1	telephone number	Yes, partially, no		$CM_{1,6,4,1}$
54.4.2	location	Yes, partially, no		$CM_{1,6,4,2}$
54.4.3	capacity	Yes, partially, no		$CM_{1,6,4,3}$

Table 6. Survey sheet to assess the Emergency Preparedness Planning Indicator—Part 6.

ID	Question	Reply Options	Source	Individual Indicator
	Main Indicator CM—Crisis Management			
	Sub Indicator CM_2—Provision of Resources			
55	Are the resources required for the substitute water supply (mobile treatment plants, mobile pipelines, transport vehicles) kept available or is access to them ensured?	Yes, partially, no	[14]	$CM_{2,1}$
56	Are the materials required for the substitute water supply (pressure increasing systems, hose connections, etc.) kept in stock or is access ensured?	Yes, partially, no	[14]	$CM_{2,2}$
	Sub Indicator CM_3—Exercises			
57	Was the interaction with the authorities and organisations involved in the event of a crisis in the water supply discussed?	Yes, partially, no	[14,17,23]	$CM_{3,1}$
58	Has the interaction with the authorities and organisations involved been practised for crisis situations in the water supply?	Yes, partially, no	[14,17,23]	$CM_{3,2}$
	Sub Indicator CM_4—Communication			
59	Is access to communication media ensured in the event of a crisis?	Yes, partially, no	[14,17,36]	$CM_{4,1}$

Table 7. Survey sheet to assess the Emergency Preparedness Planning Indicator—Part 7.

ID	Question	Reply Options	Source	Individual Indicator
	Main Indicator E—Evaluation			
	Sub Indicator E_1—Evaluation Preliminary Planning			
60	Are the awareness raising aspects regularly evaluated?	Yes, partially, no	[14,17]	$E_{1,1}$
61	Are the definitions of responsibilities regularly evaluated?	Yes, partially, no	[14,17]	$E_{1,2}$
	Sub Indicator E_2—Evaluation Risk Analysis			
62	Is the hazard analysis regularly evaluated?	Yes, partially, no	[14,17]	$E_{2,1}$
63	Is the vulnerability analysis regularly evaluated?	Yes, partially, no	[14,17]	$E_{2,2}$
64	Is the risk identification regularly evaluated?	Yes, partially, no	[14,17]	$E_{2,3}$
65	Are the risk comparison and evaluation regularly evaluated?	Yes, partially, no	[14,17]	$E_{2,4}$
	Sub Indicator E_3—Evaluation Preventive Measures			
66	Are the structural redundancies regularly evaluated?	Yes, partially, no	[14,17]	$E_{3,1}$
67	Are the interrelations of supply regularly evaluated?	Yes, partially, no	[14,17]	$E_{3,2}$
68	Are the grid construction measures regularly evaluated?	Yes, partially, no	[14,17]	$E_{3,3}$
69	Are the remote monitoring and control systems regularly evaluated?	Yes, partially, no	[14,17]	$E_{3,4}$
70	Are the general measures regularly evaluated?	Yes, partially, no	[14,17]	$E_{3,5}$
	Sub Indicator E_4—Evaluation Crisis Management			
71	Are the organisation and coordination measures regularly evaluated?	Yes, partially, no	[14,17]	$E_{4,1}$
72	Is the provision of resources regularly evaluated?	Yes, partially, no	[14,17]	$E_{4,2}$
73	Are the exercised regularly evaluated?	Yes, partially, no	[14,17]	$E_{4,3}$
74	Are the communication measures regularly evaluated?	Yes, partially, no	[14,17]	$E_{4,4}$

References

1. Sowby, R.B. Emergency preparedness after COVID-19: A review of policy statements for the U.S. water sector. *Util. Policy* **2020**, *64*, 101058. [CrossRef] [PubMed]
2. Haakh, F.; Merkel, W. Die Wasserversorgung im COVID-19 Krisenmanagement: Systemanalyse und Szenarienplanung. *Energie Wasser-Praxis* **2020**, *71*, 34–41.
3. Mays, L.W. *Water Supply Systems Security*; McGraw-Hill Professional Engineering Civil Engineering; McGraw-Hill: New York, NY, USA, 2004.
4. States, S. *Security and Emergency Planning for Water and Wastewater Utilities*; American Water Works Association: Denver, CO, USA, 2010.
5. Gopalakrishnan, K.; Peeta, S. *Sustainable and Resilient Critical Infrastructure Systems: Simulation, Modeling, and Intelligent Engineering*; Springer: Berlin/Heidelberg, Germany, 2010. [CrossRef]
6. Grigg, N.S. Water Utility Security: Multiple Hazards and Multiple Barriers. *J. Infrastruct. Syst.* **2003**, *9*, 81–88. [CrossRef]
7. Spellman, F.R. *Water Infrastructure Protection and Homeland Security*; Government Institutes: Lanham, MD, USA, 2007.
8. Mendonça, D.; Wallace, W.A. Impacts of the 2001 World Trade Center Attack on New York City Critical Infrastructures. *J. Infrastruct. Syst.* **2006**, *12*, 260–270. [CrossRef]
9. Mendonça, D.; Wallace, W.A. Adaptive Capacity: Electric Power Restoration in New York City following the 11 September 2001 Attacks. In Proceedings of the 2nd Symposium on Resilience Engineering, Juan-les-Pins, France, 8–10 November 2006.
10. Nelson, D.R.; Adger, W.N.; Brown, K. Adaptation to Environmental Change: Contributions of a Resilience Framework. *Annu. Rev. Environ. Resour.* **2007**, *32*, 395–419. [CrossRef]
11. World Health Organization. *Environmental Health in Emergencies and Disasters: A Practical Guide*; World Health Organization: Geneva, Switzerland, 2002.
12. Bross, L.; Wienand, I.; Krause, S. *Sicherheit der Trinkwasserversorgung: Teil 2: Notfallvorsorgeplanung*; Praxis im Bevölkerungsschutz; Bundesamt für Bevölkerungsschutz und Katastrophenhilfe: Bonn, Germany, 2019; Volume 15.
13. Bundesministerium des Innern, für Bau und Heimat. *Schutz Kritischer Infrastrukturen—Risiko- und Krisenmanagement · Leitfaden für Unternehmen und Behörden*; Bundesministerium des Innern, für Bau und Heimat: Bonn, Germany, 2011.
14. Wienand, I.; Hasch, M. *Sicherheit der Trinkwasserversorgung: Teil 1: Risikoanalyse*; Praxis im Bevölkerungsschutz, Bundesamt für Bevölkerungsschutz und Katastrophenhilfe: Bonn, Germany, 2016; Volume 15.
15. Bundesamt für Bevölkerungsschutz und Katastrophenhilfe. *Schutz Kritischer Infrastruktur: Risikomanagement im Krankenhaus*; Praxis im Bevölkerungsschutz; Bundesamt für Bevölkerungsschutz und Katastrophenhilfe: Bonn, Germany, 2008; Volume 2.
16. Bundesamt für Bevölkerungsschutz und Katastrophenhilfe. *Risikoanalyse im Bevölkerungsschutz: Ein Stresstest für die Allgemeine Gefahrenabwehr und den Katastrophenschutz*; Bundesamt für Bevölkerungsschutz und Katastrophenhilfe: Bonn, Germany, 2015.
17. AWWA. *M19 Emergency Planning for Water and Wastewater Utilities*, 5th ed.; American Water Works Association: Denver, CO, USA, 2018.
18. Organisation for Economic Co-operation and Development. *Handbook on Constructing Composite Indicators: Methodology and User Guide*; Organisation for Economic Co-operation and Development: Paris, France, 2008.
19. Bollin, C.; Hidajat, R. Community-Basded Risk Index: Pilot Implementation in Indonesia. In *Measuring Vulnerability to Natural Hazards. Towards Disaster Resilient Societies*; Birkmann, J., Ed.; United Nations University Press: Tokyo, Japan; New York, NY, USA, 2006; pp. 271–289.
20. Joerin, J.; Shaw, R.; Takeuchi, Y.; Krishnamurthy, R. The adoption of a climate disaster resilience index in Chennai, India. *Disasters* **2014**, *38*, 540–561. [CrossRef] [PubMed]
21. DIN EN 15975-2. *Sicherheit der Trinkwasserversorgung—Leitlinien für das Risiko- und Krisenmanagement—Teil 2: Risikomanagement*; Springer Vieweg: Berlin/Heidelberg, Germany, 2013.

22. Bross, L.; Krause, S.; Wannewitz, M.; Stock, E.; Sandholz, S.; Wienand, I. Insecure Security: Emergency Water Supply and Minimum Standards in Countries with a High Supply Reliability. *Water* **2019**, *11*, 732. [CrossRef]

23. AWWA. *G440 Emergency Preparedness Practices*; AWWA: Singapore, 2017.

24. AWWA. *J100 Risk and Resilience Management of Water and Wastewater Systems*; AWWA: Singapore, 2010.

25. DIN ISO 31000. *Risikomanagement*; Walter de Gruyter GmbH & Co KG: Berlin, Germany, 2018.

26. Boyle, D.B. Interagency Connections: Insurance Against Interruptions in Supply. *J. Am. Water Works Assoc.* **1980**, *72*, 192–195. [CrossRef]

27. Hoch, W. Planungsgrundsätze für das Bemessen von Wasserverteilungsnetzen unter Berücksichtigung der Löschwasserversorgung. In *Wassertransport und -Verteilung*; Sattler, R., Hirner, W., Eds.; DVGW Lehr- und Handbuch Wasserversorgung, Oldenbourg: München, Germany, 1999; pp. 85–123.

28. Baur, A.; Fritsch, P.; Hoch, W.; Merkl, G.; Rautenberg, J.; Weiß, M.; Wricke, B. *Mutschmann/Stimmelmayr Taschenbuch der Wasserversorgung*, 17th ed.; Springer Vieweg: Wiesbaden, Germany, 2019. [CrossRef]

29. Mehlhorn, H.; Weiß, M. Fernleitungssysteme. In *Wassertransport und -Verteilung*; Sattler, R., Hirner, W., Eds.; DVGW Lehr- und Handbuch Wasserversorgung, Oldenbourg: München, Germany, 1999; pp. 123–169.

30. Grombach, P.; Haberer, K.; Merkl, G. *Handbuch der Wasserversorgungstechnik*, 3rd ed.; Oldenbourg-Industrieverlag: München, Germany, 2000.

31. DVGW W 1050. Objektschutz von Wasserversorgungsanlagen. 2012. Available online: http://www.dwa. de/dwa/sitemapping.nsf/literaturvorschau?openform&bestandsnr=57260 (accessed on 1 September 2020).

32. Schlicht, H. Instandhaltung von Wasserverteilungsnetzen. In *Wassertransport und -Verteilung*; Sattler, R., Hirner, W., Eds.; DVGW Lehr- und Handbuch Wasserversorgung, Oldenbourg: München, Germany, 1999; pp. 373–403.

33. Morley, K.; Riordan, R. *Utilities Helping Utilities: An Action Plan for Mutial Aid and Assistance Networks for Water and Wastewater Utilities*; American Water Works Association: Singapore, 2006.

34. Doe, S.R.K.; Whitman, B.E. *Security and Emergency Management for Water Systems*, 1st ed.; Bentley Institute Press: Exton, PA, USA, 2011.

35. DVGW W 1020. Empfehlungen und Hinweise für den Fall von Abweichungen von Anforderungen der Trinkwasserverordnung; Maßnahmeplan und Handlungsplan. 2018. Available online: https://shop.wvgw. de/var/assets/leseprobe//510186_lp_W%201020_2018_03.pdf (accessed on 1 September 2020).

36. United States Environmental Protection Agency. *Effective Risk and Crisis Communication during Water Security Emergencies: Summary Report of EPA Sponsored Message Mapping Workshops*; United States Environmental Protection Agency: Washington, DC, USA, 2007.

37. Bundesministerium des Innern, für Bau und Heimat. *Leitfaden Krisenkommunikation*, 5th ed.; Bundesministerium des Innern, für Bau und Heimat: Bonn, Germany, 2014.

38. AWWA. *G430 Security Practices for Operation and Management*; AWWA: Singapore, 2015.

39. Asadzadeh, A.; Kötter, T.; Salehi, P.; Birkmann, J. Operationalizing a concept: The systematic review of composite indicator building for measuring community disaster resilience. *Int. J. Disaster Risk Reduct.* **2017**, *25*, 147–162. [CrossRef]

40. Islam, M.S.; Swapan, M.S.H.; Haque, S.M. Disaster risk index: How far should it take account of local attributes? *Int. J. Disaster Risk Reduct.* **2013**, *3*, 76–87. [CrossRef]

41. Lazarus, N.W. Coping capacities and rural livelihoods: Challenges to community risk management in Southern Sri Lanka. *Appl. Geogr.* **2011**, *31*, 20–34. [CrossRef]

42. Beccari, B. A Comparative Analysis of Disaster Risk, Vulnerability and Resilience Composite Indicators. *PLoS Curr.* **2016**, *8*. [CrossRef] [PubMed]

43. Balica, S. Approaches of understanding developments of vulnerability indices for natural disasters. *J. Environ. Eng.* **2012**, *11*, 963–974. [CrossRef]

44. DIN EN 15975-1. Sicherheit der Trinkwasserversorgung—Leitlinien für das Risiko- und Krisenmanagement—Teil 1: Krisenmanagement. 2016. Available online: https://www.boutique.afnor.org/standard/din-en-15975-1/security-of-drinking-water-supply-guidelines-for-risk-and-crisis-management-part-1-crisis-management-german-version-en-15975-120/article/852388/eu139819 (accessed on 1 September 2020).

45. AWWA. *Planning for an Emergency Drinking Water Supply*; U.S. Environmental Protection Agency's National Homeland Security Research Center: Manila, Philippines, 2011.

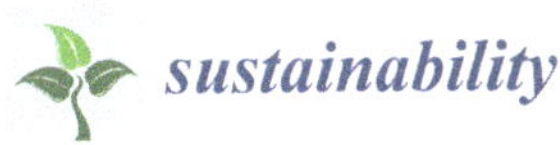 *sustainability*

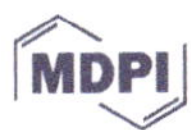

Article

Disaster Preparedness and Professional Competence Among Healthcare Providers: Pilot Study Results

Krzysztof Goniewicz [1],* and Mariusz Goniewicz [2]

[1] Department of Aviation Security, Military University of Aviation, 08-521 Dęblin, Poland
[2] Department of Emergency Medicine, Medical University of Lublin, 20-059 Lublin, Poland; mariusz.goniewicz@umlub.pl
* Correspondence: k.goniewicz@law.mil.pl

Received: 12 May 2020; Accepted: 16 June 2020; Published: 17 June 2020

Abstract: The preparedness of a hospital for mass-casualty incident and disaster response includes activities, programs and systems developed and implemented before the event. These measures are designed to provide the necessary medical care to victims of disasters, and to minimize the negative impact of individual events on medical services. Up until now, there has been no systematic survey in Poland concerning the readiness of hospitals, as well as medical personnel, to deal with mass-casualty incidents. Consequently, little is known about the knowledge, skills, and professional competences of healthcare workers. The objective of this pilot study was to start an exploration and to collect data on the competences of healthcare workers, in addition to assessing the preparedness of hospitals for mass-casualty incidents. Utilizing an anonymous survey of a random sample, 134 healthcare providers were asked to respond to questions about the competencies they needed, and hospital preparedness during disaster response. It turned out that the test subjects evaluate their own preparedness for mass-casualty incidents and disasters better than the preparedness of their current place of work. The pilot study demonstrated that a properly designed questionnaire can be used to assess the relationship between hospital and staff preparedness and disaster response efficiency. Evaluation of the preparedness and effectiveness of disaster response is a means of finding and removing possible gaps and weaknesses in the functioning and effective management of a hospital during mass-casualty incidents.

Keywords: disasters; healthcare workers; hospital preparedness; hospitals

---

1. Introduction

In a globalized world, in which crisis incidents are becoming more frequent, more devastating and have a significant impact on the health and lives of societies, the quality of healthcare services, including in particular the operational capacity of hospitals, is crucial for health security. A well-established preparedness program is a prerequisite for the effective response to emergencies of healthcare systems, including hospitals.

The preparedness of a hospital for mass-casualty incident and disaster response includes activities, programs and systems developed and implemented before the event. These measures are designed to provide the necessary medical care to victims of disasters, and to minimize the negative impact of individual events on medical services. These undertakings include, in particular, the appropriate training of medical personnel, appropriate safeguarding of logistics, and having validated emergency response procedures in place in the hospital. Evaluation of preparedness for incidents and disasters, as well as the effectiveness of response, is one way in which to locate and remove possible gaps and weaknesses in the functioning and effective management of the hospital during mass-casualty incidents (events that overwhelm the local healthcare system, where the number of casualties vastly exceeds the local resources and capabilities in a short period of time) [1–3].

Even in a well-prepared hospital, responding effectively to a disaster is a complex challenge. In the literature, there are many methods and evaluations [4–10] of the level of hospital emergency preparedness, but there is no consensus on correct and standardized methods and tools that would clearly define how individual institutions should prepare for crisis incidents [11–14]. This is largely due to the allocation of individual hospitals as well as, among others, geographical, demographic, climatic, social and economic factors, which may impact upon or be associated with the occurrence of particular events in a given region, or the response to them. It is also unclear whether individual procedures can reliably predict, in real time, the effectiveness of hospital functions [15–17]. Although many studies [18–27] have assessed the correlation between the level of hospital preparedness and disaster response, only a few functional elements have actually been assessed.

Although the World Health Organization (WHO) has developed the Hospital Safety Index (HSI) [28], a checklist of all hazards, which is a standardized, globally accepted method for assessing hospital preparedness, to date there have been no legally regulated international standards for hospital preparedness and response to crisis incidents [29–32].

Up until now, there has been no systematic survey in Poland concerning the readiness of hospitals, as well as medical personnel, to deal with mass-casualty incidents. Consequently, little is known about the knowledge, skills, and professional competences of healthcare workers [33–35]. This information is crucial for the development of effective response plans for individual hospitals, as well as for the preparation of training tailored to the needs of medical personnel [36,37]. The above-mentioned factors prompted the authors to undertake this study.

2. Aim

The main aim of the study is to investigate and to collect data on the competences of healthcare workers, in addition to assessing the preparedness of hospitals for mass-casualty incidents. An additional aim is to use the data from this initial survey to design a more comprehensive analysis of disaster preparedness (preparedness is defined by the United Nations International Strategy for Disaster Reduction as knowledge, capabilities and actions of governments, organizations, community groups and individuals "to effectively anticipate, respond to, and recover from, the impacts of likely, imminent or current hazard events or conditions), as well as new training and exercise models, which could improve the preparedness of health services for mass-casualty incidents and disasters.

3. Materials and Methods

3.1. Test Site

The study was conducted between 10 and 21 February 2020 at Public University Hospital No. 1 (polish SPSK No. 1) in Lublin. This hospital was selected as one of the largest hospitals in the Lublin region, and for this reason, it was chosen for the pilot study. SPSK No. 1 has a total of about 550 beds (including chemotherapy beds). It employs about 1600 people (including doctors, nurses and other medical personnel, as well as administration, technical, cleaning and service personnel). According to the latest data provided by the hospital, the number of hospitalizations for the academic year of 2017–2018 was about 40,000 cases, and the number of surgical procedures performed was about 19,000. The average time of hospitalization was 4.4 days.

3.2. Population Studied

The quantitative pilot study was conducted in the form of an anonymous questionnaire on a random sample of 134 healthcare workers, which account for 11.1% of the total number of employed healthcare workers at SPSK 1. More than half of them were women (56%). Men, on the other hand, constituted 44% of the research group. The respondents were mostly people with over 20 years of service (41.8%), while less frequently they had 6–10 years of service (19.4%), 0–5 years (16.4%),

11–15 years (12.7%) or 16–20 years (9.7%). Doctors (41.8%) and nurses (46.3%) represented the highest proportion of the study group, whereas 11.9% of respondents were paramedics.

3.3. Study Design

An extensive analysis of literature, and then the arrangement of the acquired knowledge through categorization and knowledge mapping, led to the development of a research tool in the form of a close-ended questions questionnaire. A qualitative method was used to verify the research tool and the questionnaire was tested on a sample of 10 people in order to check whether the respondents understood the questions it contained and whether the respondents reacted to some questions. This group was then excluded from the pilot study and their answers were not included in the final analysis. The questionnaire was designed in such a way that the time required to complete it did not exceed 15 min.

3.4. Type of Study

In the pilot study, an original questionnaire was available in both paper and online versions, and contained 18 closed questions and two additional descriptive questions. The respondents were asked about their own competences, experience, courses, and training completed, as well as knowledge about preparedness of the workplace for mass-casualty incidents. Respondents were also asked to rate their own preparedness on a scale from 1 to 10, as well as the preparedness of the hospital in which they worked, for mass-casualty incidents.

3.5. Data Analysis

Statistical analyses were conducted using IBM SPSS Statistics version 26. Frequency analyses, analysis of basic descriptive statistics, correlation analysis using Spearman's rho coefficient, the chi square test of independence, the Student's t-test for dependent samples, a one-way analysis of variance, and a Student's t-test for independent samples in addition to Mann Whitney's test were performed. The level of statistical significance was set at the classic level of $\alpha = 0.05$.

3.6. Ethical Considerations

The study is not a medical experiment and legally does not require the approval of the Bioethics Committee.

4. Results

4.1. Frequency Analysis

In response to the question about participation in a mass-casualty incident or disaster as a healthcare worker, the majority of respondents (74.6%) declared that they had not participated in such an event. More than a quarter of the respondents (25.4%) answered in the affirmative to the analyzed question.

The respondents were asked whether the facility where they currently worked has a plan for dealing with mass-casualty incidents and disasters. Most of the respondents (71.6%) answered "yes" to this question. Only 3% of the respondents answered "no" to this question. More than a quarter of the respondents (25.4%) felt they did not know the answer to this question (Table 3).

The respondents most frequently (77.6%) reported that they were familiar with the procedure for dealing with mass-casualty incidents and disasters. Only 22.4% of the research group was not acquainted with the procedure for handling such situations.

Most of the respondents (79.1%) knew who was responsible for managing mass-casualty incidents and disasters in the facility of their current workplace. On the other hand, 20.9% answered in negatively to this question.

In response to the question concerning the knowledge of the procedures to be followed in the event of evacuation during a mass-casualty incident at their workplace, the majority of respondents (87.3%) answered affirmatively. Only 12.7% of respondents did not know the procedures to be followed in this situation.

The respondents were asked whether their workplace had adequate logistical infrastructure for mass-casualty incidents. Most often (41.8%) respondents did not know whether their workplace had such a logistical infrastructure. On the other hand, 39.6% of the respondents believed their workplace to be prepared logistically for mass-casualty incidents. On the other hand, 18.7% of respondents answered negatively to this question.

More than half of the respondents (54.5%) reported a lack of organization with drills regarding disaster management at their workplace. In turn, 45.5% of the respondents stated that such activities had been organized at their workplace.

As far as the frequency of organizing drills is concerned, respondents most frequently reported that such drills were organized less frequently than once every 3 years (91.8%). Individual respondents provided the following answers: once every 3 years (3%), once every 2 years (3%) and annually (2.2%). More than half of the respondents (53.7%) had not received training related to disaster preparedness at their current workplace. However, 46.3% of respondents reported that they had received such training.

In response to the question concerning knowledge of triage, almost all respondents (99.3%) answered yes. Only one person answered negatively to this question.

4.2. Relationship between Sociodemographic Variables and Evaluation of Preparedness for Mass-Casualty Incidents and Disasters

The statistical analyses carried out checked the relationship between sociodemographic variables and the evaluation of preparedness for mass-casualty incidents and disasters. To this end, a correlation analysis using Spearman's rho coefficient and a one-way analysis of variance were performed.

Initially, the relationship between the seniority of the respondents and the evaluation of preparedness for mass-casualty incidents and disasters was tested. For this purpose, correlation analyses using Spearman's rho coefficient were performed. The results of this analysis are presented in Table 1.

Table 1. Results of the analysis of correlation between the length of service of the respondents and the evaluation of preparedness for mass-casualty incidents and disasters.

		Length of Service
Evaluation of the preparedness of the current workplace for a mass-casualty incident or disaster	Spearman's *rho*	0.19
	significance	0.033
Evaluation of one's own preparedness for mass-casualty incidents or disasters	Spearman's *rho*	0.14
	significance	0.108

According to the analyses carried out, seniority is positively linked to the evaluation of the preparedness of the current workplace for a mass-casualty incident or disaster (weak link). This shows that the longer the respondents have been working, the better do they evaluate the preparedness of the institution where they work for a mass-casualty incident or disaster.

A one-way analysis of variance was then carried out to see if occupation differentiates the evaluation of preparedness for mass-casualty incidents or disasters. The results of this analysis are presented in Figure 1.

The results indicate a statistically significant effect for assessing the preparedness of the current workplace for a mass-casualty incident or disaster. In order to investigate the exact differences, Sidak post hoc tests were performed. The test results show no statistically significant difference.

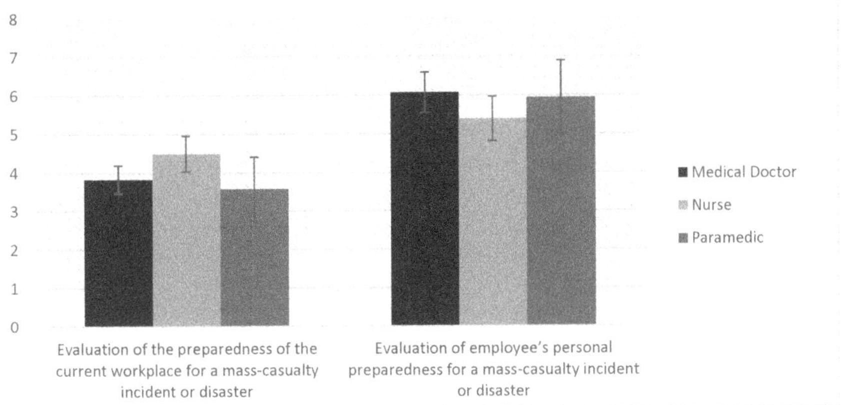

Figure 1. Average with a confidence interval of 95% for the evaluation of preparedness for mass-casualty incidents and disasters by occupation.

4.3. Differences between the Evaluation of Preparedness for a Mass-Casualty Incident or Disaster in the Current Place of Work and the Evaluation of One's Own Preparedness

In the next stage of the analyses, it was assessed whether there are differences between the evaluation of one's own preparedness and the evaluation of the current workplace's preparedness for a mass-casualty incident and disaster. For this purpose, Student's t-test was performed for dependent samples. The results of this test are presented in Table 2 and in Figure 2.

Table 2. Differences between the evaluation of preparedness for a mass-casualty incident or disaster in the current place of work, and the evaluation of one's own preparedness.

	Current Place of Work		Own		t	p	95% CI	
	M	*SD*	*M*	*SD*			*LL*	*UL*
Evaluation of preparedness for a mass-casualty incident or disaster	4.10	1.68	5.71	2.14	−9.28	<0.001	−1.95	−1.27

M—mean; *Me*—median; *SD*—standard deviation; *Bias.*—bias; *Kurt.*—kurtosis; *Min & Max.*—the lowest and highest value of distribution; *D*—Kolmogorov–Smirnov test result; *p*—significance.

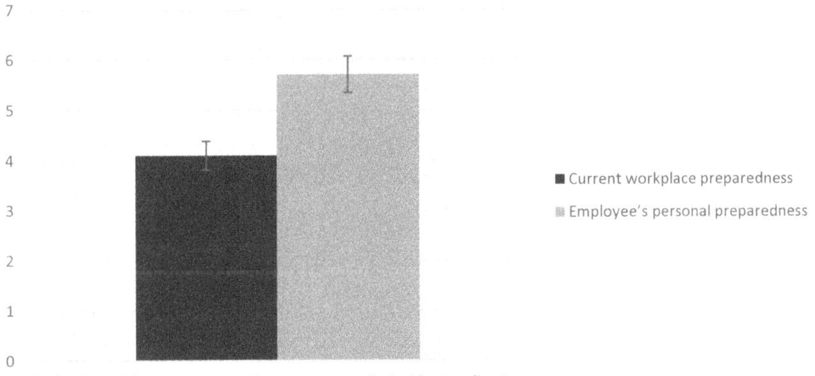

Figure 2. Average with a 95% confidence interval for the evaluation of preparedness for a mass-casualty incident or disaster for the current place of work, and one's own preparedness.

The test results indicate statistically significant differences. It turned out that the test subjects evaluate their own preparedness for mass-casualty incidents and disasters better than the preparedness of the current place of work. The strength of this effect is high.

4.4. Differences in the Evaluation of Preparedness for a Mass-Casualty Incident or Disaster Depending on Previous Participation in a Mass-Casualty Incident or Disaster as a Healthcare Professional

It was assessed whether the subjects who had previously been involved in a mass-casualty incident or disaster as a healthcare worker differ in their evaluation of preparedness for such situations from those who had not been involved in such an event. A Mann Whitney test was conducted due to the large numerical differences between the analyzed groups. The results are presented in Table 3.

Table 3. Differences between persons who have been involved in a mass-casualty incident or disaster as a healthcare worker, and persons who have not been involved in such an event in terms of their evaluation of preparedness for a mass-casualty incident or disaster.

	Have You Ever Been Involved in a Mass-Casualty Incident or Disaster as a Healthcare Professional?				*Z*	*p*
	Yes (*n* = 34)		No (*n* = 100)			
	Average Rank	*Me*	Average Rank	*Me*		
Evaluation of the preparedness of the current workplace for a mass-casualty incident or disaster	65.42	4.00	67.52	4.00	−0.28	0.783
Evaluation of one's own preparedness for a mass-casualty incident or disaster	86.12	7.00	61.17	5.00	−3.27	0.001

M—mean; *Me*—median; *SD*—standard deviation; *Bias.*—bias; *Kurt.*—kurtosis; *Min & Max.*—the lowest and highest value of distribution; *D*—Kolmogorov–Smirnov test result; *p*—significance.

The results of the tests indicate a statistically significant effect of moderate strength for the evaluation of one's own preparedness for mass-casualty incidents or disasters. As it turns out, respondents who took part in a mass-casualty incident or disaster as a healthcare worker evaluate their own preparedness much better than respondents who had not been involved in such an event.

4.5. Differences in the Evaluation of Preparedness for a Mass-Casualty Incident or Disaster Depending on the Organisation of Drills by the Institution and Whether They Were Attended by the Respondents

In order to check the differences in the evaluation of preparedness for mass-casualty incidents or disasters between respondents with different opinions concerning the organization of drills by the institution and depending on whether they took place, Student's t-tests for independent samples and Mann Whitney tests were performed. Initially, a Student's t-test for independent samples was conducted. It was decided to assess whether the respondents whose institution had organized drills regarding disaster management differed from those whose institution had not conducted such drills in relation to the evaluation of preparedness for such situations. The test results are presented in Table 2.

It was then assessed whether the evaluation of preparedness for such situations is impacted by the frequency of training on what to do in the event of a mass-casualty incident or disaster. Due to significant differences in the number of groups compared, Mann Whitney tests were performed.

The results of this test indicate a statistically significant and moderate effect for the evaluation of the preparedness of the current workplace for a mass-casualty incident or disaster. This results from the fact that the respondents, whose institution organized drills for such situations once every 3 years or more often, better evaluate the preparedness of the institution than the respondents whose institution organized trainings less frequently than once every 3 years. The results of the tests are presented in Table 4.

Table 4. Differences in the evaluation of preparedness for a mass-casualty incident or disaster, depending on the organization of drills by the institution, and whether they were attended by the respondents.

	Have There Been Any Disaster Management Drills Organized in the Facility Where you Currently Work?						95% CI	
	Yes ($n = 60$)		No ($n = 73$)		t	p		
	M	SD	M	SD			LL	UL
Evaluation of the preparedness of the current workplace for a mass-casualty incident or disaster	4.43	1.58	3.82	1.72	2.12	0.036	0.04	1.18
Evaluation of one's own preparedness for a mass-casualty incident or disaster	6.49	1.67	5.11	2.33	3.99	< 0.001	0.70	2.07
	Less than once every 3 years ($n = 123$)		Once every 3 years or more often ($n = 11$)				Z	p
	Average rank	Me	Average rank	Me				
Evaluation of the preparedness of the current workplace for a mass-casualty incident or disaster	64.28	4.00	97.18	6.00			−2.76	0.006
Evaluation of one's own preparedness for a mass-casualty incident or disaster	66.19	6.00	82.18	7.00			−1.32	0.186

M—mean; *Me*—median; *SD*—standard deviation; *Bias.*—bias; *Kurt.*—kurtosis; *Min & Max.*—the lowest and highest value of distribution; *D*—Kolmogorov–Smirnov test result; *p*—significance.

It was then assessed whether training in preparation for disasters impacts upon the evaluation of preparedness for mass-casualty incidents or disasters. Student's t-tests for independent tests were performed for this purpose.

The results of this test indicate significant differences for the evaluation of both one's own preparedness and also that of the institution. Both of these effects are of moderate strength. The analysis showed that after training, the respondents evaluate their own and the institution's preparedness for a mass-casualty incident or disaster better than the respondents without such training. Test results are presented in Figure 3.

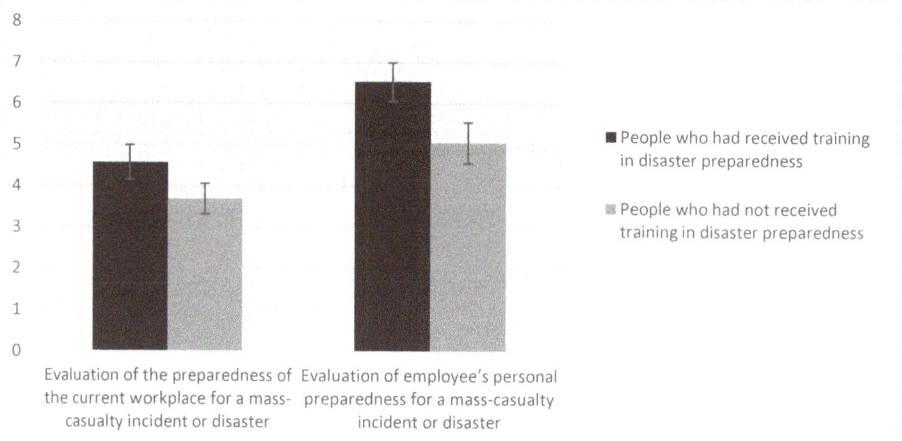

Figure 3. Average with a 95% confidence interval for evaluations of preparedness for mass-casualty incidents and disasters, categorized by participation in training related to preparation for such situations.

5. Discussion

The creation of hospital crisis management plans, evacuation plans and procedures in the event of mass-casualty incidents, and the necessity for staff to be familiar with them, is an important step towards preparing for such events. However, the lack of such plans may lead to chaos and complete disorientation [38–42].

The research shows that the majority of the respondents knew that the institution at which they currently worked had a plan for dealing with mass-casualty incidents and disasters. Moreover, over 70% of respondents reported that they knew who was responsible for the management of operations in crisis situations and were aware of the procedures to be followed during a disaster.

In mass-casualty incidents and disasters, due to the limited capacity and resources of the emergency services on site, it is not possible to provide medical assistance to all victims simultaneously. Some of them will have to wait for such assistance. In the first instance, medical assistance must be provided to victims who need it at that moment, i.e., people in immediate danger of death. This assistance must be effective. The aim is to provide maximum benefits to as many people as possible under specified conditions. The need to do what is best for victims of a mass-casualty incident or disaster makes it necessary to continuously apply medical segregation of the victims. Triage is one of the most important and often the only undertaking of rescue services providing quick control of the situation in the area of a mass-casualty incident or disaster [43].

In the study concerning triage, almost all respondents declared having the ability to conduct triage.

Each hospital should have its own evacuation plan, as every healthcare facility is different, with different architectural features, number of floors in the building, numbers of patients and their physical and mental condition, equipment, and many other features. Additionally, each event is different. Evacuation can take place in connection with a bomb threat when there are no obstacles in the form of smoke, fire, toxic products from combustion, problems with visibility, or time pressure—as happens in the case of fire. Proper evacuation of a hospital requires a well-thought-out strategy and good preparation and, in order to achieve this, drills carried out in advance [13].

The research demonstrates that the respondents are familiar with the procedures to be followed in case of evacuation in the event of a mass-casualty incident at their workplace. The developing of an evacuation plan for the healthcare facility, familiarizing the entire staff with it, and performing regular evacuation drills, are necessary to ensure the safety of patients and workers [13].

The impact of catastrophes can be avoided or reduced by adopting risk management measures, which should be implemented by taking advantage of local resources and taking appropriate actions in terms of planning, education and training [44,45].

The human factor is a significant problem in the proper, continuous preparation for emergency situations or disasters in healthcare organizations. The shortage of medical personnel [46], the overload of current work, the increasing amount of documentation, and the completion of a number of necessary formalities can make doctors reluctant to participate in such training, especially during prolonged periods of relative calm when there are no unexpected events. It can be a problem to force staff to familiarize themselves with the documentation, operating procedures and evacuation plans for mass-casualty events and disasters. In most cases, this consists of a quick, cursory, thoughtless review, because in times of prolonged security, people do not feel an approaching threat, so they do not have a strong motivation to prepare for crisis situations [47].

More than half of the respondents (54.5%) reported a lack of organization of drills concerning disaster management in their workplace. As far as the frequency of organizing drills is concerned, the majority indicated that such drills were organized less frequently than once every 3 years.

The challenges faced by the healthcare services force them to provide continuous training in the organization of responses to mass-casualty incidents and disasters, and in cooperation with other emergency services. Simulations and drills are organized from time to time, but this is not enough. It is worth remembering that every event, even seemingly simple to perform, is difficult, and not every scenario can be foreseen. There can never be too many drills. Only through continuous practice can the most appropriate procedures and skills to deal with crisis situations be developed. Besides having excellent equipment and access to appropriate personal protective equipment (e.g., in the case of a patient infected with the SARS-CoV-2 coronavirus), above all, working in accordance to safety procedures that have been prepared in advance is an example of exemplary disaster management [48].

The only drawback after the exercises is usually the lack of review and feedback for the participants. This problem was reported by the respondents in the conducted research.

Theory will never equate to practice. Only practiced procedures provide the opportunity to verify the knowledge and skills of staff, and make it possible to carry out an analysis of the speed and effectiveness of the drills, and if necessary to make corrections, eliminate errors and, above all, acquire habits that will guarantee proper behavior [49].

Each hospital should have properly prepared disaster management procedures. Such guidelines should be prepared well in advance. When a threat occurs, it should be sufficient enough to adapt them to the specific situation, so that there is no need to create everything from scratch.

Humanity has experienced many disasters and pandemics in the past, but these have been overcome (e.g., smallpox, plague, measles, polio, whooping cough, typhus, rabies and cholera).

The current pandemic has very clearly shown the speed with which even the best healthcare systems in different countries can be overwhelmed and devastated. These observations show that health should be at the top of the political agenda.

6. Limitations

The main limitation of this study was that only the employees of one hospital were studied. The COVID-19 pandemic proved to be a huge obstacle in further research. Despite these limitations, the study revealed some implementation and scientific gaps for researchers, but at the same time it is a chance to initiate discussion and become a small contribution to solving the crisis that disaster leads to. The experience gained from this study will form the basis for planned future studies with more hospitals, and a more comprehensive approach. It will also help to properly amend the questions, which will make it easier to design a future research tool.

7. Conclusions

The pilot study revealed that a properly designed questionnaire can be used to assess the relationship between hospital and staff preparedness and disaster response efficiency.

The knowledge and skills of health professionals in relation to specific events and their impact on people, as well as the appropriate treatment, are essential for the quality of healthcare services during disasters.

In order to achieve the level of preparedness and the effectiveness of the disaster response, it is necessary that every hospital has pre-prepared and validated procedures.

An experimental study involving a range of hospitals should be carried out, using more comprehensive assessment tools, to assess the correlation between the level of preparedness and performance of the hospital and the impact of the preparation of the hospital and its staff towards the survival of disaster victims.

Evaluation of the preparedness and effectiveness of disaster response is a means of identifying and removing possible gaps and weaknesses in the functioning and effective management of a hospital during mass-casualty incidents.

Author Contributions: Conceptualization: K.G.; data collection: K.G. and M.G.; formal Analysis: K.G. and M.G.; writing—original draft preparation: K.G. and M.G. All authors have read and agreed to the published version of the manuscript.

Funding: This research received no external funding.

Conflicts of Interest: The authors declare no conflict of interest.

References

1. Djalali, A.; Carenzo, L.; Ragazzoni, L.; Azzaretto, M.; Petrino, R.; Della Corte, F.; Ingrassia, P.L. Does hospital disaster preparedness predict response performance during a full-scale exercise? A pilot study. *Prehospital Disaster Med.* **2014**, *29*, 441–447. [CrossRef] [PubMed]

2. Olivieri, C.; Ingrassia, P.L.; Della Corte, F.; Carenzo, L.; Sapori, J.M.; Gabilly, L.; Segond, F.; Grieger, F.; Arnod-Prin, P.; Larrucea, X.; et al. Hospital preparedness and response in CBRN emergencies: TIER assessment tool. *Eur. J. Emerg. Med.* **2017**, *24*, 366–370. [CrossRef] [PubMed]

3. Djalali, A.; Castren, M.; Khankeh, H.; Gryth, D.; Radestad, M.; Öhlen, G.; Kurland, L. Hospital disaster preparedness as measured by functional capacity: A comparison between Iran and Sweden. *Prehospital Disaster Med.* **2013**, *28*, 454–461. [CrossRef] [PubMed]

4. Adini, B.; Laor, D.; Hornik-Lurie, T.; Schwartz, D.; Aharonson-Daniel, L. Improving hospital mass casualty preparedness through ongoing readiness evaluation. *Am. J. Med. Qual.* **2012**, *27*, 426–433. [CrossRef]

5. Cagliuso, N. Stakeholders' experiences with US hospital emergency preparedness: Part 1. *J. Bus. Contin. Emerg. Plan.* **2014**, *8*, 156–168.

6. Gillett, B.; Silverberg, M.; Roblin, P.; Adelaine, J.; Valesky, W.; Arquilla, B. Computer-facilitated assessment of disaster preparedness for remote hospitals in a long-distance, virtual tabletop drill model. *Prehospital Disaster Med.* **2011**, *26*, 230–233. [CrossRef]

7. Higgins, W.; Wainright III, C.; Lu, N.; Carrico, R. Assessing hospital preparedness using an instrument based on the Mass Casualty Disaster Plan Checklist: Results of a statewide survey. *Am. J. Infect. Control* **2004**, *32*, 327–332. [CrossRef]

8. Mortelmans, L.J.; Gaakeer, M.I.; Dieltiens, G.; Anseeuw, K.; Sabbe, M.B. Are Dutch hospitals prepared for chemical, biological, or radionuclear incidents? A survey study. *Prehospital Disaster Med.* **2017**, *32*, 483–491. [CrossRef]

9. Nekoie-Moghadam, M.; Kurland, L.; Moosazadeh, M.; Ingrassia, P.L.; Della Corte, F.; Djalali, A. Tools and checklists used for the evaluation of hospital disaster preparedness: A systematic review. *Disaster Med. Public Health Prep.* **2016**, *10*, 781–788. [CrossRef]

10. Alruwaili, A.; Islam, S.; Usher, K. Disaster Preparedness in Hospitals in the Middle East: An Integrative Literature Review. *Disaster Med. Public Health Prep.* **2019**, *13*, 806–816. [CrossRef]

11. Lazar, E.J.; Cagliuso, N.V.; Gebbie, K.M. Are we ready and how do we know? The urgent need for performance metrics in hospital emergency management. *Disaster Med. Public Health Prep.* **2009**, *3*, 57–60. [CrossRef] [PubMed]

12. Ogedegbe, C.; Nyirenda, T.; DelMoro, G.; Yamin, E.; Feldman, J. Health care workers and disaster preparedness: Barriers to and facilitators of willingness to respond. *Int. J. Emerg. Med.* **2012**, *5*, 29. [CrossRef] [PubMed]

13. Goniewicz, K.; Misztal-Okońska, P.; Pawłowski, W.; Burkle, F.M.; Czerski, R.; Hertelendy, A.J.; Goniewicz, M. Evacuation from Healthcare Facilities in Poland: Legal Preparedness and Preparation. *International J. Environ. Res. Public Health* **2020**, *17*, 1779. [CrossRef] [PubMed]

14. Beerens, R.J.J.; Tehler, H. Scoping the field of disaster exercise evaluation—A literature overview and analysis. *Int. J. Disaster Risk Reduct.* **2016**, *19*, 413–446. [CrossRef]

15. Hodge, A.J.; Miller, E.L.; Skaggs, M.K.D. Nursing self-perceptions of emergency preparedness at a rural hospital. *J. Emerg. Nurs.* **2017**, *43*, 10–14. [CrossRef]

16. Kollek, D.; Cwinn, A.A. Hospital emergency readiness overview study. *Prehospital Disaster Med.* **2011**, *26*, 159–165. [CrossRef]

17. Cocco, C.; Thomas-Boaz, W. Preparedness planning and response to a mass-casualty incident: A case study of Sunnybrook Health Sciences Centre. *J. Bus. Contin. Emerg. Plan.* **2019**, *13*, 6–21.

18. Valesky, W.; Roblin, P.; Patel, B.; Adelaine, J.; Zehtabchi, S.; Arquilla, B. Assessing hospital preparedness: Comparison of an on-site survey with a self-reported, internet-based, long-distance tabletop drill. *Prehospital Disaster Med.* **2013**, *28*, 441–444. [CrossRef]

19. Adini, B.; Goldberg, A.; Cohen, R.; Bar-Dayan, Y. Relationship between equipment and infrastructure for pandemic influenza and performance in an avian flu drill. *Emerg. Med. J.* **2009**, *26*, 786–790. [CrossRef]

20. Skryabina, E.; Reedy, G.; Amlôt, R.; Jaye, P.; Riley, P. What is the value of health emergency preparedness exercises? A scoping review study. *Int. J. Disaster Risk Reduct.* **2017**, *21*, 274–283. [CrossRef]

21. Verheul, M.L.; Dückers, M.L.; Visser, B.B.; Beerens, R.J.; Bierens, J.J. Disaster exercises to prepare hospitals for mass-casualty incidents: Does it contribute to preparedness or is it ritualism? *Prehospital Disaster Med.* **2018**, *33*, 387–393. [CrossRef] [PubMed]

22. Foote, M.; Daver, R.; Quinn, C. Using "mystery patient" drills to assess hospital ebola preparedness in new York City, 2014–2015. *Health Secur.* **2017**, *15*, 500–508. [CrossRef] [PubMed]

23. Ali, M.; Williams, M.D. No-Notice Mystery Patient Drills to Assess Emergency Preparedness for Infectious Diseases at Community Health Centers in New York City, 2015-2016. *J. Community Health* **2019**, *44*, 387–394. [CrossRef] [PubMed]

24. Djalali, A.; Ardalan, A.; Ohlen, G.; Ingrassia, P.L.; Della Corte, F.; Castren, M.; Kurland, L. Nonstructural safety of hospitals for disasters: A comparison between two capital cities. *Disaster Med. Public Health Prep.* **2014**, *8*, 179–184. [CrossRef]

25. Arab, M.A.; Khankeh, H.R.; Mosadeghrad, A.M.; Farrokhi, M. Developing a hospital disaster risk management evaluation model. *Risk Manag. Healthc. Policy* **2019**, *12*, 287. [CrossRef]

26. Shabanikiya, H.; Jafari, M.; Gorgi, H.A.; Seyedin, H.; Rahimi, A. Developing a practical toolkit for evaluating hospital preparedness for surge capacity in disasters. *Int. J. Disaster Risk Reduct.* **2019**, *34*, 423–428. [CrossRef]

27. Lennquist Montán, K.; Riddez, L.; Lennquist, S.; Olsberg, A.; Lindberg, H.; Gryth, D.; Örtenwall, P. Assessment of hospital surge capacity using the MACSIM simulation system: A pilot study. *Eur. J. Trauma Emerg. Surg.* **2017**, *43*, 525–539. [CrossRef]

28. World Health Organization; Pan American Health Organization. *Hospital Safety Index: Guide for Evaluators*, 2nd ed.; World Health Organization: Geneva, Switzerland, 2015; Available online: https://apps.who.int/iris/handle/10665/258966 (accessed on 15 June 2020).

29. Fallah-Aliabadi, S.; Ostadtaghizadeh, A.; Ardalan, A.; Fatemi, F.; Khazai, B.; Mirjalili, M.R. Towards developing a model for the evaluation of hospital disaster resilience: A systematic review. *BMC Health Serv. Res.* **2020**, *20*, 64. [CrossRef]

30. Vichova, K.; Hromada, M. The Evaluation System to Ensure the Transport of Emergency Supplies of Fuel to the Hospitals. *Transp. Res. Procedia* **2019**, *40*, 1618–1624. [CrossRef]
31. Khankeh, H.; Mosadeghrad, A.M.; Abbasabadi Arab, M. Developing accreditation standards for disaster risk management: An approach for hospital preparedness improvement–editorial. *J. Mil Med.* **2019**, *20*, 574–576.
32. Martinez, D.; Talbert, T.; Romero-Steiner, S.; Kosmos, C.; Redd, S. Evolution of the Public Health Preparedness and Response Capability Standards to Support Public Health Emergency Management Practices and Processes. *Health Secur.* **2019**, *17*, 430–438. [CrossRef] [PubMed]
33. Veenema, T.G. (Ed.) *Disaster Nursing and Emergency Preparedness*; Springer Publishing Company: Berlin, Germany, 2018.
34. Gowing, J.R.; Walker, K.N.; Elmer, S.L.; Cummings, E.A. Disaster preparedness among health professionals and support staff: What is effective? An integrative literature review. *Prehospital Disaster Med.* **2017**, *32*, 321–328. [CrossRef] [PubMed]
35. Hussein, A.; Mahmoud, N. Emergency Preparedness and Perceived Competence in Disaster. *Alex. Sci. Nurs. J.* **2016**, *18*, 1–14.
36. Goniewicz, K.; Goniewicz, M.; Burkle, F.M. The Territorial Defence Force in disaster response in Poland: Civil-military collaboration during a state of emergency. *Sustainability* **2019**, *11*, 487. [CrossRef]
37. Goniewicz, K.; Burkle, F.M. Disaster early warning systems: The potential role and limitations of emerging text and data messaging mitigation capabilities. *Disaster Med. Public Health Prep.* **2019**, *13*, 709–712. [CrossRef]
38. Delshad, V.; Borhani, F.; Khankeh, H.; Abbaszadeh, A.; Sabzalizadeh, S.; Moradian, M.J.; Behzadi, M.J.R.; Abadi, M.G.; Farzinnia, B. The effect of activating early warning system on motahari hospital preparedness. *Health Emerg. Disasters Q.* **2015**, *1*, 3–8.
39. Amiri, M.; Chaman, R.; Raei, M.; Shirvani, S.D.N.; Afkar, A. Preparedness of hospitals in north of iran to deal with disasters. *Iran. Red Crescent Med. J.* **2013**, *15*, 519. [CrossRef]
40. Daneshmandi, M.; Amiri, H.; Vahedi, M.; Farshi, M. Assessing level of Preparedness for disaster in hospitals of a selected medical sciences university-1388. *J. Mil Med.* **2010**, *12*, 167–171.
41. Aladhrai, S.A.; Djalali, A.; Della Corte, F.; Alsabri, M.; El-Bakri, N.K.; Ingrassia, P.L. Impact of the 2011 revolution on hospital disaster preparedness in Yemen. *Disaster Med. Public Health Prep.* **2015**, *9*, 396–402. [CrossRef]
42. Jama, T.J.; Kuisma, M.J. Preparedness of Finnish emergency medical services for chemical emergencies. *Prehospital Disaster Med.* **2016**, *31*, 392–396. [CrossRef]
43. Christian, M.D.; Toltzis, P.; Kanter, R.K.; Burkle, F.M.; Vernon, D.D.; Kissoon, N. Treatment and triage recommendations for pediatric emergency mass critical care. *Pediatr. Crit. Care Med.* **2011**, *12*, S109–S119. [CrossRef] [PubMed]
44. Goniewicz, K.; Khorram-Manesh, A.; Hertelendy, A.J.; Goniewicz, M.; Naylor, K.; Burkle, F.M., Jr. Current Response and Management Decisions of the European Union to the COVID-19 Outbreak: A Review. *Sustainability* **2020**, *12*, 3838. [CrossRef]
45. Goniewicz, K.; Magiera, M.; Rucińska, D.; Pawłowski, W.; Burkle, F.M.; Hertelendy, A.J.; Goniewicz, M. Geographic Information System Technology: Review of the Challenges for Its Establishment as a Major Asset for Disaster and Emergency Management in Poland. *Disaster Med. Public Health Prep.* **2020**, 1–6. [CrossRef] [PubMed]
46. Dubas-Jakóbczyk, K.; Domagała, A.; Mikos, M. Impact of the doctor deficit on hospital management in Poland: A mixed-method study. *Int. J. Health Plan. Manag.* **2018**. [CrossRef]
47. Fox, J.H.; Burkle, F.M.; Bass, J.; Pia, F.A.; Epstein, J.L.; Markenson, D. The effectiveness of psychological first aid as a disaster intervention tool: Research analysis of peer-reviewed literature from 1990–2010. *Disaster Med. Public Health Prep.* **2012**, *6*, 247–252. [CrossRef]
48. Smith, N.; Fraser, M. Straining the System: Novel Coronavirus (COVID-19) and Preparedness for Concomitant Disasters. *Am J Public Health* **2020**, *110*, 648–649. [CrossRef]
49. Goniewicz, K.; Burkle, F.M. Challenges in implementing Sendai framework for disaster risk reduction in Poland. *Int. J. Environ. Res. Public Health* **2019**, *16*, 2574. [CrossRef]

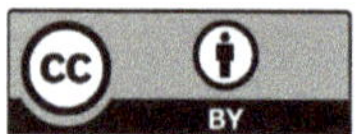

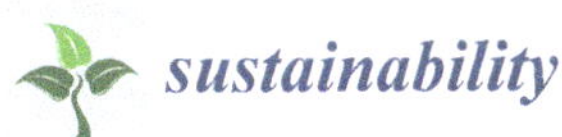 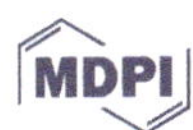

Article

Nurses' Readiness for Emergencies and Public Health Challenges—The Case of Saudi Arabia

Mohammed Ali Salem Sultan [1,2,*], **Amir Khorram-Manesh** [3,4], **Eric Carlström** [2,5],
Jarle Løwe Sørensen [5], **Hadi Jaber Al Sulayyim** [6] and **Fabian Taube** [4,7]

1   Model of Care, Directorate of Health Affairs, Najran 66255, Saudi Arabia
2   Institute of Health and Care Sciences, Sahlgrenska Academy, Gothenburg University, 413 46 Göteborg, Sweden; eric.carlstrom@gu.se
3   Institute of Clinical Sciences, Sahlgrenska Academy, Gothenburg University, 413 90 Göteborg, Sweden; amir.khorram-manesh@surgery.gu.se
4   Department of Research and Development, Swedish Armed Forces Centre for Defence Medicine, 426 76 Göteborg, Sweden; fabian.taube@amm.gu.se
5   USN School of Business, Campus Vestfold, University of South-Eastern Norway, 3603 Kongsberg, Norway; jarle.sorensen@usn.no
6   Department of Infection and Prevention and Control, Directorate of Health Affairs, Najran 66255, Saudi Arabia; hadialsleem@hotmail.com
7   Institute of Medicine, Sahlgrenska Academy, Gothenburg University, 41345 Göteborg, Sweden
*   Correspondence: mohammed.sultan@gu.se

Received: 12 July 2020; Accepted: 21 September 2020; Published: 23 September 2020

Abstract: This study was aimed at assessing the readiness of 200 emergency nurses in the southern part of Saudi Arabia in the management of public health emergencies, major incidents, and disasters by using quantitative research through a self-reporting validated questionnaire containing 10 different dimensions. All registered nurses working in emergency departments who were willing to participate, of all ages and gender groups, were included. Nurses who were not present during the study period because of vacation or maternity leave, nurses at the managerial level, and nursing aides were excluded. The participating nurses reported good knowledge in almost all investigated aspects of the theoretical dimensions of emergency management. However, they revealed perceived weaknesses in practical dimensions of emergency management and difficulties in assessing their own efforts. There was a significant correlation between qualification and the dimensions of emergency preparedness, epidemiology and surveillance, isolation and quarantine and critical resources, which indicates a need for strengthening their practical contribution as well as their theoretical knowledge. Educational initiatives combining theoretical and practical aspects of emergency management may provide an opportunity to examine nurses' knowledge, skills, and abilities continuously in an environment with no harm to patients.

Keywords: disaster; emergency; healthcare; nurse; readiness; preparedness; public health

---

1. Introduction

The increasing incidences of public health emergencies and disasters necessitate global awareness, multiagency collaboration, and emergency system readiness to respond [1]. Major incidents and disasters (MIDs) might be inevitable, but they can be mitigated by performing an appropriate risk and vulnerability assessment (RVA) as the foundation for creating a disaster response plan [2]. Risks and vulnerabilities causing a public health emergency or an MID may vary in different countries; however, the current coronavirus 2019 (COVID 19) pandemic has clearly demonstrated how a local outbreak can influence the spread of a disease and how it can result in lessons learned for global benefits. A response plan targets all possible risks, not only to enable countries to act based on their resources but also to share knowledge and compare their outcome to improve their response. Global threats can be man-made or natural (e.g., terrorism, pandemics and disasters). Vulnerabilities are the weaknesses that can be exploited by threats, and they can be dimensions which are either missing, such as strategic leadership, or of poor quality, such as the lack of proper education [3]. Although all parts of a healthcare system should be ready to manage an MID, hospital preparedness is particularly important since hospitals should serve not only the affected people but also other emergency or elective cases in need of help simultaneously. Therefore, a well-prepared hospital needs an RVA-based response plan and should facilitate educational initiatives to build up a pool of well-educated and skilled staff [4].

Because of their numbers and distribution, nurses are the largest group in the healthcare domain who face MIDs, and their knowledge and level of preparedness play a crucial role in the pre-, peri-, and post-MID periods [5] In previous studies, about 80% of Philippine nurses were found to be neither fully prepared nor knowledgeable about disaster preparedness and response, and they lacked an awareness of existing management protocols [6]. Furthermore, 65.4% of Pakistani nurses had theoretical knowledge related to disaster plans, drills, and preparedness but very little practical knowledge about MID management [7]. Finally, in Egypt and China, the majority of nurses had unsatisfactory levels of information and knowledge about disaster management and needed to join specific training programmes [8,9]. These studies reveal the importance of theoretical and practical dimensions in nurses' preparedness.

The Kingdom of Saudi Arabia (KSA) engages nearly 80% of the Arabian Peninsula, and its desert area accommodates the largest continuous sand desert in the world [10]. The KSA is a disaster-prone country with varying grades of emergencies. It has one of the world's highest mortality rates in motor vehicle crashes [11]. Terrorist incidents such as bombings have resulted in periodic internal instability as well as shifts in regional and international political dynamics [12]. Mass gatherings (Ramadan and Hajj) are two special events on the Islamic calendar that contribute to overcrowding during prayer performance and other rituals, resulting in numerous incidents [13]. Finally, many cities experience building collapses regularly as a result of mass gatherings, insufficient building safety, and a lack of control by the authorities, leading to injuries and deaths [14]. Natural disasters, such as flooding, earthquakes, and drought, occur frequently in the KSA. Floods are the most frequently experienced natural event because of unplanned urban development and improper drainage or the low ground of some high-populated areas, such as Jeddah and Mecca, which are surrounded by mountains and are easily affected by rainfall, resulting in flooding [15]. These threats make a good case for the KSA's preparedness in MIDs to be studied. One recent study from the KSA on emergency nurses' disaster preparedness showed that 28% of the nurses had inadequate knowledge [16]. The number of participants, however, was small ($n = 72$). Other studies such as the one from Australia have also confirmed these results, showing nurses' confusion about their role in MID management and their shortcomings in basic knowledge regarding standard disaster terminology and types of disasters [17]. Altogether, these studies highlight a knowledge gap in the overall preparedness of the nurses to deal with disasters.

2. Aim

This study aims to assess the theoretical and practical MID readiness of emergency nurses in the southern KSA, where MIDs frequently occur and well-educated, multinational nurses are employed to increase its response capacity.

3. Materials and Methods

3.1. Study Design

This study employed a descriptive quantitative design using a validated questionnaire to assess the knowledge and awareness among licensed nursing staff of preparedness to respond to emergencies and specific healthcare scenarios.

3.2. Questionnaire

This study used the Emergency Preparedness Information Questionnaire (EPIQ) to assess the disaster preparedness of nurses [18]. EPIQ contains a variety of topical areas, of which two are relevant for the present study, i.e., (1) the 10 specific competency dimensions related to preparedness in the case of large-scale emergency events and (2) self-assessed familiarity across these competency areas. EPIQ is the only reliable and validated tool in the literature that evaluates nurses' perceived familiarity of emergency preparedness and disaster response core competencies. It uses familiarity as an important measure of the acquisition of new information. Wisniewski et al. developed EPIQ by performing an extensive search in the literature, combined with nurses' perceptions of perceived familiarity with these capabilities. They also sought to determine preferred education methods and demographics for future educational endeavours. EPIQ has been validated by psychometric testing and used in several studies aiming to measure levels of disaster preparedness and provides a comprehensive analysis of the topic of study since it covers broad areas [19,20]. It works to individually assess all areas of healthcare and delves into in-depth information relevant to the research. Additionally, it is simple to read and interpret and provides a user-friendly interface.

EPIQ consists of 51 items divided into two parts: the first six questions relate to demographic and individual information. Secondly, 45 knowledge-based questions are distributed among the 10 emergency preparedness competency dimensions, which are (1) Emergency Preparedness Terms and Activities, (2) Incident Command System (ICS) and own role within it, (3) Ethical Issues in Triage, (4) Epidemiology and Surveillance, (5) Isolation/Quarantine, (6) Decontamination, (7) Communication/Connectivity, (8) Psychological Issues, (9) Special Populations, and (10) Accessing Critical Resources (Appendix A).

3.3. Setting

The research was conducted at the Ministry of Health's (MOH) hospitals ($n = 10$) in the Najran region, located in the southern part of the KSA.

3.4. Population and Sample

All nurses at the 10 hospitals included in the study were informed about the study by the nursing office director at each hospital. The participants were randomly included from the list of nurses working in each emergency department (ED), thus avoiding the bias of choosing a specific group. They were ensured that their participation was voluntary, they could withdraw from the study whenever they decided to, and the obtained data were handled confidentially. They received basic information about the study and its goals, and informed consent was obtained from each participant. A power analysis with a standardised statistical power of 0.80 and medium effect size of 0.5 premediated the appropriate sample size to 200 nurses. The self completion questionnaire was presented to the participants through the SurveyMonkey website.

3.5. Data Collection and Processing

Collected data were stored at the hospitals' research centres. Nurses answered the questionnaires on a specific research day to prevent response influence. The respondents were asked to provide correct information. The information provided was subject only to research, and the researcher could not disclose the respondents' identities at any time, no matter the circumstances. The included participants were registered nurses working in EDs who were willing to participate, in all age and gender groups. Nurses who were not present during the study period because of vacation or maternity leave, nurses at the managerial level, and nursing aides were excluded.

All data concerning the 10 emergency preparedness competency dimensions were analysed by the authors. The primary investigator was responsible for collecting data and categorising them for further analysis by the teammate. Each dimension consisted of a number of questions, in which participants could indicate their familiarity with a topic based on a five-point Likert scale (see results).

3.6. Ethical Approval

For this study, an ethical committee certificate of approval was obtained from the Institutional Review Board at the General Directorate of Health Affairs in the Najran region (IRB Log Number 2020-27 E—Date of approval: 1 July 2020).

3.7. Statistics

The homogeneity of the items in the subscales of the EPIQ was analysed by calculating Cronbach's alpha using Statistical Package for the Social Sciences (SPSS) software version 20. Cronbach's alpha was 0.98, which shows high internal consistency and, according to Brace, Kemp and Snelgar [21], is considered satisfactory. Other results are descriptively presented in actual numbers and percentages. A Kolmogorov–Smirnov test was used to explore normality. As a result of skewness in the data, Spearman's rho was used to test co-variation. Means were compared using the Mann–Whitney U and Kruskal–Wallis tests. Statistical significance was recognised at $p < 0.05$, and all tests were two-tailed.

4. Results

Of the 200 nurses who answered the questionnaire, 181 (90.5%) were female and 19 (9.5%) were male. A majority of the respondents (45.5%) were 22–30 years old. About 39% of the nurses were 31–40 years old, while the remaining 15.5% were 40 years old or older. About 93.5% of the nurses had a Bachelor of Science in Nursing (BSN), 6% had a Master of Science in Nursing (MSN), and 0.5% had a Doctor of Philosophy (PhD) in Nursing. Most of the practicing nurses, especially those in EDs within MOH hospitals, possessed undergraduate qualifications from MOH-certified education and training institutions. About 12% of the nurses had more than 16 years of experience within EDs, 20% had 11–15 years of experience, and 34% had 6–10 years of experience, while the remaining 34% had 1–5 years of experience.

The remaining results of the study were categorised into the following 10 dimensions, which denote the extent to which nurses are aware of disaster risks and preparedness. Each dimension consisted of several questions, in which nurses were asked to indicate their familiarity with a topic based on a five-point Likert scale as follows: very familiar (5), somewhat familiar (4), familiar to neutral (3), somewhat unfamiliar (2), and not familiar (1). The positive threshold was 'familiar to neutral' to 'very familiar'.

Table 1 shows that most of the participants had good knowledge (familiar to very familiar) in most items of these dimensions: signs and symptoms (different biological agents: 49.5%, and better for Anthrax: 75%), modes of transmission (56.5%), antidote and adverse reaction (66% and 69.5%, respectively). However, participants seemed to be uncertain about their practical capabilities, skills, and evaluations of their own actions, including necessary first aid interventions such as ventilation and oxygen administration during a public health emergency (32% and 39.5%, respectively).

Table 1. Description of 200 nurses' responses regarding familiarity with Emergency Preparedness Terms and Activities.

Items	Very Familiar	Somewhat Familiar	Familiar to Neutral	Somewhat Unfamiliar	Not Familiar	Total
1. Signs/symptoms of exposure to different biological agents	11 (5.5%)	16 (8%)	72 (36%)	82 (41%)	19 (9.5%)	100%
2. Signs/symptoms of Anthrax inhalation	26 (13%)	56 (28%)	68 (34%)	42 (21%)	8 (4%)	100%
3. Modes of transmission for different types of biological agents (anthrax, smallpox, etc.)	12 (6%)	24 (12%)	77 (38.5%)	71 (35.5%)	16 (8%)	100%
4. Match antidote and prophylactic medications to specific biological/chemical agents	9 (4.5%)	35 (17.5%)	88 (44%)	55 (27.5%)	13 (6.5%)	100%
5. Possible adverse reactions to smallpox vaccination	16 (8%)	37 (18.5%)	86 (43%)	44 (22%)	17 (8.5%)	100%
6. Basic first aid in a large-scale emergency event (including oxygen administration and ventilation)	6 (6%)	4 (2%)	48 (24%)	84 (42%)	58 (29%)	100%
7. How to evaluate the effectiveness of your own actions during a large-scale emergency	4 (2%)	11 (5.5%)	64 (32%)	92 (46%)	29 (14.5%)	100%

Table 2 shows that a majority of the nurses surveyed had good knowledge regarding what they needed to do during a large-scale emergency. They also appeared to have good knowledge about the emergency operations plan (EOP), Incident Command System (ICS), physical locations of all entities, the importance of medical decision-making, etc.

Table 2. Description of nurses' responses regarding their familiarity with the Incident Command System (ICS) and their role (*n* = 200).

Items	Very Familiar	Somewhat Familiar	Familiar to Neutral	Somewhat Unfamiliar	Not Familiar	Total
1. The content of emergency operations plan (EOP) in your agency/organisation	25 (12.5%)	84 (42%)	72 (36%)	15 (7.5%)	4 (2%)	100%
2. To which functional group in the Incident Command System (ICS) you would be assigned during a large-scale emergency event	23 (11.5%)	62 (31%)	84 (42%)	24 (12%)	7 (3.5%)	100%
3. The physical location to which you would report if a large-scale emergency event occurred	27 (13.5%)	78 (39%)	76 (38%)	14 (7%)	5 (2.5%)	100%
4. Assess and respond to site safety issues for self, co-workers and affected people during a large-scale emergency event	25 (12.5%)	77 (38.5%)	80 (40%)	13 (6.5%)	5 (2.5%)	100%
5. The strategic rationale used to develop the ICS response/action plan	13 (6.5%)	68 (34%)	89 (44.5%)	25 (12.5%)	5 (2.5%)	100%
6. Your agency's preparedness for responding to a large-scale emergency event	22 (11%)	81 (40.5%)	73 (36.5%)	18 (9%)	6 (3%)	100%
7. Differences between decision-making processes in the Incident Command System for a large-scale emergency event and non-emergency situations	24 (12%)	76 (38%)	82 (41%)	14 (7%)	4 (2%)	100%
8. Tasks which should NOT be delegated to volunteers in a large-scale emergency event	22 (11%)	65 (32.5%)	86 (43%)	21 (10.5%)	6 (3%)	100%

Table 3 shows nurses' approaches to the assessment of affected people's health following a crisis and their familiarity with ethical issues in MIDs, such as during triage. Overall, they claimed that they had good knowledge and understanding of these issues.

Table 3. Description of nurses' responses regarding their familiarity with Ethical Issues in Triage (N = 200).

Items	Very Familiar	Somewhat Familiar	Familiar to Neutral	Somewhat Unfamiliar	Not Familiar	Total
1. How to perform a rapid physical assessment of a victim of a large-scale emergency event	28 (14%)	78 (39%)	77 (38.5%)	13 (6.5%)	4 (2%)	100%
2. How to perform a rapid mental health assessment of a victim of a large-scale emergency event	25 (12.5%)	64 (32%)	86 (43%)	20 (10%)	5 (2.5%)	100%
3. How to assist with triage in a large-scale emergency event	32 (16%)	73 (36.5%)	72 (36%)	18 (9%)	5 (2.5%)	100%
4. General issues related to the proper handling of the dead during a large-scale emergency event (ethical, legal, cultural, and safety)	29 (14.5%)	65 (32.5%)	84 (42%)	19 (9.5%)	3 (1.5%)	100%

Table 4 shows nurses' knowledge in mitigating the further outbreak of a disease. Overall, most of the nurses claimed that they had good knowledge in handling the administrative measures needed in chemical, biological, radiological, and nuclear (CBRN) surveillance.

Table 4. Description of nurses' responses regarding their familiarity with Epidemiology and Surveillance (N = 200).

Items	Very Familiar	Somewhat Familiar	Familiar to Neutral	Somewhat Unfamiliar	Not Familiar	Total
1. History and assessment surveillance data for creating a high index of suspicion that a patient has been exposed to a biological agent	20 (10%)	62 (31%)	92 (46%)	21 (10.5%)	5 (2.5%)	100%
2. When to report an unusual set of symptoms to an epidemiologist	19 (9.5%)	80 (40%)	74 (37%)	23 (11.5%)	4 (2%)	100%
3. Diseases that are immediately reportable to state health departments	26 (13%)	86 (43%)	72 (36%)	13 (6.5%)	3 (1.5%)	100%
4. Ability to identify the exacerbation of an underlying disease as a result of exposure to a chemical or biological agent or to radiation	20 (10%)	67 (33.5%)	95 (47.5%)	14 (7%)	4 (2%)	100%

In Table 5, nurses evaluated their knowledge of isolation and quarantine issues. Most of the surveyed nurses seemed to have good knowledge in these areas.

Table 5. Description of nurses' responses regarding their familiarity with Isolation/Quarantine (N = 200).

Items	Very Familiar	Somewhat Familiar	Familiar to Neutral	Somewhat Unfamiliar	Not Familiar	Total
1. Isolation procedures for people exposed to biological or chemical agents	33 (16.5%)	80 (40%)	66 (33%)	17 (8.5%)	4 (2%)	100%
2. Your facility's/community's quarantine process	36 (18%)	90 (45%)	60 (30%)	10 (5%)	4 (2%)	100%

Table 6 shows that most of the nurses had good knowledge of the decontamination process in their hospitals, including the use of personal protective equipment (PPE).

Table 6. Description of nurses' responses regarding their familiarity with Decontamination (N = 200).

Items	Very Familiar	Somewhat Familiar	Familiar to Neutral	Somewhat Unfamiliar	Not Familiar	Total
1. Selection of the appropriate personal protective equipment when caring for patients exposed to chemical, biological, radiological, and nuclear (CBRN) agents	63 (31.5%)	95 (47.5%)	35 (17.5%)	4 (2%)	3 (1.5%)	100%
2. The decontamination procedures stated in your facility's emergency operations plan	36 (18%)	89 (44.5%)	61 (30.5%)	10 (5%)	4 (2%)	100%
3. The impact on the environment from a large-scale emergency event	24 (12%)	82 (41%)	72 (36%)	18 (9%)	4 (2%)	100%

Table 7 addresses the communication aspect of emergency response. A majority of the nurses had good knowledge of communication and information sharing during an emergency and of the need for debriefing and communication devices.

Table 7. Description of nurses' responses regarding their familiarity with Communication/Connectivity (N = 200).

Items	Very Familiar	Somewhat Familiar	Familiar to Neutral	Somewhat Unfamiliar	Not Familiar	Total
1. The procedure used to document provision of care in a large-scale emergency event	21 (10.5%)	77 (38.5%)	79 (39.5%)	19 (9.5%)	4 (2%)	100%
2. Chain of custody during a large-scale emergency event	15 (7.5%)	63 (31.5%)	92 (46%)	26 (13%)	4 (2%)	100%
3. Procedure for communicating critical patient information to those transporting patients	24 (12%)	86 (43%)	74 (37%)	11 (5.5%)	5 (2.5%)	100%
4. Effectively present information about degree of risk to various audiences	23 (11.5%)	60 (30%)	95 (47.5%)	17 (8.5%)	5 (2.5%)	100%
5. Identify the different abilities of key partners in your emergency operations plan (EOP)	18 (9%)	65 (32.5%)	88 (44%)	24 (12%)	5 (2.5%)	100%
6. Appropriate debriefing activities during a large-scale emergency event	19 (9.5%)	53 (26.5%)	102 (52%)	19 (9.5%)	7 (3.5%)	100%
7. Use of all types of communication devices (phone, fax, email, personal digital assistant (PDAs), etc.)	31 (15.5%)	64 (32%)	88 (44%)	13 (6.5%)	4 (2%)	100%

Table 8 shows that a majority of the nurses had good knowledge of appropriate and necessary psychological support during MIDs, claimed that they could provide health counselling/education in issues related to chemical, biological, radiological, nuclear, and explosive (CBRNE) agents, and could communicate with, identify, and evaluate youth and adults with post-traumatic stress disorder (PTSD).

Table 8. Description of nurses' responses regarding their familiarity with Psychological Issues (N = 200).

Items	Very Familiar	Somewhat Familiar	Familiar to Neutral	Somewhat Unfamiliar	Not Familiar	Total
1. Appropriate psychological support for all parties involved in a large-scale emergency event	23 (11.5%)	67 (33.5%)	88 (44%)	17 (8.5%)	5 (2.5%)	100%
2. Provide health counselling/education to patients regarding the long-term impact of chemical, biological, radiological, nuclear, and explosive (CBRNE) agents	31 (15.5%)	48 (24%)	89 (44.5%)	26 (13%)	6 (3%)	100%
3. Signs of post-traumatic stress in patients seen for routine health care following an event	21 (10.5%)	68 (34%)	86 (43%)	20 (10%)	5 (2.5%)	100%
4. How to evaluate a teenager to detect post-traumatic mental health problems	17 (8.5%)	59 (29.5%)	87 (43.5%)	28 (14%)	9 (4.5%)	100%

Table 9 shows nurses' knowledge in handling special populations affected by a disaster. A majority of nurses claimed to have good knowledge and understanding of the unique needs and expectations required for care of vulnerable groups.

Table 9. Description of nurses' responses regarding their familiarity with Special Populations (N = 200).

Items	Very Familiar	Somewhat Familiar	Familiar to Neutral	Somewhat Unfamiliar	Not Familiar	Total
1. Procedures for providing care to children/youth during a large-scale emergency event in cases in which prior consent from parent/legal guardian is possible	20 (10%)	61 (30.5%)	88 (44%)	27 (13.5%)	4 (2%)	100%
2. The appropriate care of sensitive/vulnerable patient groups during a large-scale emergency (i.e., aged, pregnant women, and the disabled)	18 (9%)	65 (32.5%)	87 (43.5%)	25 (12.5%)	5 (2.5%)	100%

Table 10 shows the ability of nurses to access critical resources during an MID. They seemed to have good knowledge and capabilities to perform necessary measures in all areas within this dimension.

Table 10. Description of nurses' familiarity responses rate of Accessing Critical Resources (N = 200).

Items	Very Familiar	Somewhat Familiar	Familiar to Neutral	Somewhat Unfamiliar	Not Familiar	Total
1. During an event, where to quickly access up-to-date resources for specific CBRNE incidents	17 (8.5%)	52 (26%)	90 (45%)	35 (17.5%)	6 (3%)	100%
2. Determine the appropriate agency to which reportable diseases are to be directed	18 (9%)	54 (27%)	91 (45.5%)	27 (13.5%)	10 (5%)	100%
3. The process for gaining access to the Strategic National Stockpile	11 (5.5%)	36 (18%)	86 (43%)	48 (24%)	19 (9.5%)	100%
4. Please provide an assessment of your overall familiarity with response activities/preparedness in the case of a large-scale emergency event	19 (9.5%)	63 (31.5%)	88 (44%)	25 (12.5%)	5 (2.5%)	100%

The results of normality, measured with the Kolmogorov–Smirnov test, indicated the data to be significantly skewed (sig. 0.00). As a result of the skewness and the fact that the data were ordinal and presented as ranks, a non-parametric test, Spearman's rho, was chosen to measure bivariate correlations. The variables of age, qualification, and experience were tested for the 10 studied dimensions of nurses' familiarity responses. Significant correlations were found in the correlations on qualification and dimensions of Emergency Preparedness (sig. 0.006), Epidemiology and Surveillance (sig. 0.008), Isolation and Quarantine (sig. 0.000) and Critical Resources (sig. 0.019). All significant correlations represented a small to moderate association (Critical Resources, 0.185–Isolation and Quarantine, 0.266) (Table 11).

Table 11. Ranks and statistics of nurses' responses regarding their familiarity with Emergency Preparedness Terms and Activities, Epidemiology and Surveillance, Isolation/Quarantine, and Accessing Critical Resources/Qualification (sign $\leq$ 0.05, N = 200).

		Emergency Preparedness	Qualification			Epidemiology and Surveillance	Qualification
Emergency preparedness	CC	1.0	0.195	Epidemiology & Surveillance Qualification	CC	1.0	0.188
	Sig.tt		0.006		Sig.tt		0.008
Qualification	CC	0.195	1.0		CC	0.188	1.0
	Sig.tt	0.006			Sig.tt	0.008	
		Isolation/ Quarantine	Qualification			Critical Resources	Qualification
Isolation/ Quarantine	CC	1.0	0.266	Critical Resources	CC	1.0	0.185
	Sig.tt		0.000		Sig.tt		0.019
Qualification	CC	0.266	1.0	Qualification	CC	0.185	1.0
	Sig.tt	0.000			Sig.tt	0.019	

CC = Correlation Coefficient, Sig.tt = Significant two-tailed.

The psychological issues dimension was significant when correlated to age (sig. 0.029), qualification (sig. 0.026), and experience (sig. 0.027). The correlations represented a small association (0.154–0.158) (Table 12).

Table 12. Ranks and statistics of nurses' responses regarding their familiarity with Psychological Issues/Age, Qualification and Experience (sign $\leq$ 0.05, N = 200).

		Psychologi-Cal Issues	Age			Psychologi-Cal Issues	Qualification			Psychologi-Cal Issues	Experience
Psychological issues	CC	1.0	0.154	Psychological issues	CC	1.0	0.158	Psychological issues	CC	1.0	0.157
	Sig.tt		0.029		Sig.tt		0.026		Sig.tt		0.027
Age	CC	0.154	1.0	Qualification	CC	0.158	1.0	Experience	CC	0.157	1.0
	Sig.tt	0.029			Sig.tt	0.026			Sig.tt	0.027	
		Psychologi-Cal Issues	Age			Psychologi-Cal Issues	Qualification			Psychologi-Cal Issues	Experience
Psychological issues	CC	1.0	0.154	Psychological issues	CC	1.0	0.158	Psychological issues	CC	1.0	0.157
	Sig.tt		0.029		Sig.tt		0.026		Sig.tt		0.027
Age	CC	0.154	1.0	Qualification	CC	0.158	1.0	Experience	CC	0.157	1.0
	Sig.tt	0.029			Sig.tt	0.026			Sig.tt	0.027	

CC = Correlation Coefficient, Sig.tt = Significant two-tailed.

5. Discussions

In this paper, we assessed the readiness of emergency nurses in the southern region of the KSA in the management of public health emergencies, major incidents, and disasters. The reasons for such evaluation were the continuous exposure of the region to both man-made and natural disasters and the advanced educational backgrounds of the nursing staff.

The results of this study indicate a good preparedness in all theoretical dimensions of MID management, including emergency preparedness terms and activities, Incident Command Systems and their role in MID management, ethical issues in triage, epidemiology and surveillance, isolation and quarantine, decontamination, communication issues, psychological issues, management of special/vulnerable populations, and assessment of critical resources. However, the nurses appeared to be uncertain about their skills and practical performance and the evaluation of their own abilities. These results are opposite to what was reported earlier from the KSA [16] and thus confirm a good theoretical knowledge and a need for practical opportunities. Bearing in mind that 93.5% of nurses had a BSN, 6% had an MSN, and 0.5% had a PhD in nursing and that most of the practicing nurses (66%) had more than five years of experience, these results might be indicative of a need for further educational initiatives to improve the skills and practical performance of all nurses working in the management of MIDs [6–9].

The quantitative nature of this study and the collected data provide an understanding of the preparedness of nurses working at MOH hospitals in the southern region of the KSA and reveal both strengths and weaknesses that can be implementable and relevant in other regions and countries.

The current COVID-19 pandemic has demonstrated difficulties in MID management, such as resource scarcity and medical decision-making, which seem to be more complicated in practice than in theory [22]. The EPIQ questionnaire enabled the researchers to capture various dimensions of disaster preparedness and response in nursing environments [23]. However, the nurses' lack of confidence in their own skills and performance should be considered a critical shortcoming. Several studies have shown that healthcare workers who are confident in their own level of competence are more likely to react effectively in real crises than those who are not [24–28]. Nurses' theoretical knowledge, such as their ability to identify the signs and symptoms associated with highly infectious biological and chemical agents, is essential for enhancing disaster preparedness; however, this theoretical knowledge should be incorporated in practical performance to yield a robust preparedness. Proper education and training in an environment where nurses can act without hesitation, make mistakes with no harm to patients, and establish contact with necessary agencies without getting rejected will enable them to attain the required knowledge and skills to identify and report signs and symptoms that are unclear and to treat and intervene with necessary and evaluable measures [4,29–32]. Such performance and collaborative action will ensure their confidence in their response activities as key players in an MID.

Nurses' emergency preparedness is determined by their familiarity with their organisation's emergency operations plan (EOP), which allows them to follow the recommended procedures for crisis intervention from a healthcare perspective [33]. Nurses' knowledge of the ethical, legal, cultural, psychological, and safety dimensions of emergency response is critical for effective intervention and recovery [23,34]. Planning to address the needs of special populations is a strategic dimension of emergency response and recovery initiatives [17]. Effective communication during an emergency is essential for ensuring nurses' collaboration with other stakeholders involved in a crisis event. The epidemiology and surveillance aspects of disaster management require streamlined communication among various departments and agencies [17].

Most of the nurses in this study reported knowledge of and familiarity with all aforementioned dimensions. However, since MIDs are rare events, they have no chance to evaluate their theoretical and practical abilities in a real situation. Simulation exercises may offer a chance to examine these abilities in a safe environment with no harm to patients [4,35,36]. These exercises may also offer an opportunity to raise their awareness about pandemics, quarantine, isolation, the use of PPE, and other critical resources to foster recovery and minimise the spread of highly infectious diseases. A majority of nurses in this study understood the methods for isolation but lacked adequate knowledge concerning the community quarantine process and the impact it may have on the mental health of both affected people and workers. This finding supports earlier findings by McCarthy [23,37], which as part of building modern contemporary emergency nurses, argued the need for nurses to increase their understating of procedures performed and competency in practice. This shortcoming would be addressed in collaborative simulation exercises [4].

In this study, there was a significant correlation between qualification and the dimensions of emergency preparedness, epidemiology and surveillance, isolation and quarantine, and critical resources. These findings are in accordance with Gladston, who reported a significant correlation between nurses' perceptions and qualifications [38], and similar to studies showing statistically significant associations between the dimensions of psychological issues and age, qualification and experience [38–41].

6. Limitations

This study focussed on nursing staff working in emergency departments only and did not consider other nurses' roles and responses. The sample consisted overwhelmingly of women. The small number of male nurses was not a representative sample of the male population of nurses in the region. The non-parametric correlations provided some useful data possible to generalise to a broader population. However, when comparing means, the results were mainly non-significant. Repeated non-parametric tests on the data (Mann–Whitney U and Kruskal–Wallis Test) indicated the need for an extended study. Data for this study were collected in the Najran region only, which is one of 13 regions in Saudi Arabia, so there was a limitation to the ability to generalise the results to all parts of Saudi Arabia. Furthermore, this study focussed on nurses working in MOH hospitals, while nurses working in other agencies, such as Saudi Arabian Oil Company (ARAMCO) Medical Services, Security Forces hospitals, National Guard hospitals, and the Armed Forces Hospitals of Saudi Arabia were not included. Finally, self-reported surveys by nature have bias: response recall, the possibility that questions will be misinterpreted, and the possibility that respondents' perceived knowledge may not be what they actually know.

7. Conclusions

The aim of this study was to evaluate the theoretical and practical readiness of nurses in MID management. The results indicate that nurses working in Najran EDs in the southern part of the KSA have good theoretical knowledge but lack confidence in their practical performance. Several studies have shown the significance of self-confidence in healthcare workers' responses to real crises [24–28]. Since theoretical knowledge should go hand in hand with practical knowledge to achieve successful outcomes in MIDs, bolstering practical emergency preparedness exercises, for example, with scenario-based simulation exercises [4] may enhance nurses' readiness for crisis response.

Author Contributions: Conceptualization: M.A.S.S., A.K.-M.; Data curation: M.A.S.S., H.J.A.S.; Formal analysis: M.A.S.S., H.J.A.S., A.K.-M., E.C., J.L.S., and F.T.; Investigation: M.A.S.S.; Methodology: M.A.S.S., E.C., A.K.-M.; Project administration: M.A.S.S.; Resources: M.A.S.S.; Supervision: A.K.-M.; Validation: E.C., J.L.S. and F.T.; Writing—original draft: M.A.S.S.; Writing—review and editing: A.K.-M., E.C., J.L.S., and F.T. All authors have read and agreed to the published version of the manuscript.

Funding: This research received no external funding.

Acknowledgments: All authors would like to thank James W. Peltier for providing us the questionnaire.

Conflicts of Interest: Authors declare no conflicts of interest.

Appendix A Questionnaire

The questionnaire is divided into two parts. The first six questions related to demographic and individual information, while the remaining 45 knowledge-based questions are distributed in the 10 emergency preparedness competency dimensions.

Appendix A.1 PART I

Demographics

Kindly tick the box where necessary

1. State your age □ 22–30 years □ 31–40 years □ > 40 years

2. State your gender □ Male □ Female

3. What is your academic degree? □ BS □ MS □ PhD

4. What is your nursing experience? □ 1–5 years □ 6–10 □ 11–15 □ > 16

5. What is your experience in the ED? □ 1–5 □ 6–8□ > 9

6. What is your marital status? □ Single □ Married □ Divorced □ Widow/widower

Appendix A.2 PART II

Table A1. Emergency Preparedness Information Questionnaire (EPIQ).

S. No	Components	Not Familiar		Somewhat Unfamiliar		Familiar to Neutral		Somewhat Familiar		Very Familiar	
I	**Emergency Preparedness Terms and Activities**	N	%	N	%	N	%	N	%	N	%
1	Signs/symptoms of exposure to different biological agents										
2	Signs/symptoms of Anthrax inhalation										
3	Modes of transmission for different types of biological agents (anthrax, smallpox, etc.)										
4	Match antidote and prophylactic medications to specific biological/chemical agents										
5	Possible adverse reactions to smallpox vaccination										
6	Basic first aid in a large-scale emergency event (including oxygen administration and ventilation)										
7	How to evaluate the effectiveness of your own actions during a large-scale emergency										
II	**Incident Command System (ICS) and your role within it**	N	%	N	%	N	%	N	%	N	%
8	The content of emergency operations plan (EOP) in your agency/organisation										
9	To which functional group in the Incident Command System (ICS) you would be assigned during a large-scale emergency event										
10	The physical location to which you would report if a large-scale emergency event occurred										
11	Assess and respond to site safety issues for self, co-workers and affected people during a large-scale emergency event										
12	The strategic rationale used to develop the ICS response/action plan										
13	Your agency's preparedness for responding to a large-scale emergency event										
14	Differences between decision-making processes in the Incident Command System for a large-scale emergency event and non-emergency situations.										
15	Tasks which should NOT be delegated to volunteers in a large-scale emergency event										

Table A1. *Cont.*

S. No	Components	Not Familiar		Somewhat Unfamiliar		Familiar to Neutral		Somewhat Familiar		Very Familiar	
III	**Ethical Issues in Triage**	N	%	N	%	N	%	N	%	N	%
16	How to perform a rapid physical assessment of a victim of a large-scale emergency event										
17	How to perform a rapid mental health assessment of a victim of a large-scale emergency event										
18	How to assist with triage in a large-scale emergency event										
19	General issues related to the proper handling of the dead during a large-scale emergency event (ethical, legal, cultural and safety)										
IV	**Epidemiology and Surveillance**	N	%	N	%	N	%	N	%	N	%
20	History and assessment surveillance data for creating a high index of suspicion that a patient has been exposed to a biological agent										
21	When to report an unusual set of symptoms to an epidemiologist										
22	Diseases that are immediately reportable to state health departments										
23	Ability to identify the exacerbation of an underlying disease as a result of exposure to a chemical or biological agent or to radiation										
V	**Isolation/Quarantine**	N	%	N	%	N	%	N	%	N	%
24	Isolation procedures for people exposed to biological or chemical agents										
25	Your facility's/community's quarantine process										
VI	**Decontamination**	N	%	N	%	N	%	N	%	N	%
26	Selection of the appropriate personal protective equipment when caring for patients exposed to CBRN agents										
27	The decontamination procedures stated in your facility's emergency operations plan										
28	The impact on the environment from a large-scale emergency event										

Table A1. *Cont.*

S. No	Components	Not Familiar		Somewhat Unfamiliar		Familiar to Neutral		Somewhat Familiar		Very Familiar	
VII	**Communication/Connectivity**	N	%	N	%	N	%	N	%	N	%
29	The procedure used to document provision of care in a large-scale emergency event										
30	Chair of custody during a large-scale emergency event										
31	Procedure for communicating critical patient information to those transporting patients										
32	Effectively present information about degree of risk to various audiences										
33	Identify the different abilities of key partners in your emergency operations plan (EOP)										
34	Appropriate debriefing activities during a large-scale emergency event										
35	Use of all types of communication devices (phone, fax, email, personal digital assistant (PDAs), etc.)										
VIII	**Psychological Issues**	N	%	N	%	N	%	N	%	N	%
36	Appropriate psychological support for all parties involved in a large-scale emergency event										
37	Provide health counselling/education to patients regarding the long-term impact of CBRNE agents										
38	Signs of post-traumatic stress in patients seen for routine health care following an event										
39	How to evaluate a teenager to detect post-traumatic mental health problems										

Table A1. *Cont.*

S. No	Components	Not Familiar		Somewhat Unfamiliar		Familiar to Neutral		Somewhat Familiar		Very Familiar	
		N	%	N	%	N	%	N	%	N	%
IX	**Special Populations**	N	%	N	%	N	%	N	%	N	%
40	Procedures for providing care to children/youth during a large-scale emergency event in cases in which prior consent from parent/legal guardian is possible										
41	The appropriate care of sensitive/vulnerable patient groups during a large-scale emergency (i.e., aged, pregnant women and the disabled)										
X	**Accessing Critical Resources**	N	%	N	%	N	%	N	%	N	%
42	During an event, where to quickly access up-to-date resources for specific CBRNE incidents										
43	Determine the appropriate agency to which reportable diseases are to be directed										
44	The process for gaining access to the Strategic National Stockpile										
45	Please provide an assessment of your overall familiarity with response activities/preparedness in the case of a large-scale emergency event										

References

1. Skliarov, S.; Kaptan, K.; Khorram-Manesh, A. Definition and General Principles of Disasters. In *Handbook of Disaster and Emergency Management*; Khorram-Manesh, A., Ed.; Kompendiet: Göteborg, Sweden, 2017; Chapter 1; pp. 17–22.
2. Khorram-Manesh, A.; Nyberg, L. Risk and Vulnerability Analysis. In *Handbook of Disaster and Emergency Management*; Khorram-Manesh, A., Ed.; Kompendiet: Göteborg, Sweden, 2017; Chapter 4, pp. 35–37.
3. Khorram-Manesh, A. Flexible surge capacity—Public health, public education, and disaster management. *Health Promot. Perspect.* **2020**, *10*, 175–179. [CrossRef] [PubMed]
4. Khorram-Manesh, A.; Berlin, J.; Carlström, E. Two Validated Ways of Improving the Ability of Decision-Making in Emergencies; Results from a Literature Review. *Bull. Emerg. Trauma* **2016**, *4*, 186–196. [PubMed]
5. Schultz, C.H.; Koenig, K.L.; Whiteside, M.; Murray, R. Development of National Standardized All-Hazard Disaster Core Competencies for Acute Care Physicians, Nurses, and EMS Professionals. *Ann. Emerg. Med.* **2012**, *59*, 196–208. [CrossRef] [PubMed]
6. Labrague, L.J.; Yboa, B.C.; McEnroe-Petitte, D.M.; Lobrino, L.R.; Brennan, M.G.B. Disaster Preparedness in Philippine Nurses. *J. Nurs. Sch.* **2016**, *48*, 98–105. [CrossRef] [PubMed]
7. Shabbir, R.; Afzal, M.; Sarwar, H.; Gilani, S.A.; Waqas, A. Nurses knowledge and practices regarding disasters management and emergency preparedness. *Saudi J. Med. Pharm. Sci.* **2017**, *3*, 464–476.
8. Khalil, N.S.; Atia, A.S.M.; Moustafa, M.F.; Soliman, H.T.T. Emergency nurses' knowledge and practice regarding preparedness of disaster management at a university hospital, Egypt. *Nurs. Healthc. Int. J.* **2019**, *3*, 1–12.
9. Xu, Y.; Zeng, X.; Yehua, X.; Xia, Z. Necessity for disaster-related nursing competency training of emergency nurses in China. *Int. J. Nurs. Sci.* **2016**, *3*, 198–201. [CrossRef]
10. Emil, M.; Sultan, M.; Sefry, S.; Ahmed, M.; AboAbdallah, M.; Chouinard, K.; Krawczyk, M. Reconstruction of the paleohydrological setting of the Rub Al Khali, Saudi Arabia. In Proceedings of the American Geophysical Union Fall Meeting Abstracts, San Francisco, CA, USA, 9–13 December 2013.
11. Hassan, H.M.; Al-Faleh, H. Exploring the risk factors associated with the size and severity of roadway crashes in Riyad. *J. Saf. Res.* **2013**, *47*, 67–74.
12. Alamri, Y.A. Emergency Management in Saudi Arabia: Past, Present and Future. In *Comparative Emergency Management: Understanding Disaster Policies, Organizations, and Initiatives from Around the World*; McEntire, D.A., Ed.; Federal Emergency Management Agency: Washington, DC, USA, 2010; p. 21.
13. Fadhlullah, S.Y.; Ismail, W. A Statistical Approach in Designing an RF-Based Human Crowd Density Estimation System. *Int. J. Distrib. Sens. Netw.* **2016**, *12*, 8351017. [CrossRef]
14. Rahman, J.; Thu, M.; Arshad, N.; Van Der Putten, M. Mass Gatherings and Public Health: Case Studies from the Hajj to Mecca. *Ann. Glob. Health* **2017**, *83*, 386–393. [CrossRef]
15. Global Facility for Disaster Reduction and Recovery GFDRR. 2020. Saudi Arabia. Available online: https://www.gfdrr.org/en/saudi-arabia (accessed on 11 April 2020).
16. AlShehri, B. Emergency nurses' preparedness for disaster in the Kingdom of Saudi Arabia. *J. Nurs. Educ. Pr.* **2017**, *7*, e013563. [CrossRef]
17. Hammad, K.; Arbon, P.; Gebbie, K.M. Emergency nurses and disaster response: An exploration of South Australian emergency nurses' knowledge and perceptions of their roles in disaster response. *Australas. Emerg. Nurs. J.* **2011**, *14*, 87–94. [CrossRef]
18. Wisniewski, R.; Dennik-Champion, G.; Peltier, J.W. Emergency Preparedness Competencies. *JONA J. Nurs. Adm.* **2004**, *34*, 475–480. [CrossRef] [PubMed]
19. Garbutt, S.J.; Peltier, J.W.; Fitzpatrick, J.J. Evaluation of an instrument to measure nurses' familiarity with emergency preparedness. *Mil. Med.* **2008**, *173*, 1073–1077. [CrossRef] [PubMed]
20. McKibbin, A.E.; Sekula, K.; Colbert, A.M.; Peltier, J.W. Assessing the Learning Needs of South Carolina Nurses by Exploring Their Perceived Knowledge of Emergency Preparedness: Evaluation of a Tool. *J. Contin. Educ. Nurs.* **2011**, *42*, 547–558. [CrossRef] [PubMed]
21. Brace, N.; Kemp, R.; Snelgar, R. *SPSS for Psychologists: A Guide to Data Analysis Using SPSS for Windows*, 3rd ed.; Lawrence Erlbaum Associates Publishers: New York, NY, USA, 2006.

22. Goniewicz, K.; Khorram-Manesh, A.; Hertelendy, A.J.; Goniewicz, M.; Naylor, K.; Burkle, F.M. Current Response and Management Decisions of the European Union to the COVID-19 Outbreak: A Review. *Sustainability* **2020**, *12*, 3838. [CrossRef]

23. McCarthy, G.; Cornally, N.; Mahoney, C.O.; White, G.; Weathers, E. Emergency nurses: Procedures performed and competence in practice. *Int. Emerg. Nurs.* **2013**, *21*, 50–57. [CrossRef]

24. Li, H.-Y.; Bi, R.-X.; Zhong, Q.-L. The development and psychometric testing of a Disaster Response Self-Efficacy Scale among undergraduate nursing students. *Nurse Educ. Today* **2017**, *59*, 16–20. [CrossRef]

25. Al Thobaity, A.; Williams, B.; Plummer, V. A new scale for disaster nursing core competencies: Development and psychometric testing. *Australas. Emerg. Nurs. J.* **2016**, *19*, 11–19. [CrossRef]

26. Lee, Y.; Lee, M.; Park, S. Development of the disaster nursing competency scale for nursing students. *J. Korean Soc. Disaster Inform.* **2013**, *9*, 511–520.

27. Valentine, M.A.; Nembhard, I.M.; Edmondson, A.C. Measuring teamwork in health care settings: A review of survey instruments. *Med. Care.* **2015**, *53*, e16–c30. [CrossRef] [PubMed]

28. Regan, S.; Laschinger, H.K.; Wong, C.A. The influence of empowerment, authentic leadership, and professional practice environments on nurses' perceived interprofessional collaboration. *J. Nurs Manag.* **2016**, *24*, E54–E61. [CrossRef] [PubMed]

29. Al Khalaileh, M.A.; Bond, E.; Alasad, J.A. Jordanian nurses' perceptions of their preparedness for disaster management. *Int. Emerg. Nurs.* **2012**, *20*, 14–23. [CrossRef]

30. Fung, O.W.M.; Loke, A.Y.; Lai, C.K.Y. Disaster preparedness among Hong Kong nurses. *J. Adv. Nurs.* **2008**, *62*, 698–703. [CrossRef]

31. Veenema, T.G.; Griffin, A.; Gable, A.R.; MacIntyre, L.; Simons, R.N.; Couig, M.P.; Walsh, J.J.; Lavin, M.C.C.; Dobalian, A.; Larson, E. Nurses as Leaders in Disaster Preparedness and Response-A Call to Action. *J. Nurs. Sch.* **2016**, *48*, 187–200. [CrossRef] [PubMed]

32. Alim, S.; Kawabata, M.; Nakazawa, M. Evaluation of disaster preparedness training and disaster drill for nursing students. *Nurse Educ. Today* **2015**, *35*, 25–31. [CrossRef]

33. Ireland, M.; Ea, E.; Kontzamanis, E.; Michel, C. Integrating Disaster Preparedness into a Community Health Nursing Course: One School's Experience. *Disaster Manag. Response* **2006**, *4*, 72–76. [CrossRef] [PubMed]

34. Ibrahim, F.A.A. Nurses Knowledge, Attitudes, Practices and Familiarity Regarding Disaster and Emergency Preparedness—Saudi Arabia. *Am. J. Nurs. Sci.* **2014**, *3*, 18–25. [CrossRef]

35. Chapman, K.; Arbon, P. Are nurses ready? Disaster preparedness in the acute setting. *Australas. Emerg. Nurs. J.* **2008**, *11*, 135–144. [CrossRef]

36. Weiner, E.; Irwin, M.; Trangenstein, P.; Gordon, J. Emergency preparedness curriculum in nursing schools in the United States. *Nurs. Educ. Perspect.* **2006**, *26*, 334–339.

37. Volkman, J.C.; Rebmann, T.; Hilley, S.; Alexander, S.; Russell, B.; Wagner, W. Infection prevention disaster preparedness planning for long-term care facilities. *Am. J. Infect. Control* **2012**, *40*, 206–210. [CrossRef] [PubMed]

38. Gladston, S.; Nayak, R. Disaster preparedness among nurses working in a paediatric acute care setting of a tertiary hospital, south India. *IOSR J. Nurs. Health Sci.* **2017**, *18*, 25–35.

39. Al-Hunaishi, W.; Hoe, V.C.; Chinna, K. Factors associated with healthcare workers willingness to participate in disasters: A cross-sectional study in Sana'a, Yemen. *BMJ Open* **2019**, *9*, e030547. [CrossRef]

40. Bella Magnaye, R.N.; Muñoz, M.S.; Muñoz, M.A.; Muñoz, R.G.; Muro, J.H. The role, preparedness and management of nurses during disasters. *Int. Sci. Res. J.* **2011**, *3*, 269–294.

41. Tzeng, W.-C.; Feng, H.-P.; Cheng, W.-T.; Lin, C.-H.; Chiang, L.-C.; Pai, L.; Lee, C.-L. Readiness of hospital nurses for disaster responses in Taiwan: A cross-sectional study. *Nurse Educ. Today* **2016**, *47*, 37–42. [CrossRef]

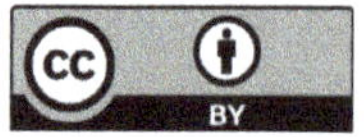

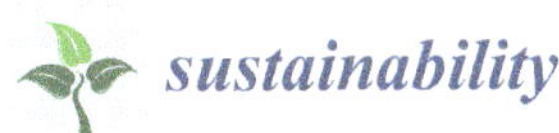 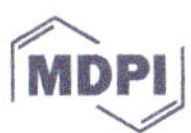

Article

A Study on the Job Retention Intention of Nurses Based on Social Support in the COVID-19 Situation

Young-Jae Kim [1], So-Young Lee [2] and Jeong-Hyung Cho [1,*]

[1]   Department of Physical Education of Chung-Ang University, Seoul 06974, Korea; yjkim@cau.ac.kr
[2]   Department of Nursing of Jungwon University, Chungbuk 28024, Korea; soyoung.lee@jwu.ac.kr
*   Correspondence: cheer1007@naver.com; Tel.: +82-2-820-5386

Received: 5 July 2020; Accepted: 30 August 2020; Published: 4 September 2020

Abstract: This study investigated how social support influences the job engagement and job retention intention of nurses struggling in the continuing scenes of the COVID-19 pandemic. To this end, 382 nurses were the participants, data from 377 of whom were analyzed in total, with the following results. First, it showed that nurses' job engagement and job retention intention were high, depending on their age and work experience. Second, in terms of the factors related to COVID-19, the group with experience in nursing patients infected with COVID-19 and nurses working in COVID-19 divisions had low job retention intention. Lastly, it appeared that there were differences in job engagement and job retention intention depending on the category and type of social support. These results suggest that social support should be provided strategically to ensure nurses' job retention.

Keywords: COVID-19; nurse; job engagement; social support

1. Introduction

Since the first outbreak of COVID-19 in December 2019 [1], there are now (7 May 2020) approximately 3,871,312 infected and 272,856 deaths as a result of the COVID-19 pandemic [2]. The rapid spread of COVID-19 around the world has caused serious damage to each nation, including fatal risks, unemployment, and deteriorating work–life balance [3–5]. Accordingly, a state of emergency was declared worldwide because of COVID-19, and efforts are being exerted to overcome the current situation [6]. This includes nurses taking care of COVID-19 patients at the scenes of COVID-19 infections, where they have to wear protective equipment for many hours, leaving marks on their faces [7]. However, as COVID-19 has been ongoing for a long time, nurses are facing hardships in carrying out their jobs [8,9]. In every country, nurses are being praised for their efforts, and countless encouraging messages are relayed to medical workers through mass media. For example, Banksy, an anonymous England-based street artist, sent a painting to Southampton General Hospital that memorialized nurses as children's heroes [10]. In addition, people are spreading encouraging dance challenge videos with the theme of "support for the nurses" through social networking services' platforms [11]. These efforts recognize that nurses are the most directly exposed to COVID-19 and that their work has increased dramatically during the pandemic; in so doing, they bring greater awareness to the situation, and nurses around the world have praised these efforts [12].

This social support (i.e., encouragement sent to nurses) is possible because many people can relate to the sacrifices and service of the nurses in the COVID-19 pandemic despite the risks. Social support has a positive effect on subjects' mental health; in particular, it influences job-related stress reduction and can even enhance self-esteem [13]. In addition, as technology develops, social knowledge is being created through the means of social networks [14].

In a study by Lee and Yoon [15], it was found that nurses who received social support had reduced depression and high self-resilience. Furthermore, social support reduces nurses' emotional labor and burnout [16]. Since the COVID-19 situation absolutely requires the staffing of nurses, it is imperative to study the effectiveness of nurses' current social support. Social support is conceptually defined as providing individuals with resources in either tangible or intangible forms, which are typically divided into the categories of emotional, instrumental, or informational support, and appraisal [17]. Additionally, social support is characterized by mutuality, that is, an exchange in resources between individuals or between an individual and a group. Sullivan [18] stated that people want to have positive relationships with others and feel accepted, so efforts are made for social interaction. Social support appears differently as individuals face more difficult situations. Krause [19] stated that in this sense, social support could be harmful, although most cases of social support are considered positive. For example, social support can have positive effects such as reducing stress and improving self-esteem, but alcohol consumption and stress may increase [20,21]. Precedent studies conducted on social support show that it was used as a measure of social resources to control the stress that results from the working environment [22,23]. Munro's research [24], which targeted 60 Australian nurses, showed that social support has a negative relationship with initial stress. Moreover, Lee Young Mi [15] stated that nurses' social support appears differently depending on general characteristics, and job satisfaction is higher when social support is recognized. Recent studies show that social workers' turnover is positively affected by social support [25], and a study of nurses said that social support helps them cope with the working environment and thrive [13].

Therefore, it is necessary to investigate how social support influences job retention for nurses who are managing duties that are more difficult than usual in the pandemic situation. However, according to research results related to nurses in the context of the COVID-19 epidemic, the nurses' working environment is dangerous and more exhausting than usual [26–28]. A study by Maben and Bridges [29] suggested that nurses need psychological and mental health support. In addition, only studies about the high job stress of nurses in pandemic outbreak situations and turnover intention are in progress [30,31], and there is insufficient practical research into how social support recognized by nurses is connected to job retention. In response, this study aims to investigate how social support affects job engagement and how the job retention intention of nurses is affected by social support in the continuing COVID-19 situation.

2. Materials and Methods

2.1. Participants

The sample of this study included nurses who had a national nursing certificate. In addition, only nurses currently on duty were allowed to participate; this was assured through screening questions administered before they participated in the questionnaire. Data were collected from 11–24 May 2020, when confirmed cases of COVID-19 were < 10 patients a day, but then suddenly started increasing to 20–30 patients. The size of the samples used in the study was calculated using the G*power 3.0 program (Heinrich-Heine-Universität Düsseldorf, Düsseldorf, Germany), and, as a result of calculating by applying 0.15 moderate effect size, 0.05 level of significance and 0.85 statistical power, at least 314 participants were required. In this study, participants who were voluntarily willing to participate were selected, and 382 participants joined in total. Among them, the data of 377 participants were used. Responses that had the same number of answers and those in which the respondent had the highest job rank but lowest earned income were excluded from the data. For the survey, a Google online questionnaire was made and distributed to the participants via email out of consideration for COVID-19. This study was conducted with the approval of the Institutional Review Board of Chung-Ang University (1041078-202005-HRSB-124-01).

2.2. Measurement

2.2.1. Job Engagement

To measure job engagement, this study used the tool developed by Kim [32], which was a modified translation of the Utrecht Work Engagement Scale (UWES) developed by Schaufeli and Bakker [33] accompanied by Kim's supplements. This tool consists of 17 questions in three sub-areas: energy (six questions), sacrifice (five questions), and immersion (six questions). Typical questions include "When I wake up in the morning, I want to go to work," "I can work for a long time at a time," and "I feel proud of my work." The questionnaire consisted of a five-point scale in which one point represents strongly disagree and five points indicates strongly agree. The higher score on the five-point Likert scale signifies a higher level of job engagement. In this study, Cronbach's α was 0.91, and the sub-areas were 0.87 for energy, 0.84 for sacrifice, and 0.82 for immersion. The exploratory factor analysis for Job Engagement is given in Table 1.

Table 1. Results of Exploratory Factor Analysis (EFA) for Job Engagement Scale.

Items	EFA		
	1	2	3
Energy 4	0.835		
Energy 3	0.808		
Energy 1	0.800		
Energy 6	0.706		
Energy 2	0.696		
Energy 7	0.583		
Energy 5	0.565		
Sacrifice 3		0.870	
Sacrifice 4		0.745	
Sacrifice 1		0.540	
Sacrifice 2		0.518	
Immersion 1			0.780
Immersion 2			0.712
Immersion 3			0.594
Cronbach's α	0.866	0.842	0.817
Eigenvalue	4.111	2.702	1.920
Variance (%)	29.363	19.303	13.714
Variance Cumulated (%)	29.363	48.666	62.380
KMO = 0.835, χ^2 = 1408.494, df = 66, $p < 0.001$			

2.2.2. Job Retention Intention

As the measurement tool for job retention intention, this study used questions from the Theory of Planned Behavior (TPB) developed by Ajzen [34] that measured behavioral intention. The Theory of Planned Behavior consists of a structure with four independent factors including attitudes about behavior, subjective norm, perceived behavioral control, and behavioral intention. In this study, only the three questions related to behavioral intention were used. Job engagement questions consisted of "I will continue my career next month," "I will continue my career after six months," and "I will continue my career after a year." The questionnaire consisted of a five-point scale with one point indicating strongly disagree and five points meaning strongly agree. The behavioral intention factor is composed of a five-point Likert scale, and in this study, the higher the score, the greater the nurse's intention to keep the job. The reliability analysis, Cronbach's α, was found to be 0.87.

2.2.3. Social Support

This study organized questions based on the content and composition of social support in the studies of Shirey [14] and Choo [35], who studied nurses. Social support consisted of three questions in total: "experience of social support," "social support categories," and "types of social support." The questions were as follows: "Have you ever received or seen social support to nurses during COVID-19? Who did you receive social support from? What type of social support did you receive?" The social support questions are all composed of nominal measures.

2.3. Data Analysis

To achieve the study purpose, all the analyses for this study were performed using SPSS Ver. 25.0 (IBM, Armonk, NY, USA) after encoding and data cleaning. In order to examine socio-demographic factors, frequency analysis and descriptive analysis were conducted, and to obtain reliability and validity of the measuring instrument, Cronbach's α and exploratory factor analysis were carried out. Lastly, a *t*-test and one-way ANOVA were executed to investigate differences in job engagement and job retention intention depending on the independent variables (characteristics of the subjects and types of social support).

3. Results

Table 2 presents the characteristics of the nurses involved in this study. Females participated more than males, and females showed a higher level of job engagement and job retention intention than males as well. The group of the nurses aged 41 or over showed the highest level of job engagement and job retention intention, and married respondents showed a higher level of job engagement and job retention intention. The group of nurses working for general hospitals occupied the largest proportion of the participants, but the group of those working for health centers and communities showed a higher level of job engagement and job retention intention. The group of head nurses displayed a higher level of job engagement, and the group of charge nurses displayed a higher level of job retention intention. In relation to COVID-19-related characteristics, the nurses with experience in caring for COVID-19 patients had a higher level of job engagement.

Table 3 shows the results of nurses' job engagement. While the differences in job engagement followed by social support were not statistically significant, the group that recognized it (M = 3.392, SD = 0.639) showed a high result (F = 2.145, $p > 0.05$). In the case of the detailed differences that appeared depending on the category of support, the group that received support from family displayed the highest level of engagement (M = 3.541, SD = 0.578), and the group supported by work colleagues (M = 2.998, SD = 0.657) scored the lowest (F = 3.463, $p < 0.001$). In terms of the types of social support, social support group through the mass media (M = 3.454, SD = 0.654) showed the highest job engagement (F = 0.380, $p > 0.05$).

Table 4 shows the differences in the job retention intention of nurses followed by social support. The job retention intention of nurses based on social support was highest for the group that could not recognize social support (M = 3.952, SD = 1.001), but there was no significant difference (F = 2.918, $p > 0.05$). For the detailed differences followed by the support categories, the group that recognized national encouragement (M = 4.174, SD = 0.968) recorded the highest scores for job retention intention, and the group that recognized encouragement by the company (M = 3.577, SD = 0.929) recorded the lowest (F = 2.997, $p > 0.05$). Lastly, in terms of the types of social support, the group that recognized encouragement through mass media (M = 4.227, SD = 0.972) had the highest job retention intention (F = 3.389, $p < 0.05$).

Table 2. Demographic Characteristics and Scores by Variables ($n = 377$).

Variable	n	%	Job Engagement			Job Retention Intention		
			M	SD	F/t	M	SD	F/t
Gender								
Male	39	10.3	3.431	0.674	0.521	3.803	0.843	0.487
Female	338	89.7	3.350	0.667		3.922	1.022	
Age (years)								
≤25	18	4.8	3.511	0.495		3.648	0.918	
26–30	115	30.5	3.089	0.699		3.655	1.020	
31–35	114	30.2	3.368	0.630	9.713 ***	3.733	0.985	9.785 ***
36–40	65	17.2	3.460	0.602		4.220	0.907	
≥41	65	17.2	3.672	0.609		4.430	0.865	
Married								
Yes	145	38.5	3.529	0.677	16.127 ***	4.160	0.943	15.275 ***
No	232	61.5	3.251	0.617		3.752	1.011	
Income (USD)								
≤$1500	44	11.7	3.358	0.766		4.030	1.198	
$1501–2500	185	49.1	3.296	0.669	2.797 *	3.733	0.984	6.514 ***
$2501–3500	104	27.6	3.359	0.620		3.948	0.990	
>$3500	44	11.7	3.617	0.625		4.439	0.673	
Type of workplace								
Senior general hospital	121	32.1	3.345	0.660		3.961	0.989	
General hospital	159	42.2	3.321	0.627	0.927	3.712	0.974	6.621 ***
Health center and community	97	25.7	3.436	0.738		4.168	1.015	
Nursing position								
General nurse	296	78.5	3.277	0.660		3.810	1.012	
Charge nurse	56	14.9	3.525	0.572	14.689 ***	4.279	0.898	6.758 ***
Head nurse	25	6.6	3.948	0.611		4.253	0.898	
Nursing experience (years)								
<1	37	9.8	3.180	0.791		3.297	1.102	
1–3	71	18.8	3.291	0.575		3.770	0.767	
3–5	81	21.5	3.403	0.606	2.867 *	3.843	0.897	9.294 ***
Between 5–10	103	27.3	3.283	0.694		3.890	1.143	
>10	85	22.5	3.539	0.675		4.380	0.860	
COVID-19 nursing experience								
Yes	44	11.7	3.478	0.623	1.598	3.674	0.935	2.764
No	333	88.3	3.342	0.672		3.940	1.101	
Service in COVID-19 related division								
Yes	45	11.9	3.170	0.797	4.064 *	3.688	1.013	2.480
No	332	88.1	3.383	0.645		3.939	1.001	
Total	377	100	3.358	0.667		3.909	1.004	

* $p < 0.05$, *** $p < 0.001$.

Table 3. Result of one-way analysis of variance about job engagement.

Item	Frequency (n)	Average	Standard Deviation	Mean Square	F	Probability	Observed Power	Post Verification
Experience of social support ($n = 377$)								
Yes	260	3.392	0.639	0.954	2.145	0.144	0.309	
No	117	3.283	0.724					
Social support categories ($n = 260$)								
Family [a]	93	3.541	0.578					
Friend [b]	50	3.336	0.674					
Colleague [c]	20	2.998	0.657	1.364	3.463	0.009	0.855	a > c
Country [d]	82	3.363	0.663					
Company [e]	15	3.333	0.498					
Types of social support ($n = 260$)								
Mass media [α]	63	3.454	0.654					
Analog media [β]	40	3.323	0.455					
Social network service [γ]	52	3.365	0.662	0.156	0.380	0.768	0.124	
Conversation and encouragement [δ]	105	3.394	0.682					

Note: [a] Family, [b] Friend, [c] Colleague, [d] Country, [e] Company, [α] Mass media, [β] Analog media, [γ] Social network service, [δ] Conversation and encouragement.

Table 4. Results of one-way analysis of variance about job retention intention.

Item	Frequency (n)	Average	Standard Deviation	Mean Square	F	Probability	Observed Power	Post Verification
Experience of social support (n = 377)								
Yes	260	3.814	1.009	1.531	1.519	0.219	0.233	
No	117	3.952	1.001					
Social support categories (n = 260)								
Family [a]	93	4.017	0.904					
Friend [b]	50	3.713	1.130					
Colleague [c]	20	3.616	1.082	2.918	2.997	0.019	0.794	
Country [d]	82	4.174	0.968					
Company [e]	15	3.577	0.929					
Types of social support (n = 260)								
Mass media [α]	63	4.227	0.972					
Analog media [β]	40	3.600	0.777					
Social network service [γ]	52	3.891	0.930	3.311	3.389	0.019	0.762	α > β
Conversation and encouragement [δ]	105	3.952	1.090					

Note: [a] Family, [b] Friend, [c] Colleague, [d] Country, [e] Company, [α] Mass media, [β] Analog media, [γ] Social network service, [δ] Conversation and encouragement.

4. Discussion

This study explored the job engagement and job retention intention of nurses who are nursing patients despite the risks in the long-term COVID-19 pandemic situation. There were differences in the nurses' job engagement and job retention intention depending on their social characteristics. A specific discussion of these findings follows.

First, the participants recorded higher job engagement and job retention intention depending on their age and work experience. The research findings support the results of previous research on the job engagement of nurses and organizational citizenship behavior, which revealed that a higher age leads to increased job engagement, organizational citizenship behavior, and career involvement [36]. Organizational citizenship behavior contributes to the maintenance and reinforcement of social and psychological contexts that support task performance for organizations above a minimum demand for duties, and it is necessary for medical treatment jobs. Medical organizations require close communication and cooperation between employees, and flexible job performance skills. This competence is complementary to "job engagement" with regard to carrying out duties with a positive attitude [37,38]. Nursing duties generally involve working in teams across three shifts to carry out continuous nursing duties. Therefore, in such a difficult situation as a pandemic, team formation that includes a nurse who is older and more experienced could help heighten nurses' job engagement and job retention intention.

For COVID-19-related factors, job retention intention was low for the group who had experience taking care of patients infected with COVID-19 and the nurses working in COVID-19-related divisions. This result is similar to that of previous research, which has shown that exposure to environmental risks negatively influences the choice of sustainable jobs [39]. Before nurses in South Korea select their jobs, they take the oath of the Nightingale Pledge. This is because health and medical care are difficult and require sacrifices [40]. However, the study result implies that nurses' work ethic as professionals could diminish in situations similar to the COVID-19 pandemic in which their own lives are at risk. The decrease in the job retention intention of nurses signifies the decline of the nursing workforce, which is a large barrier to overcoming the COVID-19 situation. Accordingly, it has been suggested that measures are needed to heighten the job retention intention of nurses who work in COVID-19-related divisions, or care for patients infected with COVID-19. In particular, it should be taken into account that working in a stressful working environment (e.g., emergency department) or organizational variables (e.g., bad working environment) may lead to a low intention to retain the job.

Lastly, there are differences in job engagement and job retention intention based on the categories and types of social support. This result is consistent with the research results that state that social support reduces job stress [41] and helps overcome disasters [42]. In addition, research targeted at nurses reports that the level of burnout decreases as social support increases [43]. Even in this study, the group that received support from their family in the same context showed the highest job engagement and job retention intention. Currently, nurses are struggling psychologically with the exposure of their families to potential COVID-19 infection [44]. Therefore, family support could have increased importance for them because family members' support can reduce concerns about infecting family members because of their work. Regarding types of social support, support through mass media showed high job engagement and job retention intention. The mass media applies the most direct decisive measures to people and society [45]. It has been reported that providing information about individuals in mass media positively influences their self-esteem, image, and sense of belonging [46]. The research finding of this study has the same context, as it suggests that the group that recognizes social support through mass media has high job engagement and job retention intention. As the world continues to battle the pandemic, we need to support nurses who are treating COVID-19 patients with continuous messages of encouragement through the media.

This study identified the differences in nurses' job engagement and job retention intention through their social characteristics and social support to ensure the necessary job retention to cope with the COVID-19 situation. Nevertheless, this study has the following limitations: First, the continuing COVID-19 situation could cause varied job retention intentions depending on the level of fatigue and risks felt by nurses, so careful consideration is required in interpretation. Second, social support could vary according to method and meanings, depending on individuals' cultural differences. Third, this study was conducted in the context of COVID-19, a global infectious disease. Therefore, it is necessary to take care when extending interpretations to ordinary situations. Fourth, this study was conducted as a basic study due to the special circumstances of COVID-19. In future studies, a study including a control group should be conducted to increase the effectiveness. Lastly, this study identifies differences as a cross-sectional study, so it does not represent causal relations.

5. Conclusions

This study shows that the differences in job engagement and job retention intention of nurses working on the frontlines of the COVID-19 situation depend on their social characteristics and support. Differences in job engagement and job retention intention are based on nurses' individual characteristics and working environments, so these characteristics must be considered in operations for nurses to continue in their jobs. In particular, the job retention intention of nurses working in COVID-19-related divisions was low; this issue should be taken into careful consideration. Low job retention intention could cause significant damage to the nursing workforce, and it should be recognized that this may cause hardships in overcoming the COVID-19 pandemic. To win against COVID-19 and adequately prepare for a future COVID-19 pandemic situation, press media targeting nurses (e.g., news, articles, and documentaries) should become more active and family support should be provided.

Author Contributions: Conceptualization, Y.-J.K. and S.-Y.L.; Methodology, J.-H.C.; Validation, Y.-J.K., S.-Y.L. and J.-H.C.; Formal Analysis, J.-H.C.; Investigation, S.-Y.L. and J.-H.C.; Data Curation, J.-H.C. and Y.-J.K.; Writing—Original Draft Preparation, S.-Y.L.; Writing—Review and Editing, S.-Y.L. and Y.-J.K. All authors have read and agreed to the published version of the manuscript.

Funding: This research received no external funding.

Conflicts of Interest: The authors declare no conflict of interest.

References

1. Cirrincione, L.; Plescia, F.; Ledda, C.; Rapisarda, V.; Martorana, D.; Moldovan, R.E.; Theodoridou, K.; Cannizzaro, E. COVID-19 Pandemic: Prevention and protection measures to be adopted at the workplace. *Sustainability* **2020**, *12*, 3603. [CrossRef]
2. Worldometer. Coronavirus Cases. COVID-19 Coronavirus Pandemic. Available online: https://www.worldometers.info/ (accessed on 7 May 2020).

3. Kim, Y.J.; Cho, J.H. Correlation between preventive health behaviors and psycho-social health based on the leisure activities of South Koreans in the COVID-19 crisis. *Int. J. Environ. Res. Public Health* **2020**, *17*, 4066. [CrossRef]

4. Kutikov, A.; Weinberg, D.S.; Edelman, M.J.; Horwitz, E.M.; Uzzo, R.G.; Fisher, R.I. A war on two fronts: Cancer care in the time of COVID-19. *Ann. Intern. Med.* **2020**, *172*, 756–758. [CrossRef] [PubMed]

5. Pirouz, B.; Haghshenas, S.; Haghshenas, S.S.; Piro, P. Investigating a serious challenge in the sustainable development process: Analysis of confirmed cases of COVID-19 (new type of coronavirus) through a binary classification using artificial intelligence and regression analysis. *Sustainability* **2020**, *12*, 2427. [CrossRef]

6. Cohen, J.; Kupferschmidt, K. Countries test tactics in 'war' against COVID-19. *Science* **2020**, *367*, 1287–1288. [CrossRef]

7. Huang, L.; Lin, G.; Tang, L.; Yu, L.; Zhou, Z. Special attention to nurses' protection during the Covid-19 epidemic. *Crit. Care* **2020**, *24*. [CrossRef] [PubMed]

8. Hewings-Martin, Y. 'It's Really a Hard Time Right Now, Says Chicago Nurse Looking after COVID-19 Patients. *Medical News Today*. Available online: https://www.medicalnewstoday.com/articles/its-really-a-hard-time-right-now-says-chicago-nurse-looking-after-covid-19-patients (accessed on 28 April 2020).

9. Nowell, A. Hospice Nurse Describes how Covid-19 Has Changed her Work. *Wigan Today*. Available online: https://www.wigantoday.net/health/hospice-nurse-describes-how-covid-19-has-changed-her-work-2886454 (accessed on 20 June 2020).

10. Sukheja, B. Good News: Five Heartwarming Stories to Cheer the Mood Amid COVID-19 Crisis. *R. Republic World*. Available online: https://www.republicworld.com/entertainment-news/whats-viral/five-heartwarming-stories-to-cheer-up-amid-covid-19-lockdown.html (accessed on 7 May 2020).

11. Jones, L.A. Dancing Philly Nurses 'Level Up' Video Goes Viral, Garners Heartfelt Thanks from Celebs. Billy Penn. Available online: https://billypenn.com/2020/04/07/dancing-philly-nurses-level-up-video-goes-viral-garners-heartfelt-thanks-from-celebs/ (accessed on 7 April 2020).

12. Juan, G.S.; Sara, D.S.; Macarena, R.M.; Mónica, O.M.; Juan, J.G.I.; Carlos, R.F. Sense of coherence and psychological distress among healthcare workers during the COVID-19 pandemic in Spain. *Sustainability* **2020**, *12*, 6855. [CrossRef]

13. Shirey, M.R. Social support in the workplace: Nurse leader implications. *Nurs. Econ.* **2004**, *22*, 313.

14. Nichole, E.; Kevin, B.W. Social network sites as vehicles for effective/ineffective social support. In *Social Support and Health in the Digital Age*; Lexington Books: Rowman & Littlefield: Lanham, MD, USA, 2019.

15. Lee, A.S.; Yoon, C.K. Influence of ego-resilience and social support on the depression of hospital nurses. *Korean J. Occup. Health Nurs.* **2012**, *21*, 46–54. [CrossRef]

16. Kim, I.S. The role of self-efficacy and social support in the relationship between emotional labor and burn out, turn over intention among hospital nurses. *J. Nurs. Adm.* **2009**, *15*, 515–526.

17. Langford, C.P.H.; Bowsher, J.; Maloney, J.P.; Lillis, P.P. Social support: A conceptual analysis. *J. Adv. Nurs.* **1997**, *25*, 95–100. [CrossRef] [PubMed]

18. Sullivan, H.S. *The Interpersonal Theory of Psychiatry*; Perry, H.S., Gawel, M.L., Eds.; Norton: New York, NY, USA, 1953.

19. Krause, N. Chronic financial strain, social support, and depressive symptoms among older adults. *Psychol. Aging* **1987**, *2*, 185. [CrossRef] [PubMed]

20. Hagihara, A.; Tarumi, K.; Nobutomo, K. Positive and negative effects of social support on the relationship between work stress and alcohol consumption. *J. Stud. Alcohol* **2003**, *64*, 874–883. [CrossRef] [PubMed]

21. Jenkins, R.; Elliott, P. Stressors, burnout and social support: Nurses in acute mental health settings. *J. Adv. Nurs.* **2004**, *48*, 622–631. [CrossRef]

22. Laschinger, H.K.S.; Havens, D.S. The effect of workplace empowerment on staff nurses' occupational mental health and work effectiveness. *J. Nurs. Adm.* **1997**, *27*, 42–50. [CrossRef]

23. Laschinger, H.K.S.; Finegan, J.; Shamian, J.; Wilk, P. Workplace empowerment as a predictor of nurse burnout in restructured healthcare settings. *Longwoods Rev.* **2003**, *1*, 2–11.

24. Munro, L.; Rodwell, J.; Harding, L. Assessing occupational stress in psychiatric nurses using the full job strain model: The value of social support to nurses. *Int. J. Nurs.* **1998**, *35*, 339–345. [CrossRef]

25. Kim, H.; Stoner, M. Burnout and turnover intention among social workers: Effects of role stress, job autonomy and social support. *Adm. Soc. Work* **2008**, *32*, 5–25. [CrossRef]

26. Jackson, D.; Bradbury-Jones, C.; Baptiste, D.; Gelling, L.; Morin, K.; Neville, S.; Smith, G.D. Life in the Pandemic: Some reflections on nursing in the context of COVID-19. *J. Clin. Nurs.* **2020**, *29*, 2041–4043. [CrossRef]

27. Liu, Z.; Han, B.; Jiang, R.; Huang, Y.; Ma, C.; Wen, J.; Ma, Y. Mental health status of doctors and nurses during COVID-19 epidemic in China. *SSRN* **2020**. [CrossRef]

28. Wu, Y.; Wang, J.; Luo, C.; Hu, S.; Lin, X.; Anderson, A.E.; Qian, Y. A comparison of burnout frequency among oncology physicians and nurses working on the front lines and usual wards during the COVID-19 epidemic in Wuhan, China. *J. Pain Symptom Manag.* **2020**, *60*, 60–65. [CrossRef] [PubMed]

29. Maben, J.; Bridges, J. Covid-19: Supporting nurses' psychological and mental health. *J. Clin. Nurs.* **2020**, *29*, 2742–2750. [CrossRef] [PubMed]

30. Chang, C.S.; Du, P.L.; Huang, I.C. Nurses' perceptions of severe acute respiratory syndrome: Relationship between commitment and intention to leave nursing. *J. Adv. Nurs.* **2006**, *54*, 171–179. [CrossRef]

31. Maunder, R.; Hunter, J.; Vincent, L.; Bennett, J.; Peladeau, N.; Leszcz, M.; Sadavoy, J.; Verhaeghe, R.; Steinberg, L.M.; Mazzulli, T. The immediate psychological and occupational impact of the 2003 SARS outbreak in an teaching hospital. *Can. Med. Assoc. J.* **2003**, *168*, 1245–1251.

32. Kim, W.H.; Park, J.G.; Kwon, B. Work engagement in South Korea: Validation of the Korean version 9-item Utrecht work engagement scale. *Psychol. Rep.* **2017**, *120*, 561–578. [CrossRef]

33. Schaufeli, W.B.; Bakker, A.B.; Salanova, M. The measurement of work engagement with a short questionnaire: A cross-national study. *Educ. Psychol. Meas.* **2006**, *66*, 701–716. [CrossRef]

34. Ajzen, I. From intentions to actions: A theory of planned behavior. In *Action-Control: From Cognition to Behavior*; Springer: New York, NY, USA, 1985. [CrossRef]

35. Choo, E.H.; Baek, Y.M. Who supports MeToo movement, and how are they mobilized? Focusing on the different media mobilization mechanism between women and men. *Korean Soc. J. Commun. Stud.* **2018**, *62*, 37–65.

36. Song, E.J.; Kim, M.J.; Koh, M.S. Moderating effects of career commitment in the relationship between work engagement and organizational citizenship behaviors of the clinical nurses. *J. Korean Acad. Nurs. Adm.* **2019**, *25*, 167–174. [CrossRef]

37. Chae, M.O. Ego resilience, career decision-making self-efficacy and job seeking stress of senior nursing students. *J. Digit. Converg.* **2019**, *17*, 229–238. [CrossRef]

38. Kim, H.S.; Park, S.Y. The relationship between social network and organizational commitment and job satisfaction: Focused on mediating effects of job engagement. *Soc. Sci. Stud.* **2011**, *35*, 203–231.

39. Middermann, L.H.; Kratzer, J.; Perner, S. The impact of environmental risk exposure on the determinants of sustainable entrepreneurship. *Sustainability* **2020**, *12*, 1534. [CrossRef]

40. Luo, E. Increasing cost efficiency in health care without sacrificing the human touch. *AMA J. Ethics* **2015**, *17*, 1059–1063. [CrossRef] [PubMed]

41. La Rocco, J.M.; Jones, A.P. Organizational conditions affecting withdrawal intentions and decisions as moderated by work experience. *Psychol. Rep.* **1980**, *46* (Suppl. S3), 1223–1231. [CrossRef]

42. Wilkin, J.; Biggs, E.; Tatem, A.J. Measurement of social networks for innovation within community disaster resilience. *Sustainability* **2019**, *11*, 1943. [CrossRef]

43. Yom, Y.H.; Kim, H.J. Effects of compassion satisfaction and social support in the relationship between compassion fatigue and burnout in hospital nurses. *J. Korean Acad. Nurs.* **2012**, *42*, 870–878. [CrossRef] [PubMed]

44. Sun, N.; Wei, L.; Shi, S.; Jiao, D.; Song, R.; Ma, L.; Liu, S. A qualitative study on the psychological experience of caregivers of COVID-19 patients. *Am. J. Infect. Control* **2020**, *48*, 592–598. [CrossRef] [PubMed]

45. Ball-Rokeach, S.J.; DeFleur, M.L. A dependency model of mass-media effects. *Commun. Res.* **1976**, *3*, 3–21. [CrossRef]

46. Rui, J.R.; Stefanone, M.A. Strategic image management online: Self-presentation, self-esteem and social network perspectives. *Inf. Commun. Soc.* **2013**, *16*, 1286–1305. [CrossRef]

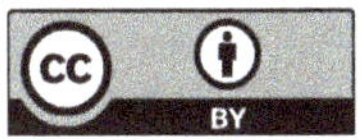

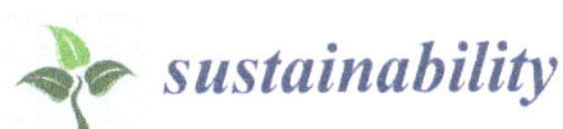 *sustainability*

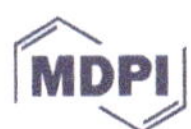

Article

Inter-Organisational Exercises in Dry and Wet Context—Why Do Maritime Response Organisations Gain More Knowledge from Exercises at Sea Than Those on Shore?

Eric Carlström [1,2,*], Leif Inge Magnussen [2], Elsa Kristiansen [2], Johan Berlin [3] and Jarle Løwe Sørensen [2]

[1] Institute of Health and Care Sciences, Sahlgrenska Academy, University of Gothenburg, SE-405 30 Goteborg, Sweden

[2] USN School of Business, University of South-Eastern Norway, P.O. Box 235, 3603 Kongsberg, Norway; leif.magnussen@usn.no (L.I.M.); elsa.kristiansen@usn.no (E.K.); jarle.sorensen@usn.no (J.L.S.)

[3] Department of Social and Behavioural Studies, University West, SE-461 86 Trollhättan, Sweden; johan.berlin@hv.se

* Correspondence: eric.carlstrom@gu.se; Tel.: +46-7027-38126

Received: 12 June 2020; Accepted: 10 July 2020; Published: 12 July 2020

Abstract: This is a study of inter-organisational exercises arranged by on-shore organisations (ONSOs) and off-shore organisations (OFFSOs). The aim was to compare findings from trained emergency staffs' perceptions of the impact of exercises. The data were retrieved from surveys conducted by the research team in conjunction with exercises. The surveys included staff from the coast guard, sea rescue, police department, fire department and ambulance services. A total of 94 professional emergency personnel participated in the ONSO exercises and 252 in the OFFSO exercises. The study was based on the suggestion that collaborative elements during an inter-organisational exercise promote learning, and learning is important to make the exercises useful. Collaboration proved to be a predictor for some of the items in learning, and learning was a predictor for some of the items in utility. There was, however, a stronger covariation between collaboration, learning and utility in the OFFSOs exercises than in the ONSOs. One reason might be the different cultures of emergency staff involved in on-shore and off-shore organisations. The OFFSOs' qualifications may be dominated by seamanship, together with professional practice, and all parties are expected to act as first responders. ONSOs, on the other hand, practice exercises from a strict professional and legal perspective.

Keywords: exercises; learning; inter-organisational; off-shore; on-shore; emergencies

1. Introduction

Strategic sustainability infers a built-in resistance to the prominence and effects of crisis events. A common way to maximise society sustainability is by maintaining the emergency response via regular exercises. Inter-organisational exercises are supposed to help authorities to become better at handling accidents, crises and disasters. Exercises involving different emergency services are carried out with the purpose of strengthening the inter-organisational ability to deal with difficult events that require extensive resources in a short time. There are, however, few studies of the efficiency of inter-organisational exercises in terms of learning and utility. One exception is Scandinavia, where inter-organisational exercises at sea and ashore have been studied [1–5]. The concept of inter-organisational exercises, as it is used in Scandinavia, describes exercises aiming to prevent organisational fragmentation, and develop integration and distribution of tasks [6,7].

In this article, we compare data from nine exercises (three ONSOs and six OFFSOs) from five published studies in order to find similarities and differences in terms of learning and utility. Comparing inter-organisational exercises arranged by on-shore and off-shore organisations can reveal context specific challenges and differences in learning outcomes. When extrapolated, it can pin-point strengths and weaknesses in different contexts of emergency preparedness. Such knowledge can, in turn, offer suggestions on how to improve the outcome from exercises and emergency response.

During the management of a societal crisis, the need for collaboration between emergency services has been actualised. As a result of criticism towards the management of rescue work during the 2011 attacks on the government blocks in Oslo and the Labour Parties Youth League summer camp on the island of Utoya, Norway in 2012, an extra principle was added to the national emergency preparedness legislation. It was the principle of collaboration, which was supposed to facilitate inter-organisational actions during emergencies [8]. In Sweden, as well as in Norway, where the data for this study were collected, the governments emphasise the importance of exercises to develop collaboration on different societal levels. In particular, inter-organisational collaboration is highlighted as a particularly important task to be practiced, specifically by getting employees to take the initiative to help each other across organisational boundaries [9–12]. This is especially true during time constraining emergencies [13,14].

In several studies, the inclusion of collaborative elements in exercises has proved to contribute to learning, and learning contributes to usefulness in real life situations. However, the studies show that even if there was a significant learning effect because of collaboration, the impact was, in some cases, moderate [13,15,16] and emergency staff have difficulties in learning from past mistakes [17]. Even if emergency response organisations are supposed to collaborate, they tend to prioritise the specific tasks they are trained for, instead of seeing the big picture [18]. Staff may engage in tasks they are accustomed to but are inactive when unaccustomed tasks need to be performed [19]. This is contradictory to collaboration, i.e., only focusing on one's own responsibilities, but being prepared to take initiatives beyond [20].

Here, learning is studied at the collective level [21]. Different patterns of action are built within the organisations, where individuals share experiences, learn from each other, and develop common approaches [22]. Learning occurs from communication across borders, different organisational agendas, the use of common resources and the different skills of collaborating professionals. According to Stein, the knowledge can be shared by permeable boundaries, ensuring multifunctional networks and integration. Demarcated boundaries and hierarchical grouping where activities are distributed into segmented tasks, on the other hand, may prevent knowledge sharing [21]. Institutional learning is accomplished by repeated action patterns, which over time create institutions that are stable in nature [23]. In this study, learning is considered to be the effect of a successful inter-organisational exercise, and learning is assumed to have impact on actual practice. Successful exercises, in terms of learning, may integrate professions at the fictive accident site [24]. Therefore, learning may occur when new patterns of thought are constructed and considered useful [25,26]. During exercises, learning is assumed to stand for change and development [27] and contribute to being open to different options and encourages initiatives to collaborate with others to achieve improved results [28]. According to Stein, inter-organisational learning builds trust, team building and coherence crossing professional borders [21]. Hence, learning can facilitate the development of routines, rules and models that have influence on daily work [29,30]

2. Maritime and Land-Based Collaboration

The collaborative culture seems to be different between emergency staff in maritime versus land-based contexts. Collaboration in the maritime context crosses national and cultural borders and is, in contrast to land-based, regulated by bi- and multi-lateral agreements and treaties. One such example of collaboration is in the high north area, where resources for search and rescue missions are lacking. Even if some areas, such as coastal Norway close to the mainland, are well-developed, distant areas are wastelands that are occasionally trafficked by crowded cruise vessels and oil installations.

The risks related to going aground or collisions with ice, or fire are not in accordance with the number of available rescue services, especially in remote areas. Disasters in wastelands and distant maritime areas put collaboration over organisational and national borders to the test [31]. Rescue missions at sea are, however, performed by all available actors and not just those who are specialised in emergency response. Long distances and severe weather conditions have forced different parties to collaborate, regardless of whether they are publicly financed rescue services, voluntary financed services (e.g., Red Cross and Society for Sea Rescue), fishing fleets or the merchant navy [32].

Several catastrophes have led to updated and sharpened legislations in the maritime context. This was intensified after a series of shipping accidents with grave environmental damages during late 1960s and early 1970s. The subsequent investigations concluded that the main cause of these accidents was human errors, resulting from poor training and lack of inter-organisational competencies [33]. Subsequently, maritime mass-casualty disasters like the Scandinavian Star disaster in 1990 [34], the Estonia disaster in 1994 [35] and the Costa Concordia wreckage in 2012 [36] shed light on the need to put more efforts in inter-organisational education and training. Hence, the maritime domain started harmonising and regulating its educational standards worldwide.

The International Maritime Organisation (IMO)—a technical agency of the United Nations—was introduced in 1959 to harmonise standards of international maritime activities, including training and qualification of mariners who navigate ships. In 1978, the IMO launched its first educational standards—the Standards of Training, Certification and Watch Keeping for Seafarers (STCW). It was considered a breakthrough, as there were practically no international standards in maritime exercises [37]. However, the STCW did not succeed in harmonizing the already established national standards around the world. Several revisions seeking to repair the shortcomings of its predecessors were made, and new conventions were prepared including the recent Manilla amendments, STCW 2010. STCW 2010 highlighted and homogenised concepts of intra-organisational exercises for mariners. The STCW standardised security exercises in different scenarios such as attacks by pirates and operations in polar waters [38].

With regard to collaboration during emergencies in land-based contexts, there are no such standards as those provided by IMO. Some standardisation in crisis organisations and crisis work can be seen within certain covenants like the European Union. Nonetheless, there is still a lack of international as well as national standards in inter-organisational exercises. At the country level, there is some fragmentation. It has been reported about intra-organisational autonomy during emergency response operations from Sweden and Norway. The official evaluation following the 2011 terrorist attacks in Norway found, among other conclusions, that the emergency response had been insufficient, and that inter-organisational collaboration efforts in particular had been inadequate [10]. An article titled "Why is collaboration minimized at the accident scene?" reported on the difference between rhetoric and practice in connection with accident work. Collaboration is seen as a rhetorical ideal rather than something that is carried out in real life accident work. The results from the study showed that police force, fire fighters and prehospital healthcare staff have an intention to develop excellent forms of collaboration at the accident scene but avoid this because of asymmetries in standards and lack of incentives [39]. A study from a tunnel exercise in Norway showed a risk for competition within organisations with unclear hierarchies. A lack of clarity in the distribution of roles and power struggles was identified as potential risks affecting the handling of emergencies [40]. Short distances and high accessibility can also be reasons why land-based emergency staff can uphold a degree of autonomy. In contrast to operations at sea, land-based operations can most often be reached by all the required resources within reasonable time and normally do not need to rely on each other's willingness to cross professional borders [41]. Information exchange during land-based emergency response operations is also known to uphold a certain degree of autonomy. Each organisation in the response network has operational field units at different levels, different functional command structures, separate back offices and intraorganisational radio communications channels [42,43].

Scandinavian countries like Norway and Sweden have a lot of similarities and few differences. Because of a long border between Norway and Sweden, partly in populated areas, they have agreements on sharing resources and coordinating actions during emergencies. The response organisations of the two countries perform common inter-organisational exercises; moreover, the radiocommunication systems, "Nødnett" in Norway and "Rakel" in Sweden, have been connected since 2016 (MSB 2018). The open borders between the countries have a long tradition, based on similar languages, constitutional monarchies, democracy and governments appointed by a parliament in both countries. They share national emergency preparedness principles of responsibility, equality and proximity in their respective legislations [8].

The dependence between organisations at incident locations is well known, which justifies the need for inter-organisational exercises to be conducted regularly [39,44]. Obviously, there are similarities and differences between OFFSOs and ONSOs' collaborative strategies during emergencies. After decades of naval disasters, OFFSOs have developed harmonised standards, while, in the ONSO context, the routines are still fragmented. The ONSO context seems to be more affected by the perception of collaboration as a rhetorical ideal while OFFSOs are characterised by a willingness to cross organisational boarders. We still do not know if collaboration exercises differ in their impact on OFFSOs and ONSOs. Despite a lack of studies [45], inter-organisational exercises arranged by off-shore organisations (OFFSOs) as well as on-shore organisations (ONSOs) are practised at considerable cost, with the supposition that they contribute to learning and utility in real life disasters [3]. We aim to find similarities and differences in the outcome from inter-organisational exercises, in terms of learning and utility, in the maritime versus land-based contexts. The study is supposed to reveal context-specific challenges, weaknesses and differences in traditions of emergency preparedness in order to suggest how to improve the outcome from inter-organisational exercises [46].

3. Methods

Five studies from a Norwegian/Swedish research team was chosen to compare inter-organisational exercises arranged by ONSOs and OFFSOs. One of the studies provided data from three ONSO exercises. Four studies contained data from six OFSO exercises, four of the OFSO exercises were pooled into two datasets. The questionnaire used to collect data during all included exercises was the collaboration, learning and utility instrument (CLU) measuring collaboration, perceived learning and utility from 1 (strongly disagree) to 5 (strongly agree) on a Likert scale [1–5] (see the Supplementary Materials). The CLU scale has been applied in similar studies of crisis exercises [1,4,47,48]. Primarily, it was developed by a team of academic instrument-developers together with emergency practitioners from response organisations. The development was made in different steps based on Stein's [21] learning theories, which have their out spring from Klabber's [49] perspectives on how institutions learn, Meyer and Rowan's 1977 decoupling theory [50], Berlin and Carlström's theories on sequential, parallel and synchronous collaboration [51]. The collaboration dimension encompassed questions about the collaborative characteristics of an exercise. The learning dimension elaborated lessons learnt from collaboration during the exercises. The utility dimension determined if the exercise was perceived to be useful during real emergencies. In addition, questions were elaborated about experience and affiliation.

The CLU surveys were all distributed and collected from emergency personnel in connection with inter-organisational exercises at the included ONSOs exercises. Regarding the OFFSOs exercises, the survey was e-mailed to the participants from an e-mail list. The homogeneity of the 17 items showed a Cronbach's α of between 0.68 and 0.88. Statistical significance was established at $p = 0.05$, and all tests were two-tailed [52]. The analysis stems primarily from descriptive data and regressions (bivariate and multiple). Data were imported and analysed in Statistical Packages for the Social Sciences (SPSS) version 24.0.

3.1. The Context of the Survey

The studied inter-organisational exercises were full-scale field exercises. All the organisations that normally participated in the scenario, e.g., coast guard, sea rescue, police department, fire department and ambulance services, were engaged in each exercise. Moreover, the exercises aimed to improve inter-organisational collaboration, crossing organisational boundaries during accidents and disasters. The exercises took place in different parts of Norway and Sweden (Table 1).

Table 1. Distribution of respondents in the on-shore organisation (ONSO) and off-shore organisation (OFFSO) exercises.

Published	Exercise/Scenario	Exercise Arrangement	Number of Organisations Involved in the Exercise	Number of Participants in the Study	Declined to Participate in the Study
[1]	Car ferry accident handled by ONSOS	ONSO	3	39	2
[1]	Fire at school	ONSO	4	28	1
[1]	Fire at work	ONSO	4	27	3
SUBTOTAL ONSOS:			11	94	5
[48]	1. Maritime oil spill 2. Maritime search and rescue	OFFSO	21	79	336
[4]	1. Fire at passenger ferry 2. Maritime search and rescue	OFFSOS	22	53	11
[50]	Maritime search and rescue	OFFSO	8	30	32
[49]	Maritime search and rescue	OFFSO	27	90	472
SUBTOTAL OFFSOS:			78	252	852
TOTAL ALL:			89	346	857

3.2. Procedures

The survey included staff in different positions, for example, operational staff in the field, and staff officers from levels of management. Informed consent was obtained from the organisers, and each respondent was provided with written information. They were informed about confidentiality and the opportunity to withdraw from participation in the survey at any time. The data were collected with informed verbal consent.

Self-administered questionnaires collecting data were distributed. The questionnaires were coded for each exercise, and the completed questionnaires were collected anonymously by the authors. The questionnaires from the ONSOs were in paper form, and the later was outlined as web-based documents, while the questionnaires of the OFFSOs were web based.

4. Results

4.1. Participants

A total of 94 participants responded to the ONSO paper form survey and 252 to the web-based OFFSO survey.

The response rate was 95% for the ONSO survey and 49% for the OFFSO survey. The participants of the ONSOs and the OFFSOs had previously participated in 1 to 12 exercises (ONSOs M = 2.87, SD = 2.24; OFFSOs M = 3.53, SD = 1.64) before the study. Their age ranged from 25 to 49 years for the ONSOs and 18–55 for the OFFSOs. In the ONSO survey, all participants (100%) belonged to the public sector (police personnel, fire fighters and ambulance services). For the OFFSO survey, 86% belonged to the public sector, 10% to private sector and 4% to volunteer sector.

4.2. Collaboration

A majority of the ONSOs (75.6%, M = 4.07, SD = 0.72) and even more of the OFFSOs (88.1%, M = 4.44, SD = 0.87) considered the exercises to be focused on collaboration. Less than half of the ONSOs (41.4%, M = 3.13, SD = 1.11) and 63.5% of the OFFSOs (M = 4.00, SD = 1.19) experienced that the collaboration began without an unnecessary waiting time. Additionally, 42.6% (M = 3.34, SD = 0.98) of the ONSOs and 57.2% (M = 3.97, SD = 1.22) of the OFFSOs considered that the exercises encompassed alternative strategies to collaborate. Moreover, 53.2% (M = 3.70, SD − 1.01) of the ONSOs and 79.7% (M = 4.40, SD = 0.99) of the OFFSOs considered that staff who needed to practice collaboration were engaged in the exercises. Discussions took place after the practical activities in the studied exercises; however, 33% of the ONSOs thought these discussions were insufficient, and they wanted more seminar activities after the practical actions (M = 3.17, SD = 1.00). In contrast, 29.8% of the OFFSOs considered the discussions to be insufficient, while 20.6% remained neutral (M = 3.42, SD = 1.42). Out of all the ONSO respondents, 44.6% did not consider the exercises to be those they usually practiced (M = 2.82, SD = 1.30), while only 5.2% of the OFFSOs considered the same (M = 4.46, SD = 0.93). The mean for all items within the collaboration dimension was 3.52 (SD = 1.01) for the ONSOs and 4.06 (SD = 0.64) for the OFFSOs (Figure 1).

4.3. Learning

The majority of the ONSO and the OFFSO respondents replied that they learnt new things to a certain degree during the exercises (ONSOs M = 3.66, SD = 1.28; OFFSOs M = 4.16, SD = 1.16). Nearly half of the ONSOs (45.7%, M = 3.26, SD = 1.34) and more than half of the OFFSOs (66.6%, M = 3.84, SD = 1.14) considered themselves to have learnt new things about the organisations involved in the exercise. Less than a quarter of the ONSOs (21.4%, M = 2.72, SD = 1.03) and under half of the OFFSOs (42.5%, M = 3.22, SD = 1.30) learnt something about the concepts and acronyms used by the organisations involved as well as their communication patterns (ONSOs 22.4%, M = 2.74, SD = 1.05; OFFSOs 60.3%, M = 3.72, SD = 1.19). Quite a few of the ONSOs (17%, M = 2.79, SD = 0.88) and half of the OFFSOs (47.9%, M = 3.72, SD = 1.19) considered themselves to have learnt about prioritising activities. The mean for all items within the learning dimension was 3.03 (SD = 0.97) for the ONSOs and 3.67 (SD = 0.93) for the OFFSOs (Figure 1).

4.4. Utility

Most of the ONSO and the OFFSO respondents (84.1% and 77.7%) considered the exercises to be useful during actual emergency work (ONSOs M = 4.45, SD = 0.90; OFFSOs M = 4.20, SD = 1.11). Furthermore, they regarded the inter-organisational exercises as having an impact on their everyday work (ONSOs 61.7%, M = 3.69, SD = 1.16; OFFSOs 44.0% M = 3.26, SD = 1.22). It should be noted here that 27.4% of the OFFOS remained neutral. The exercises were considered to be more valuable for the command officers (ONSOs 58.5%, M = 3.54, SD = 1.30; OFFSOs 50.4%, M = 3.68, SD = 1.18) than for the operative staff in the field (ONSOs 30.8%, M = 2.97, SD = 1.22; OFFSOs 29.3%, M = 3.21, SD = 1.23). The mean for all items within the utility dimension was 3.66 (SD = 1.08) for the ONSOs and 3.59 (SD = 0.71) for the OFFSOs (Figure 1).

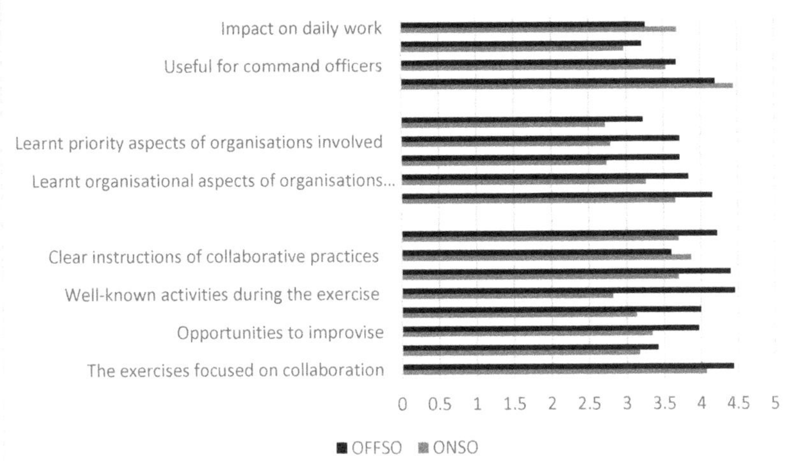

Figure 1. Mean values for the 94 ONSO and 252 OFFSO emergency personnel answering the collaboration, learning and utility instrument (CLU) scale, distributed in the dimensions utility (four items), learning (five items) and collaboration (eight items).

4.5. Bivariate Regressions

The causal effects of collaboration, learning and utility in the ONSO and OFFSO contexts were tested in a number of bivariate regressions. The collaborative dimension of the exercises was significantly correlated to the mean learning score across most of the items associated with the learning measurements in both exercise contexts. The strongest significant correlation on ONSOs was found between the item 'well-known activities during the exercise' and learning ($R = 0.48$), with this item explaining a significant proportion of variance in the mean learning score ($R^2 = 0.23$, $F = 27.67$, $p < 0.00$). The strongest significant correlation on OFFSOs was the item 'my point of view was regarded' and learning ($R = 0.40$), with this item explaining a significant proportion of variance in the mean learning score ($R^2 = 0.16$, $F = 48.86$, $p < 0.00$) (Table 2).

Table 2. Bivariate regression of items in the collaborative dimension of learning (sig. $= p < 0.05$).

Bivariate Regression ONSO N = 94 OFFSO N = 252						
Dependent Variables: Learning **Independent Variables: Collaborative** **Characteristics of Exercises**						
		Pearson R	R-square	F-Value	T-Value	Sig.
1. The exercises focused on collaboration	ONSO	0.27	0.08	7.31	5.03	0.00
	OFFSO	0.33	0.10	30.92	5.56	0.00
2. Discussions immediately after the exercise	ONSO	0.22	0.05	4.55	9.90	0.03
	OFFSO	0.16	0.02	7.08	2.66	0.01
3. Opportunities to improvise	ONSO	0.21	0.04	4.18	9.19	0.04
	OFFSO	0.24	0.05	15.93	3.99	0.00
4. Collaboration was initiated immediately	ONSO	0.39	0.16	16.81	10.19	0.00
	OFFSO	0.18	0.03	8.90	2.98	0.00
5. Well-known activities during the exercise	ONSO	0.48	0.23	27.67	13.73	0.00
	OFFSO	0.11	0.01	3.46	−1.85	0.06
6. Staff that needed to exercise participated	ONSO	0.27	0.07	7.37	7.99	0.00
	OFFSO	0.14	0.01	5.11	2.26	0.02
7. Clear instructions of collaborative practices	ONSO	0.43	0.19	21.33	8.69	0.00
	OFFSO	0.26	0.06	17.47	4.18	0.00
8. My point of view was regarded	ONSO	0.42	0.18	19.85	6.02	0.00
	OFFSO	0.40	0.16	48.86	6.99	0.00

Some of the items in the learning dimension were significantly correlated to the usefulness items. The strongest significant correlation of ONSOs was found between the item 'learnt new things' and usefulness (R = 0.47, R^2 = 0.22, F = 26.35, $p < 0.00$). A somewhat weaker correlation was found for the OFFSOs for the same item (R = 0.35, R^2 = 0.11, F = 31.99, $p < 0.00$) (Table 3).

Table 3. Bivariate regression of items in the learning dimension of utility (sig. = $p < 0.05$).

Bivariate Regression ONSO N = 94 OFFSO N = 252						
Dependent Variable: Utility Independent **Variables: Learning Characteristics of Exercises**						
		Pearson R	R-Square	F-Value	T-Value	Sig.
1. Learnt new things	ONSO	0.47	0.22	26.35	13.32	0.00
	OFFSO	0.35	0.11	31.99	5.65	0.00
2. Learnt organisational aspects of organisations involved	ONSO	0.30	0.09	8.89	16.58	0.00
	OFFSO	0.32	0.10	27.44	5.23	0.00
3. Learnt communicational aspects of organisations involved	ONSO	0.24	0.06	5.58	15.71	0.02
	OFFSO	0.29	0.08	21.82	4.67	0.00
4. Learnt priority aspects of organisations involved	ONSO	0.15	0.02	2.09	13.48	0.15
	OFFSO	0.31	0.09	25.64	5.06	0.00
5. Learnt new concepts	ONSO	0.14	0.02	1.89	16.04	0.17
	OFFSO	0.25	0.06	16.24	4.03	0.00

4.6. Multiple Regressions

Significant variables from the bivariate regressions were tested separately for the ONSOs and the OFFSOs in multiple regressions. In the case of ONSOs, the collaborative features together predicted 53% (R^2 = 0.53) of learning and for the OFFSOs, they predicted 25% (R^2 = 0.25) of the variance in learning. This meant that 47% and 75% of the predicted variance was non-unaccounted for in the case of ONSOs and OFFSOs, respectively. In the case of ONSOs, four variables were still significant: 'opportunities to improvise', 'well-known activities during the exercise', 'clear instructions for collaborative practices during the exercises' and 'my points of view were regarded'. The OFFSOs showed one still significant variable: 'my points of view were regarded'. The remaining variables displayed somewhat lower t-values and lacked significance on their own (Table 4).

Table 4. Significant variables of a multiple regression of items in the collaboration dimension of learning, (sig. = $p < 0.05$).

Multiple Regression ONSO N = 94 OFFSO N = 252					
Dependent Variable: Learning **Independent Variables: Collaborative Characteristics of Exercises**					
ONSO R = 0.73 R-SQUARE = 0.53					
	Bivariate St.Beta.	Multi.regr.St.Beta.	Diff.	T-value	Sig.
3. Opportunities to improvise	0.21	0.04	4.18	9.19	0.04
5. Well-known activities during the exercise	0.48	0.23	27.67	13.73	0.00
7. Clear instructions for collaborative practices.	0.43	0.19	21.33	8.69	0.00
8. My point of view was regarded	0.42	0.18	19.85	6.02	0.00
OFFSO R = 0.52 R-SQUARE = 0.25					
8. My point of view was regarded	0.40	0.29	0.11	4.78	0.00

In the next multiple regression, it was found that the items of learning predicted 26% (R^2 = 0.26) of the variance in usefulness in the ONSO and the OFFSO context. This meant that 74% of the predicted variance was still missing in the regressions. One variable was still significant, 'learnt new things' in the ONSO and the OFFSO contexts and 'learnt new concepts' in the OFFSO context. The other variables displayed moderate t-values and lacked significance on their own (Table 5).

Table 5. Significant variables of a multiple regression of items in the learning dimension of usefulness (sig. = $p < 0.05$).

Multiple Regression ONSO N = 94 OFFSO N = 252					
Dependent Variable: Utility. Independent Variable: Learning Characteristics of Exercises					
ONSO R = 0.50 R-SQUARE = 0.26	Bivariate St.Beta.	Multi.regr.St.Beta.	Diff.	T-value	Sig.
1.Learnt new things	0.46	0.46	0.00	4.21	0.00
OFFSO R = 0.52 R-SQUARE = 0.26					
1. Learnt new things	0.47	0.32	0.15	4.71	0.00
5. Learnt new concepts	0.63	0.13	0.50	2.04	0.04

5. Discussion

The OFFSOs considered the exercises to be focused on collaboration to a higher degree (88.1%) than the ONSOs (75.6%). In all items of collaboration, the OFFSOs scored a stronger result except on the item, 'if the actions were those they usually practiced'. Only 5.2% of the OFFSOs did not consider the actions to be those they usually practiced (ONSOs, 44.6%). A similar relation was found within the learning dimension. The majority replied they learnt new things, but the mean for all items within the learning dimension was higher for the OFFSOs (3.67) than for the ONSOs (3.03). The OFFSOs reported they learnt about communication patterns such as concepts and acronyms (60.3%) as well as prioritising (47.9%) to a higher degree than the ONSOs (22.4% and 17%). However, both OFFSOs and ONSOs showed equal results in the utility dimension. A few more participants in the ONSOs dimension perceived the exercises to be more useful during real life events than the OFFSOs (84.1% and 77.1%, respectively).

The multivariate regressions proved that collaboration had a higher degree of explanatory impact on learning for the ONSOs ($R^2 = 0.53$) than the OFFSOs ($R^2 = 0.25$). The impact of learning on the utility dimension was similar at sea and on dry land ($R^2 = 0.26$). The still significant items contributing to learning was 'my point of view was regarded' (OFFSOs and ONSOs). Additionally, 'well-known activities', 'clear instructions' and 'opportunity to improvise' had impact on learning in the ONSOs context.

The results of the study boil down to the finding that communication, learning new things and different points of view are regarded as important to achieve learning and utility from inter-organisational exercises. This calls for communicative and interactive processes during exercises [43]. There are, however, obstacles to achieving such a process. ONSOs repeat well-known activities and are known to be organisationally differentiated. OFFSOs seem to be more integrated than ONSOs, but they are restricted by international regulations. Furthermore, inter-organisational exercises often seem to strictly follow a predetermined manuscript, not allowing much room for improvisation. Consequently, exercises tend to restrict the learning and to be repetitive, drill-like and intra-organisational because of the lack of timeouts, spontaneous assessments and inter-organisational discussions, allowing for reflections on alternative ways to handle tricky situations [24,25,53]. The bivariate regressions, however, display that well-known activities had some impact on learning, especially in the ONSOs context ($R^2 = 0.23$ and OFFSO, $R^2 = 0.03$). A potential explanation can be the use of instrumental learning objectives, leaving little opportunity for improvisation [54]. This means that it is important to exercise well-known and repetitive everyday scenarios, and that new strategies may be developed to improve emergency responses. The result suggests that none of these extremes, (the unknown versus the familiar) can be excluded from inter-organisational exercises [42].

Lessons can be learned from inter-organisational exercises, both on- and offshore if they make room for the participants to talk informally before and after the training. In a recent study, the labelled side effect of the collaborative exercise was highlighted as more important than intra-organisational practices [40]. The opportunity to get to know each other and discuss structures improved collaboration in real life emergencies. This means that even though the inter-organisational exercise per se seems to have poor results, it might lead to the creation of a collaborative culture among the participants. The ability to form and develop relationships might be more valuable than the planned formal learning.

The reason for the surprisingly high degree of learning from OFFSOs exercises, in terms of communication patterns, may be traced to the fact that crisis management in the maritime context is a high-tech sector. Due to several digital and analogous communication and positioning systems as well as international and national regulations, the complexity in training for an accident, or a disaster at sea will be very educational, even if the techniques and scenarios have been practised before. Moreover, if the size of the exercise is too big, it can hamper the possibility for learning, as different actors may focus more on their individual goals and solve discipline-specific tasks rather than on cross-border collaboration and the sharing of resources [40].

Another reason for the stronger learning outcomes in the maritime context may be different cultures at sea and on dry land. ONSOs practise manoeuvres unique to their intra-organisational context, e.g., weapons, advanced medical equipment, fire and rescue equipment from a strict professional and legal perspective. The OFFSOs qualifications, on the other hand, may primarily be dominated by seamanship together with professional practice. The seamanship is a common necessity for all collaborating OFFSOs, whereas the different professions, to some extent, are limited within the physical boundaries of the ship itself. A second factor that is important for the evolvement of cultural bonds is a tradition of spontaneous communication between crews at sea. On dry land, we have bystanders, i.e., the public, and first responders, but in the maritime context all parties are expected to act as first responders, regardless of whether they are publicly financed rescue services. In densely populated areas on land, it is easier to hide behind the crowd during an emergency than it is at sea. Petrenj studied collaboration during accidents on land and highlighted that the main obstacles to collaboration was a lack of incentives and ambiguity in roles and expectations [55]. In the maritime context, actors have proven to be aware of a common and core value of understanding and agreement [56]. Such a value can offer synergies focused on the big picture rather than just prioritising specific tasks they are trained for [19]. In contrast to ONSOs, collaboration at sea seems to be part of the preparedness for everyday work and the ethos of seamanship.

5.1. Practical Implications

This study shows collaboration and learning may be obtained from exercises based on already well-known activities. In this study, well-known activities were combined with opportunities as independent factors for learning. These results can inspire exercise planners to combine the unknown with familiar scenarios. The results may also encourage planners to use timeouts, seminars and repetitions of actions in order to elaborate highly efficient types of inter-organisational collaboration. The use of scripts may hamper learning and utility. This can be addressed by increased the focus on improvisation, together with a new training methodology. Crossing organisational borders during exercises can contribute to a culture that stimulates collaboration, learning and utility in actual emergency work.

5.2. Limitations

There are limited studies on exercises and even fewer conducting meta-analysis of exercises. This study is based on five studies on nine exercises and the ONSOs were collected from only one study. In order to verify the results, several more context specific explorations have to be performed. Furthermore, studies on inter-organisational exercises on land and in the maritime context should be extended to other areas such as the aerospace industry and other security-intensive contexts. Even though Norway and Sweden, where the data for this study were collected, have a lot of similarities, exercises from different cultural contexts can provide important results, contributing to the understanding of how to improve learning and utility from inter-organisational exercises.

The poor participation for the OFFSO survey may be due to a lack of research interest among participants, but also the lack of influence of big scale exercises. It can also be related to intra-organisational focus- and sector-specific objectives. Another reason may be the web-based questionnaires. Compared to paper questionnaires, web-based questionnaires have proven to be less responsive in the Scandinavian context [57].

Supplementary Materials: The following are available online at http://www.mdpi.com/2071-1050/12/14/5604/s1, Figure S1: CLU-instrument.

Author Contributions: Conceptualization, all; methodology, E.C. and J.L.S.; writing—original draft, E.C.; writing—review and editing, all; supervision, E.C. All authors have read and agreed to the published version of the manuscript.

Funding: This research received no external funding.

Conflicts of Interest: The authors declare no conflict of interest.

References

1. Berlin, J.; Carlström, E. Collaboration Exercises. What Do They Contribute?: A Study of Learning and Usefulness. *J. Contingencies Crisis Manag.* **2015**, *23*, 11–23. [CrossRef]
2. Berlin, J.; Carlström, E. Learning and usefulness of collaboration exercises: A study of the three level collaboration (3LC) exercises between the police, ambulance, and rescue services. *Int. J. Mass Emergencies Disasters* **2015**, *33*, 428–467.
3. Kristiansen, E.; Löve-Sörensen, J.; Carlström, E.; Magnussen, L.I. Time to rethink Norwegian maritime collaboration exercises. *Int. J. Emerg. Serv.* **2017**, *6*, 14–28. [CrossRef]
4. Magnussen, L.I.; Carlström, E.; Sörensen, J.L.; Torgersen, G.E.; Hagenes, E.F.; Kristiansen, E. Learning and Usefulness stemming from collaboration in a maritime crisis management exercise in Northern Norway. *Disaster Prev. Manag.* **2018**, *27*, 129–140. [CrossRef]
5. Sorensen, J.; Magnussen, L.-I.; Torgersen, G.-E.; Christiansen, A.M.; Carlström, E. Old dogs new tricks? A Norwegian study on whether previous collaboration exercise experience impacted participants' perceived exercise effect. *Int. J. Emerg. Serv.* **2018**, *8*, 122–133. [CrossRef]
6. Axelsson, R.; Bihari-Axelsson, S. Integration and collaboration in public health: A conceptual framework. *Int. J. Health Plan. Manag.* **2006**, *21*, 75–88. [CrossRef]
7. Berlin, J.; Carlström, F. The Dominance of Mechanistic Behaviour: A Critical Study of Emergency Exercises. *Int. J. Emerg. Manag.* **2013**, *9*, 327–350. [CrossRef]
8. Norwegian Ministry of Justice and Public Security. Emergency Preparedness Principles. Available online: https://www.regjeringen.no/no/tema/samfunnssikkerhetog-beredskap/innsikt/hovedprinsipper-i-beredskapsarbeidet/id2339996/ (accessed on 30 April 2020).
9. MSB. *Så Bygger vi Säkerhet i Norden: Ett Svenskt Myndighetsperspektiv*; Myndigheten för Samhällsskydd och Beredskap: Stockholm, Sweden, 2011.
10. Norwegian Official Report. NOU 2012. Report from the July 22 Commission. Available online: https://www.regjeringen.no/contentassets (accessed on 6 June 2020).
11. Skr. *Strengthened Collaboration: Improved Safety, Stated by the Swedish Government*; Regeringskansliet/Försvarsdepartementet: Stockholm, Sweden, 2009.
12. Swedish Civil Contingencies Agency. *Civil Emergency Planning/Crisis Management in Sweden*; Myndigheten för Samhällsskydd och Beredskap: Stockholm, Sweden, 2018.
13. Berlin, J.; Carlström, E. Collaboration Exercises: The Lack of Collaborative Benefits. *Int. J. Disaster Risk Sci.* **2014**, *5*, 192–205. [CrossRef]
14. Van Wart, M.; Kapucu, N. Crisis Management Competencies. The Case of Emergency Managers in the USA. *Public Manag. Rev.* **2011**, *13*, 489–511. [CrossRef]
15. Aedo, I.; Bañuls, V.A.; Canós, J.-H.; Díaz, P.; Hiltz, S.R. Information Technologies for Emergency Planning and Training. In Proceedings of the 8th International ISCRAM International Conference on Information Systems for Crisis Response and Management Conference, Lisbon, Portugal, 8–11 May 2011.
16. Drennan, L.; McConnell, A. *Risk and Crisis Management in the Public Sector*; Routledge: New York, NY, USA, 2007.

17. Deverell, J. *Crisis-Induced Learning in Public Sector Organisations*; Elanders: Stockholm, Sweden, 2012.

18. Christensen, T.; Laegrid, T.; Rykkja, L. After a Terrorist Attack: Challenges for Political and Administrative Leadership in Norway. *J. Contingencies Manag.* **2013**, *21*, 167–177. [CrossRef]

19. Scholtens, A. Controlled Collaboration in Disaster and Crisis Management in the Netherlands, History and Practice of an Overestimated and Underestimated Concept. *J. Contingencies Manag.* **2008**, *16*, 195–207. [CrossRef]

20. Groenendaal, J.; Helsloot, I.; Scholtens, A. A Critical Examination of The Assumptions Regarding Centralized Coordination in Large-Scale Emergency Situations. *Homel. Secur. Emerg. Manag.* **2013**, *10*, 113–135. [CrossRef]

21. Stein, J. How Institutions Learn: A Socio-Cognitive Perspective. *J. Econ. Issues* **1997**, *3*, 729–740. [CrossRef]

22. Corbacioglu, S.; Kapucu, N. Organisational learning and selfadaption in dynamic disaster environment. *Disasters* **2011**, *30*, 212–233. [CrossRef]

23. Bush, P.D. The Theory of Institutional Change. *J. Econ. Issues* **1987**, *21*, 1075–1116. [CrossRef]

24. Moynihan, D.P. From intercrisis to intracrisis learning. *J. Contingencies Crisis Manag.* **2009**, *17*, 189–198. [CrossRef]

25. Gredler, M. *Evaluating Games and Simulations, a Process Approach*; Kogan Page: London, UK, 1992.

26. Moynihan, D.P. Learning under Uncertainty: Networks in Crisis Management. *Public Adm. Rev.* **2008**, *68*, 350–361. [CrossRef]

27. Sommer, M.; Braut, G.S.; Njå, O. A Model for Learning in Emergency Response Work. *Int. J. Emerg. Manag.* **2013**, *9*, 151–169. [CrossRef]

28. Nemeth, C.; Wears, R.L.; Patel, S.; Rosen, G.; Cook, R. Resilience is not control: Healthcare, crisis management, and ICT', Cognition. *Technol. Work* **2011**, *13*, 189–202. [CrossRef]

29. Sullivan, H.; Williams, P.; Jeffares, S. Leadership for Collaboration. *Public Manag. Rev.* **2012**, *14*, 41–66. [CrossRef]

30. Torres, R.T.; Preskill, H. Evaluation and organisational learning: Past, present, and future. *Am. J. Eval.* **2001**, *22*, 387–395. [CrossRef]

31. Marchenko, N.A.; Borch, O.J.; Markov, S.V.; Andreassen, N. Maritime Safety in the High North:Risk and Preparedness. In Proceedings of the Twenty-Sixth International Offshore and Polar Engineering Conference, Rhodes, Greece, 26–27 July 2016.

32. Carlström, E.; Sörensen, J. Forberedt pa krise. In *Samvirke: En Larebok i Beredskap*; Kristiansson, E., Magnussen, L.I., Carlström, E., Eds.; Universitetsforlaget: Oslo, Norway, 2017; pp. 45–58.

33. Emad, G.; Roth, W. Policy as Boundary Object: A New Way to Look at Educational Policy Design and Implementation. *Vocat. Learn.* **2008**, *2*, 19–35. [CrossRef]

34. Almersjö, O.; Ask, E.; Brokopp, T.; Brandsjö, K.; Hedelin, A.; Jaldung, H.; Lundin, T. Branden på Scandinavian Star den 7 April 1990. In *SOS-Rapport 1993:3*; Socialstyrelsen: Stockholm, Sweden, 1993.

35. Cornwell, B.; Harmon, W.; Mason, M.; Merz, B.; Lampe, M. Panic or Situational Constraints? The Case of the M/V Estonia. *Int. J. Mass Emergencies Disasters* **2001**, *19*, 5–26.

36. Alexander, D.E. The 'Titanic Syndrome': Risk and Crisis Management on the Costa Concordia. *J. Homel. Secur. Emerg. Manag.* **2011**, *9*. [CrossRef]

37. Zec, D.; Komadina, P.; Pritchard, B. Toward a global standard MET system: An analysis of the strengths and weaknesses of present MET systems. In Proceedings of the 1st International Association of Maritime Universities, Inaugural General Assembly & Congress, Istanbul, Turkey, 26–29 June 2000.

38. IMO. The STCW Convention & Code 2010 Manila Amendments. 2019. Available online: http://www.imo.org/en/OurWork/HumanElement/TrainingCertification/Pages/STCW-Convention.aspx (accessed on 1 August 2019).

39. Berlin, J.; Carlström, E. Why is collaboration minimised at the accident scene? A critical study of a hidden phenomenon. *Disaster Prev. Manag.* **2011**, *20*, 159–171. [CrossRef]

40. Kristiansen, E.; Håland Johansen, F.; Carlström, E. When it matters most. Collaboration between first responders in incidents and exercises. *J. Contingencies Crisis Manag.* **2018**, *27*, 72–78. [CrossRef]

41. Carlström, E.; Fredén, L. The First Single Responders in Sweden: Evaluation of a pre-hospital single staffed unit. *Int. Emerg. Nurs.* **2017**, *32*, 15–19. [CrossRef]

42. Comfort, L.K.; Kapucu, N. Inter-Organisational Coordination in Extreme Events: The World Trade Center Attacks, September 11, 2001. *Natl. Hazards* **2006**, *39*, 309–327. [CrossRef]

43. Wolbers, J.; Groenewegen, P.; Mollee, J.; Bím, J. Incorporating Time Dynamics in the Analysis of Social Networks in Emergency Management. *Homel. Secur. Emerg. Manag.* **2013**, *10*, 1–31. [CrossRef]

44. Borodzicz, E.P.; Van Haperen, K. Individual and group learning in crisis situations. *J. Contingencies Crisis Manag.* **2002**, *10*, 139–147. [CrossRef]

45. Sinclair, H.; Doyle, E.E.; Johnston, D.M.; Patton, D. Assessing Emergency Management Training and Exercises. *Disaster Prev. Manag.* **2012**, *21*, 507–521. [CrossRef]

46. McConnell, A.; Drennan, L. Mission Impossible? Planning and Preparing for Crisis. *J. Contingencies Crisis Manag.* **2006**, *14*, 59–70. [CrossRef]

47. Sorensen, J.L.; Magnussen, L.-I.; Torgersen, G.-E.; Christiansen, A.; Carlström, E. Perceived Usefulness of Maritime Cross-Border Collaboration Exercises. *Arts Soc. Sci. J.* **2019**, *9*. [CrossRef]

48. Sorensen, J.L. Norwegian Maritime Crisis Collaboration Exercises: Are they Useful? Ph.D. Thesis, Graduate Faculty of the School of Business and Technology Management, Northcentral University, San Diego, CA, USA, 2017.

49. Klabbers, J. *The Exercises Planners Guide*; HMSO: London, UK, 1999.

50. Meyer, J.W.; Rowan, B. Institutionalized organizations: Formal structure as myth and ceremony. *Am. J. Sociol.* **1977**, *83*, 340–363. [CrossRef]

51. Berlin, J.; Carlström, E. *Samverkan på Olycksplatsen: Om Organisatoriska Barriäreffekter*; University West: Trollhättan, Sweden, 2009.

52. Altman, D.G. *Practical Statistics for Medical Research*; Chapman and Hall: New York, NY, USA, 1991.

53. Landgren, J. Spontant organiserad samverkan kompenserar för de centrala aktörernas misslyckande. In *Samverkan för Säkerhets Skull, Myndigheten för Samhällsskydd och Beredskap*; Nilsson, N.-O., Ed.; Myndigheten för Samhällsskydd och Beredskap: Stockholm, Sweden, 2011.

54. Magnussen, L. Didactics and Innovation in Collaboration for the Unforeseen in Training Practice Preparation. In *Interaction: 'Samhandling' Under Risk: A Step Ahead of the Unforeseen*; Torgersen, G.-E., Ed.; Cappelen Damm Akademisk: Oslo, Norway, 2018; pp. 339–353.

55. Petrenj, B.; Letterie, E.; Trucco, P. Towards enhanced collaboration and information sharing towards Critical Infrastructure resilience: Current barriers and emerging capabilities. In Proceedings of the 4th Annual International Conference on Next Generation Infrastructures, Washington, DC, USA, 16–19 November 2011.

56. Rykkja, L.H. Övelser i sammfunnsikkerhet som styrnings-och samordningsverktöy. *Nord. Organ.* **2011**, *12*, 2–25.

57. Ebert, J.F.; Huibers, L.; Christensen, B.; Christensen, M.B. Paper- or Web-Based Questionnaire Invitations as a Method for Data Collection: Cross-Sectional Comparative Study of Differences in Response Rate, Completeness of Data, and Financial Cost. *J. Med. Internet Res.* **2018**, *20*, e24. [CrossRef] [PubMed]

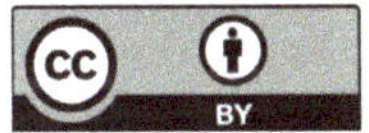

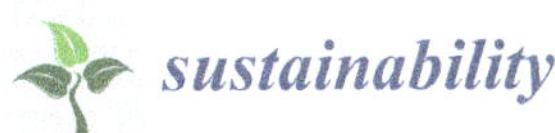 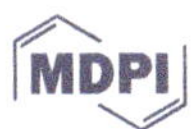

Article

Expansive Learning Process of Exercise Organizers: The Case of Major Fire Incident Exercises in Underground Mines

Sofia Karlsson [1,*], Britt-Inger Saveman [1], Magnus Hultin [2], Annika Eklund [3] and Lina Gyllencreutz [1]

[1] Department of Surgical and Perioperative Sciences, Surgery, Umeå University, 901 87 Umeå, Sweden; britt-inger.saveman@umu.se (B.-I.S.); lina.gyllencreutz@umu.se (L.G.)

[2] Department of Surgical and Perioperative Sciences, Anesthesiology and Intensive Care Medicine, Umeå University, 901 87 Umeå, Sweden; magnus.hultin@umu.se

[3] Department of Health Sciences, Section for Advanced Nursing, University West, 461 86 Trollhättan, Sweden; annika.eklund@hv.se

[*] Correspondence: sofia.karlsson@umu.se

Received: 10 June 2020; Accepted: 16 July 2020; Published: 18 July 2020

Abstract: A major fire incident in a Swedish underground mine made the personnel from the mining company and the rescue service realize their limited preparedness. It was the beginning of a collaboration project that included the development of a new exercise model for a more effective joint rescue operation practice. The aim of this study was to explore the collaborative learning process of exercise organizers from the rescue service, mining companies, the emergency medical service, a training company, and academia. The analysis was performed through the application of the theory cycle of expansive learning to the material consisting of documents from 16 collaboration meetings and 11 full-scale exercises. The learning process started by the participants questioning the present practice of the rescue operation and analyzing it by creating a flow chart. An essential part of the process was to model new tools in order to increase the potential for collaboration. The tools were examined and tested during collaboration meetings and implemented during full-scale exercises. The exercise organizers reflected that the process led to organizational development and a better understanding of the other organizations' perspectives. Consequently, a tentative model for developing the learning process of exercise organizers was developed.

Keywords: collaboration; cycle of expansive learning; full-scale exercises; major incident; organizational learning; preparedness; underground mine

---

1. Introduction

Although there is always some probability of an emergency, it is impossible to know when and where they may occur [1]. In 2013, a major fire incident occurred in one of the Swedish underground mines—a specifically challenging environment to establish a rescue operation. A mineworker had to seal himself into the vehicle in which he was working to protect himself from the smoke. Two other mineworkers decided to rescue their missing colleague and entered the smoke but became disoriented and had to enter a rescue chamber [2].

During fires, self-escape and rescue operations in the complex smoke-filled underground mining environment are difficult [3]. To reduce the risk of mortality and morbidity of severely injured mineworkers, they have to be rescued and receive medical care as quickly as possible [4]. However, to reduce the risk of becoming injured themselves, Swedish rescue service personnel in a recent study stated that they only perform life-saving rescue operations underground [5]. The rarity of major fire emergencies in underground mineral and metalliferous mines makes the experience of performing rescue operations limited [3]. Rescue operations in the underground environment require the use of specific methods and tactics performed by experienced personnel with adequate equipment [6]. While other mining countries utilize specialized mine rescue teams, most mining companies in Sweden are assisted by the local rescue service during rescue operations into the mine [7]. The rescue service personnel are assisted by trained mining company guides during reconnaissance, rescue, and smoke-diving operations [8]. Therefore, the rescue operation relies on effective collaboration between participating organizations. Although the fire in 2013 resulted in a collaboration between the rescue service and mining companies in developing rescue operation plans and training together after the incident, the emergency medical service (EMS) was not included in the collaboration [5]. The EMS personnel are responsible for the care of the injured mineworkers, and not being included led them to feel insecure in their role as responders and becoming passive actors in the rescue operation [9]. Around one half of the Swedish EMS personnel with a mine in their catchment area considered themselves unprepared to respond to underground mine emergencies [10].

The rescue operation during the Swedish mine fire of 2013 was subsequently evaluated by the rescue service, and it was concluded that the rescue service had not been sufficiently prepared to perform a smoke-diving operation into the mine [2]. In order to improve the preparedness of the organizations, development of the rescue operation practice for major underground mine fires was required. A collaboration project with exercise organizers from the rescue service, EMS, mining companies, a training company, and academia was initiated with the overall objective to improve the current rescue operation practice and organizational preparedness by composing learning material for the participating organizations. The participating exercise organizers had to critically study their own organization and their role in the rescue operation in order to develop a new rescue operation practice, which was tested during full-scale exercises. It was deemed relevant to explore the iterative changes both within and between the organizations in a structured way. Thus, the present study had the aim to explore the learning process in the collaboration between the organizers in underground mine exercises. The study retrospectively analyzed the material from the collaboration meetings and full-scale exercises conducted within the collaboration project. The material was deductively analyzed and presented in accordance with the cycle of expansive learning in order to present learning activities following a process-oriented approach.

1.1. Organizational Learning Through Exercises

Emergency exercises are used as preparation and learning for future emergencies [1]. During emergency exercises, the existing response plans, procedures, and skills, as well as the effectiveness and dynamics of the responding organizations, are evaluated [11,12]. Nonetheless, the progress and outcomes of full-scale exercises may be difficult to predict and control [13]. The managers of the emergency organizations, namely the Rescue Service Incident Commander, Ambulance Incident Commander, and Medical Incident Commander [14], need to know what needs to be done and how to effectively work together, thus they have to practice decision making and communication [15–17]. In order to manage the complex emergency situation, they have to be flexible and negotiate [11,13,16]. However, all of the involved emergency organizations have their own objectives and tasks [13], which might lead them to work independently and only sporadically brief each other of the current situation instead of working closely together and taking joint decisions [18]. Full-scale exercises can even be said to be inadequate tools for learning [19,20] and contribute to building intra-organizational skills rather than inter-organizational collaboration [21]. If the organizations lack knowledge about each other's roles, responsibilities, and tactics, this might negatively affect the efficacy and outcome of the rescue operation [22,23]. Still, full-scale exercises may also contribute to organizational learning because the participants build informal relationships with each other and thus learn the other organizations' languages which can be useful for the inter-organizational collaboration during real emergencies [24].

In full-scale exercises, learning can encompass the individual, the group, and the organizational levels simultaneously [13], and both the participants and the exercise organizers engage in the learning process [16]. After an exercise, learning can be facilitated by allowing the participants to constructively reflect on their preparedness, the process, and the lessons learned [11,16]. However, there are few studies that report on continued learning which occurs over time through participation in various activities, e.g., exercises and meetings [25]. Full-scale exercises can even be stated to only reproduce existing knowledge due to using expected scenarios and the utilization of a stable way to make decisions [26]. Full-scale exercises are also too focused on standardization and individual learning within organizations [19]. Thus, the inclusion of more collaborative elements, without finished solutions into the full-scale exercises could contribute to organizational learning [19,27].

Organizational learning also includes learning among the exercise organizers, their learning process including figuring out possible solutions to the scenarios and challenges they create [16]. The exercise organizers also learn by observing the exercise process to be able to modify the scenario and refine the exercise management structure and procedures [13,16].

1.2. Theoretical Framework

The complex nature of incidents in underground mines means none of the exercise organizers can develop exercise models alone. However, the learning process of jointly developing an exercise model can be assumed to be dynamic but challenging due to different prioritizations, concepts, tools, and primary tasks. Therefore, the theory of expansive learning was identified as a relevant framework for the present study. The cycle of expansive learning has been applied in a wide range of contexts, including health care and education contexts [28]. However, to the best of our knowledge, no previous study has applied the cycle of expansive learning to the learning of full-scale exercise organizers. The theory of expansive learning has been developed within the cultural-historical activity theory (CHAT) in which individuals are understood as part of a multi-voiced activity system with its own set of rules, division of labor, community, mediating artifacts, and objects [29]. This means that the exercise organizers have their own organizational culture with diverse ways of understanding potential challenges and solutions.

The focus of expansive learning is on changes in the object of activity, as exemplified by new practices and working methods [28]. Expansive learning occurs when the content being learned is not pre-existent but is created in collaboration among representatives from several organizations. Expansive learning can be described as a cyclical process, as presented in Figure 1, with the following phases: (1) questioning, (2) analysis, (3) modeling the new solution, (4) examining the new model, (5) implementing the new model, (6) reflection on the process, and (7) consolidating the new practice [29]. A collaborative effort is necessary to induce change, which starts when the representatives question the present practice of the activity systems and the common management of the object [29]. The representatives analyze the current practice to find the root cause of the experienced contradiction and to find solutions to the challenges through modeling [29]. Instead of adopting new tools or practices as such, the process of implementation means a continuous re-creation and expansion of the activity [30], which over time can change organizational boundaries [31].

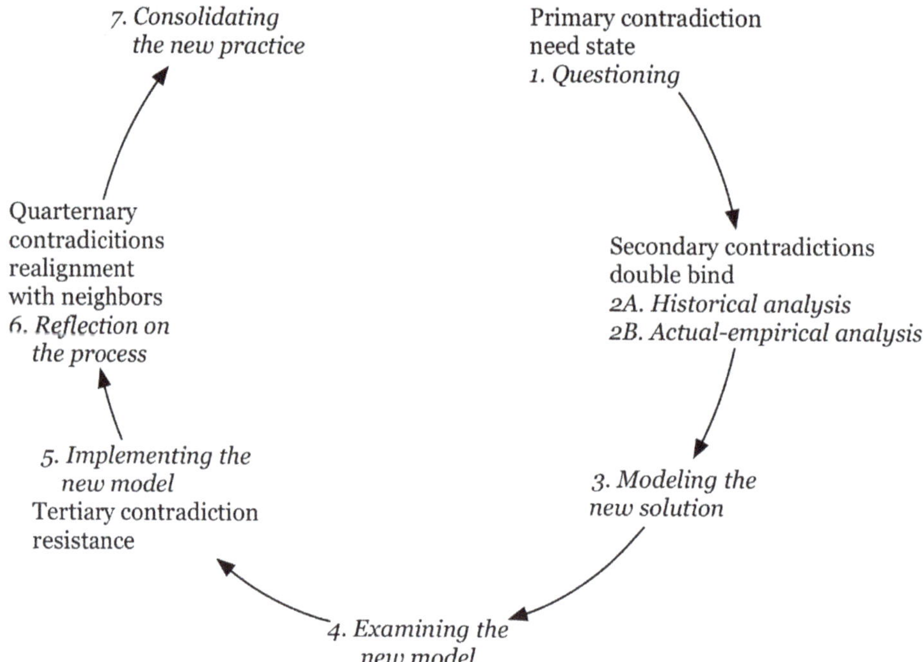

Figure 1. Cycle of expansive learning [29]. Reprinted by permission of the publisher Taylor & Francis Ltd., http://www.tandfonline.com.

2. Materials and Methods

2.1. Setting

A collaborative project was initiated in late 2016 by researchers at Umeå University to improve collaboration during rescue operations in underground mines. Sixteen exercise organizers with relevant experience of full-scale exercises and influence over both exercises and the organizational practices participated, including one rescue service manager, two managers and two operative personnel from the EMS, three managers from two mining companies, one manager and three educators from a company working with training, and three researchers and one teacher from Umeå University. During this project the group of exercise organizers met regularly both for conducting collaboration meetings and for meetings focusing on planning, conducting, and reviewing the full-scale exercises. This made the project adaptable, through the process of planning, acting, observing, and reflecting [32], where new solutions could be developed to respond to the challenges encountered during the exercises.

2.2. Material

The design of this study was a retrospective case study. The material for this study was based on a total of 144 documents from 11 full-scale underground mining exercises as well as documentation from 16 collaboration meetings; Figure 2 shows a timeline of the full-scale exercises and collaboration meetings. The individuals participating in the collaboration meetings were the same individuals planning, executing, and evaluating the exercises. The full-scale exercise participants' perspectives were included within the exercise organizers' evaluations of the full-scale exercises. After each exercise, the exercise participants were asked to reflect on the exercise and to come up with suggestions for further improvements.

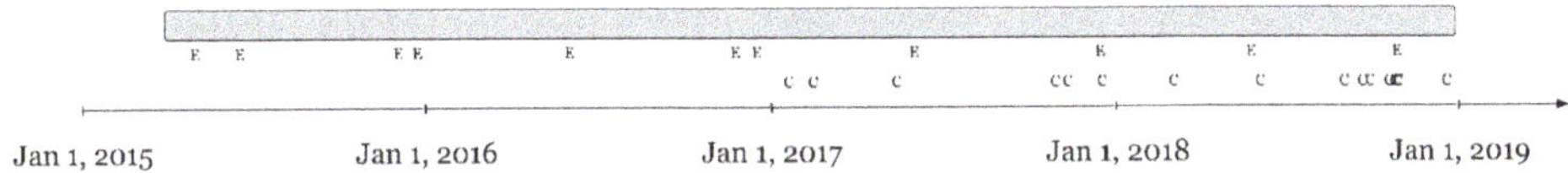

Jan 1, 2015   Jan 1, 2016   Jan 1, 2017   Jan 1, 2018   Jan 1, 2019

Figure 2. Timeline of collaboration meetings (C) and full-scale exercises (E).

The documentation from the full-scale exercises included a total of 106 documents about planning, logbooks, observation protocols, and evaluations. All of the organizations contributed with material during the full-scale exercises as follows: the rescue service, 30 documents; EMS, 24 documents; the mining companies, 14 documents; the training company, 10 documents; and Umeå University, 28 documents. The full-scale exercises were carried out from April 2015 to October 2018. The collaboration meetings were carried out between January 2017 and December 2018 and resulted in a total of 38 documents. These documents were, for example, documentation of what was discussed during the collaboration meetings.

2.3. Analysis

First, all of the material was read several times in chronological order to get an understanding of the whole material. Then all material relating to the aim was identified. The inclusion criterion was descriptions of collaboration between at least two of the organizations. Excluded text did not relate directly to collaboration, for example, technical aspects of the rescue process. The cycle of expansive learning was operationalized as an analytical tool [29,33,34]. The analysis was performed as an iterative process. At first, the material was sorted in the cycle of expansive learning per exercise/meeting, which resulted in several cycles of expansive learning. For example, steps (3) modeling the new solution, (4) examining the new model, and (5) implementing the new model were revisited several times because the exercise organizers tested a new practice or tool during the exercises and then had to modify the tool or practice or the exercise organizers found a new knowledge gap or limitation that they had to develop a new tool or practice for. To condense the richness of the material, the analysis continued by sorting the material based on the content and message of the text independent of which exercise/meeting the text originally derived from into the cycle of expansive learning. By doing so, the seven phases of the model could be illustrated in a logical way in the manuscript.

2.4. Ethics

All of the exercise organizers who contributed with material granted permission that the material could be used in this study. The study is exempt from the Swedish Act concerning the Ethical Review of Research Involving Humans [35]. The Helsinki Declaration [36] was followed. In the final manuscript, an effort was made to ensure that the identity of the exercise organizers or participants of the exercises could not be discerned.

3. Results

In the result section, the exercise organizers' learning process is illustrated by the seven phases of the cycle of expansive learning, as illustrated in Figure 3.

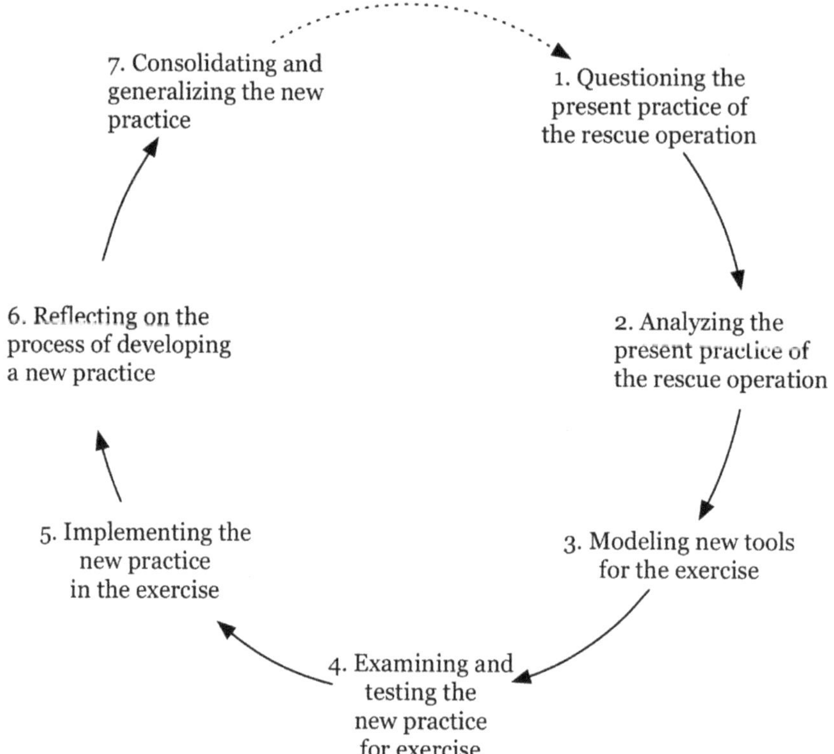

Figure 3. Cycle of expansive learning of exercise organizers as they developed the rescue operation practice as inspired by Engeström [29].

As can be discerned from the results, the learning process of the exercise organizers did not follow the cycle of expansive learning from start to finish, and the cycle was looped in various ways. The primary explanation is that the process was iterative, consisting of different types of activities (e.g., meetings and exercises), and continued over a fairly long time. As time went on, more and more data were produced from the various exercise organizers. During the first six full-scale exercises, the rescue service and mining companies together produced a total of 18 documents, while exercises 7–10 included 41 documents produced by various exercise organizers. The documentation peaked during the last reported exercise of this study; namely, during the 11th exercise, all of the exercise organizers contributed with a total of 47 documents. During the process, there was not only an increase in the number of documents, but their quality and the complexity of information also increased. The first exercise documents mainly consisted of technical reports, but as the learning process continued, the organizations also started to consider organizational and collaboration aspects.

3.1. Questioning the Present Practice of the Rescue Operation

Questioning the present practice of the rescue operation began during and after the aforementioned major fire incident in one of the Swedish underground mines. The evaluation performed by the rescue service indicated that the rescue service lacked knowledge about suitable tactics and methods for rescuing someone in a mining environment. To develop knowledge and tactics to work under these circumstances, a collaboration between the rescue service and mining companies was initiated by, for example, performing full-scale exercises together. However, the EMS was still a missing actor in this collaborative initiative, which led to EMS personnel being uncertain of how to manage these kinds of incidents. Therefore, the university partners questioned the lack of a comprehensive strategy for managing underground major fires in collaboration including all central actors.

3.2. Analyzing the Present Practice of the Rescue Operation

In order to analyze the present practice of the rescue operation, the exercise organizers created a flow chart together based on their experiences from full-scale exercises and real events. This flow chart visualized each organization's practices and activities from the incident occurring through to the last injured mineworker being transported to the hospital. This flow chart was further used as a tool to analyze collaborative challenges and to find solutions. Identified collaborative challenges included that the rescue service was perceived as having the main responsibility of the rescue operation and that each organization mainly considered their own organizational tasks. How the environment or the task at hand would necessitate modifications of the rescue operation was less discussed, and the mining organizations, for example, considered that their task was to accommodate the needs of the rescue service. Further, the EMS worked according to a pre-hospital management concept that assumes direct access to the injured and therefore were not prepared for rescue operations in which they might not have the possibility to access the injured for several hours.

3.3. Modeling New Tools for the Exercise

During the iterative process of meetings and exercises, the exercise organizers continually tried to find solutions to the identified problems with the rescue operation practice. They gradually created several tools—including a modified first-aid course for the mineworkers, an emergency management template, and an educational video—in order to facilitate the participants' ability to collaborate during the full-scale exercises.

The tool of a modified first-aid course, with a checklist for the systematic examination of an injured peer and guidelines for care and communicating injury information, was developed. The exercise organizers developed the modified first-aid course because they recognized the necessity of the mineworkers to be qualified specifically in how to care for severely injured peers underground until being rescued. The mineworkers had taken a commercial first-aid course, but the environment and their prolonged responsibility for their peers called for the development of the course. The modified first-aid course was also developed due to the exercise organizers realizing that, in order to make the exercise rescue operation of the injured mineworkers more realistic, a medical dimension needed to be added to the rescue service focus. The rescue service focus during the exercises was noticed in the unrealistic acting of the mineworkers. They waited passively until being rescued and were walking even though they were supposed to act as though they had fractures in their lower extremities. Thus, when the mineworkers were educated in the modified first-aid course they became active participants in the exercises. The injured mineworkers were instructed to not only call in the alarm of the incident but also start to act as they would in a real fire emergency. They self-escaped to a rescue chamber and there they would be helped by a peer. This meant that the mineworkers had to give first aid and care for the injured mineworker until being rescued as they would in a real event.

The exercise organizers also developed a tool of a joint emergency management template due to the realization that when the complexity of the scenarios increased, the rescue operation managers had difficulties in creating a shared situational awareness. They observed that this also became obvious to the managers themselves, who drew up a simple table to get an overview of the injured and injuries. Therefore, the exercise organizers gathered and, in several iterations, developed an emergency management template in order to increase transparency and to create common situational awareness among the managers of the rescue operation. The emergency management template tool was also complemented with a course for the managers of the mining organization.

The tool of an e-learning educational video, in order to create a common understanding of each other's structures, terminologies, and tasks during a major fire incident, was also developed by the exercise organizers. They had observed that the managers of the rescue operation did not collaborate in an optimal way and even made mistakes during the full-scale exercises. For example, during one of the exercises, the EMS managers were directed by the mining managers to the casualty collecting point and therefore were delayed in reaching the emergency operations center where the other organizations' managers were located. The mining managers had limited knowledge about the EMS organization and management structure and did not know that the first arriving EMS unit primarily has a managerial responsibility. The exercise organizers thus realized that the organizations' lack of knowledge about each other's tasks limited their collaboration.

3.4. Examining and Testing the New Practice for Exercise

The exercise organizers constantly evaluated and developed the tools during the progress of the project. For example, they developed the emergency management template when they observed that the rescue operation managers made different interpretations about what they were supposed to write on the template. The introduction of smaller rehearsal exercises focusing on the responsibilities of the managers of the rescue operation also made it possible for the exercise organizers to solve some of the identified challenges prior the full-scale exercise, for example, that there were too many people in the rescue operations center, which led to a noisy environment. The exercise organizers, therefore, instructed the rescue operations managers to start using headsets with their communication devices and also started to consider which managers needed to be in the rescue operations center and who could work in adjacent rooms.

The exercise organizers examined the new solutions for the rescue operation comprehensively and critically. They worked toward reducing the time of the rescue operation in order to make sure the injured mineworkers reached definite care as soon as possible. The exercise organizers also discussed whether the EMS personnel could enter the mine during a fire. This discussion related to the conflict between the safety of the EMS personnel and the medical needs of the injured mineworkers. The exercise organizers solved this by arguing that the managers would have to consider the circumstances of each specific incident. They further argued that if it is impossible for the EMS personnel to enter the mine, they are nevertheless responsible for the injured mineworkers and should be actively involved in the planning of the rescue operation.

3.5. Implementing the New Practice in the Exercise

The full-scale exercises were planned and performed in-between the collaboration meetings, which made it possible for the exercise organizers to test and modify the new tools, practices, and equipment for the rescue operation. The implementation of new tools and practices was an iterative process, where the implementation of one tool or practice led to certain improvements and highlighted new challenges that called for the development of yet another solution. For example, the development and implementation of the modified first-aid course led to more complex injury scenarios, which led to the development of the emergency management template. During the course of the project, the exercise organizers continued their learning process, and the scenarios of the exercises rapidly increased in complexity. The participants of the exercises, being educated in the new tools and practices between exercises, managed the increased difficulty of the scenarios. Initially, the smoke-divers aimed at rescuing confined uninjured mineworkers from one rescue chamber. Later exercises included scenarios with a long-distance smoke-diving operation involving prioritization of two rescue chambers with severely injured mineworkers within them while the Medical Incident Commander communicated with the mineworkers who were helping their injured peers.

3.6. Reflecting on the Process of Developing a New Practice

During the course of the project, the exercise organizers also started to change focus—from primarily prioritizing their own organizational objectives, they started to see how their organizational objectives contributed to the collaborative process necessary during the full-scale mining exercises.

This was evident in the evaluation reports of the exercises. In the beginning, there were few and very technical rescue service evaluation reports of the exercises. In the last of the included exercises in this study, a broad range of evaluation reports from all of the organizations, evaluating both technical, operational, and organizational aspects, were included. One of the most important realizations was that the exercises, while becoming more complex, also directed more of the attention toward the injured/non-injured mineworkers. The exercise organizers started to think, for example, about what to do if there were several injured mineworkers located at different places in the smoke-filled mine. Who should be prioritized and why? The exercise organizers realized the importance that all three organizations shared the discussion on priorities and that the prioritization was done in collaboration. The mining management has to contribute with their knowledge about the mine layout, the rescue service has to combine this knowledge with their practical knowledge about the feasibility of the rescue operation, and the EMS should give their medical prioritization of the injured and be able to explain the medical consequences of the different rescue operation choices.

The prioritization discussion highlights the possibly extensive time it will take until the injured mineworkers are rescued during major fire exercises. The tool of a modified first-aid course was also developed because the exercise organizers realized that the uninjured peers in the same rescue chamber have to be able to take care of the injured mineworkers until being rescued. The uninjured peers are thus a resource for the EMS managers if the mining communication system is operational. The Medical Incident Commander gathers information from and helps the uninjured peer in a structured way but is also able to prioritize between the injured mineworkers. This was an issue during some of the exercises, and the exercise organizers stated that the uninjured mineworkers had to give all the information and the Medical Incident Commander did not ask enough or the right questions. Therefore, the EMS exercise organizers had to modify their protocol of questions to match the modified first-aid education given to the mineworkers. However, the exercise organizers also highlighted the need of the uninjured mineworkers to receive psychological support and information about the progress of the rescue operation from the EMS.

The benefit of performing full-scale exercises was also that the exercise organizers learned the practicalities and logistics of performing a rescue operation in an extreme environment. They had to continually evaluate the necessary equipment and resources. An example of equipment that was developed and refined throughout all of the 11 exercises is a rescue carriage, which could transport both the rescue services' equipment and immobilized injured mineworkers in the smoke-filled tunnels. Another challenging aspect of the rescue operation concerned communication. Because the common emergency organization communication system was not operable in underground mines, they adopted the mining communication system. However, the exercise organizers then observed that this led to operative and collaborative issues during the exercises, e.g., the number of necessary radio frequencies.

3.7. Consolidating and Generalizing the New Practice

During the progress of the project, the exercise organizers adjusted the rescue operation practice for major fires in underground mines. They developed new knowledge and tools regarding what worked during the full-scale exercises and implemented those during the next exercise, or adjusted aspects that they evaluated needed improvement. Therefore, the rescue operation practice for major fires in underground mines was constantly changing and improving, becoming more and more comprehensive. The process also led to organizational development. The exercise organizers from the mining companies had to develop their own emergency command structure, with the preparedness to answer all of the requests from the emergency organizations and at the same time having the overall responsibility for their personnel and the mine. The exercise organizers from the rescue service also had to develop their own practices and to develop plans to conduct the rescue operation as effectively as possible by, for example, utilizing reconnaissance teams from the part-time rescue service arriving first to the mine. The complex rescue operation tended to make the planning process too excessive, which slowed the progress. The exercise organizers from the EMS also had to create new practices, develop mining rescue operation plans and adapt their management structure to conform to the complexity of the environment, for example, the location of the Medical Incident Commander was evaluated by the exercise organizers. The Medical Incident Commander should be as close to the injured mineworkers as possible but loses touch with the progress of the rescue operation when located in the mine. Therefore, the Medical Incident Commander was located in an adjacent room to the emergency operation center in order to be able to stay in touch with the progress of the rescue operation as well as with the mineworkers helping the injured.

4. Discussion

In this study, the learning process of the exercise organizers of major fire emergencies in underground mines was examined through the use of the cycle of expansive learning [29]. The results in this study presented the process that started with the major underground mine fire incident in 2013 and up to the end of 2018. During this period of time, the exercise organizers not only realized the difficulty of managing major fire incident scenarios but also made progress in improving the rescue operation practice. This was a continuous process and is an example of expansive learning [29] because the methodology of performing exercises in underground mines was not pre-existent in this context.

In this study, analyzing the material according to the cycle of expansive learning, the results showed that collaboration meetings in combination with the full-scale exercises developed the foundation for a new exercise concept. This is in line with other authors' [37] argument that exercises can be positive learning opportunities for organizations. A positive learning opportunity can be facilitated if the involved managers question the current emergency management practices and work toward developing a new and more comprehensive approach [37].

The results showed that the exercise organizers were influenced to identify collaboration challenges within the current response during the collaboration meetings. In line with what other authors [22] report, the exercise organizers in the present study had to be interested in understanding the other organizations' tasks and responsibilities during rescue operations. The collaboration meetings improved the participants' understanding of the complex situation, allowing them to discuss challenges and find solutions as also described by others [1,22]. Thus, including collaboration meetings between the full-scale exercises can motivate the exercise organizers to consider full-scale exercises from the other organizations' perspectives.

The results also indicated that the collaboration meetings in combination with the full-scale exercises also were helpful for the exercise organizers to practically examine the tools and practices they had developed. This can be compared with the implementation of collaborative elements into exercises, such as the reflection seminars, to facilitate learning as recommended by other authors [22]. In this study, the combination of collaboration meetings and practical exercises influenced the exercise organizers to identify needs and challenges of various activities, as well as possibilities to develop and test new tools to support collaboration and the development of new knowledge of how to conduct rescue operations in underground mines. Thus, a productive approach for sustainable organizational learning, as in our study, is the combination of the collaboration meetings where the tools are modeled and examined and thereafter implemented in full-scale exercises. The tools evolve as they are implemented [30], which was also the case in our study. The exercise organizers evaluated and modified the implemented tools iteratively during the following collaboration meetings and full-scale exercises. Thus, even though significant time and resources were spent on this iterative process, this process may still induce a sustainable organizational learning process.

The results of this study showed that the increased realism and complexity of the full-scale exercises resulted in the exercise organizers realizing that there was a need for the development of new solutions for the rescue operation. The exercise organizers did not have a finished instruction for how the participants ought to respond in order to rescue the injured mineworkers, except for following the practices of their respective organizations. This meant that the exercise organizers had the opportunity to observe the participants as they responded to the presented challenges. The exercise organizers could thereafter further develop the ideas of the participants and develop tools to facilitate the rescue response. Furthermore, the participants were educated in the new tools and practices between exercises, which also helped the participants manage the increasing difficulty of the scenarios. This is in contrast to the results of other authors [19] who mentioned that, in general, participants who attended several exercises considered that they did not learn anything new during the exercises. However, the participants of the exercises in this study also had great power to influence the development process, and the exercise organizers did not just observe the participants, but they also asked the participants to evaluate the exercises and to reflect on identified issues. This is supported by other authors [19] who recommend that exercise organizers focus on collaborative learning during exercises, where the participants are forced to improvise when they encounter variations of the scenario and the unforeseen.

4.1. Learning the Importance of Including the Mining Organization as an Equal Responder in the Rescue Operation

As a result of the learning process of the exercise organizers, the mining organization became an active participant of the exercise rescue operation practice. The exercise organizers realized that the mining organization has an important responsibility in the exercise rescue operation because fire incidents are located within a complex industrial context that the emergency organizations are not accustomed to. This complexity might necessitate collaboration [18,38]. However, in our study, the exercise organizers also recognized that the mining personnel were not as accustomed to managing emergencies as the rescue service and EMS personnel were. Thus, all of the developed collaboration tools can support the workers and managers within the mining organization. The modified first-aid course prepares the mineworkers for helping severely injured peers and for keeping the EMS managers informed during major incidents. The emergency management template aids the mining managers as active participants during the rescue response, and the educational video informs the mineworkers of the organizational structure and responsibilities of the rescue service and EMS. This can be compared to another exercise study [39], which showed that the organizations involved in a rescue operation at an elderly care center had different understandings of the emergency situation and that the rescue operation experiences of the police and rescue service personnel were complemented by the contextual experience of the elderly care personnel. However, the management of the rescue operation was, in general, handed over to the emergency organizations [39]. In our study, this was exemplified in the analysis of the present practice of the rescue operation by the mining personnel thinking that their main objective was to accommodate the needs of the rescue service and thus handed over most of the responsibility to the emergency organizations.

In the study mentioned above [39], the rescue operation was analyzed to have been more efficient if the emergency organizations had collaborated more with the elderly care personnel and had adapted their practices to the situation. The findings in our study showed similar outcomes. In the beginning, the mining organization mainly considered their responsibility to be to accommodate the rescue service's needs, but in the new consolidated practice for rescue operations, the mining organization had their own management structure and equal responsibility for the rescue operation. This is supported by other authors [21] who state that giving each organization specific meaningful tasks can increase organizational involvement in full-scale exercises. The increased participation of the mining organization perhaps also led to one of the most important realizations of this study. The exercise organizers reflected on the change of focus of the exercises, from the perspective of the rescue service in just carrying out a rescue operation to taking the perspective of the injured into consideration.

4.2. Methodological Considerations

This study had several benefits and limitations. The most important benefit of the study was the illustration that the learning process of the exercise organizers led to sustainable organizational change. Other benefits of the study included the comprehensive material gathered from all of the exercise organizers and from several consecutive exercises and collaboration meetings. This is an example of triangulation of the gathered material that increases the credibility of the study [40,41]. The specified inclusion and exclusion criteria, i.e., collaboration and the application of the theory in the analysis, accounted for the confirmability of the study [40,41]. Using the theory of expansive learning as a theoretical framework for the study helped to visualize and organize the learning process of the exercise organizers. The application of the cycle of expansive learning has not previously been used to analyze the iterative learning of exercise organizers, and this study can thus be seen as a contribution to the research field. By using the theory of expansive learning, it is also possible that the transferability and dependability of the study were increased [40–42].

The limitations of the study included the risk of confirmation bias [42], meaning only including information that is in accordance with the theory. To minimize the risk for this, the research team thoroughly discussed the application of the theory on the comprehensive available material for this study. When the material was analyzed in chronological order the cycle of expansive learning can be argued to loop several times in various ways, for example, when a new tool was implemented during a full-scale exercise and later consolidated while at the same time new challenges were identified. Nevertheless, this process would have been too tedious to report and the material was therefore divided based on the content and meaning of the text and on the learning of the participants. Although this approach was used, progress can still be discerned when reading the results section.

5. Conclusions

In this study, a tentative model for the development of a learning process of the organizations' exercise organizers during a set of collaboration meetings and full-scale exercises was developed, which was illustrated through the cycle of expansive learning. Through a combination of collaboration meetings and full-scale exercises, the exercise organizers were able to iteratively question and analyze the current practice of the rescue operation; to develop, test, and implement new practices and tools; to reflect on the process; and to consolidate the new practice. During the learning process, several of the steps of the cycle of expansive learning were revisited. Thus, the iterative combination of collaboration meetings and full-scale exercises led to sustainable organizational change. The strength of the combination of collaboration meetings and full-scale exercises was that the exercise organizers learned to visualize and take the other organizations' perspectives. The iterative process in which the lessons learned from one full-scale exercise were implemented during the next also meant that the exercise organizers did not have to start from the beginning each time they planned a new full-scale exercise, which in itself reduces the costs and time of full-scale exercise planning. Thus, the use of a combination of collaboration meetings and full-scale exercises with the steps of the cycle of expansive learning in mind could well be utilized in the learning process of exercise organizers as they develop their rescue operation practice. More research is needed to determine if this is an efficient way of developing the learning of exercise organizers in order to develop both the full-scale exercise practice and their organizational preparedness.

Author Contributions: Conceptualization, S.K., B.-I.S., M.H., A.E., and L.G.; methodology, S.K., B.-I.S., M.H., A.E., and L.G.; validation, S.K., B-I.S., M.H., A.E., and L.G.; formal analysis, S.K.; investigation, S.K., B.-I.S., and L.G.; resources, S.K., B.-I.S., and L.G.; data curation, S.K.; writing—original draft preparation, S.K.; writing—review and editing, S.K.; visualization, S.K. and M.H.; supervision, B.-I.S., M.H., A.E., and L.G.; project administration, S.K., B.-I.S., M.H., A.E., and L.G.; funding acquisition, B.-I.S. All authors have read and agreed to the published version of the manuscript.

Funding: Support for this project was received from the Swedish National Board of Health and Welfare along with the European Regional Development Fund under the Safety & Security Test Arena Project.

Acknowledgments: The authors would like to express their appreciation to all exercise organizers of this study as well as all the participants of the full-scale exercises and the funders of the research.

Conflicts of Interest: The authors declare no conflict of interest. The funders had no role in the design of the study; in the collection, analyses, or interpretation of data; in the writing of the manuscript, or in the decision to publish the results.

References

1. Borell, J.; Eriksson, K. Learning effectiveness of discussion-based crisis management exercises. *Int. J. Disaster Risk Reduct.* **2013**, *5*, 28–37. [CrossRef]
2. Marklund, J.; Haarala, D. *Incident investigation of mine fire 2013-08-25. (Fördjupad Olycksundersökning Gruvbrand 2013-08-25, Swe)*; Skellefteå kommun Räddningstjänsten: Skellefteå, Sweden, 2014.
3. Hansen, R. Overview of fire and smoke spread in underground mines. In Proceedings of the Fourth International Symposium on Tunnel Safety and Security, Frankfurt am Main, Germany, 17–19 March 2010.
4. National Association of Emergency Medical Technicians (U.S.). *PHTLS—Prehospital Trauma Life Support*, 9th ed.; Jones & Bartlett Learning: Burlington, MA, USA, 2020; p. 31.
5. Karlsson, S.; Gyllencreutz, L.; Engström, G.; Björnstig, U.; Saveman, B.-I. Preparedness for mining injury incidents: Interviews with Swedish Rescuers. *Saf. Sci. Monit.* **2017**, *20*, 1–10.
6. Ingason, H.; Vylund, L.; Lönnermark, A.; Kumm, M.; Fridolf, K.; Frantzich, H.; Palm, A.; Palmkvist, K. *Tactics and Methodology during Fires in Underground Constructions (TMU) Summarizing Report (Taktik och Metodik vid brand i Undermarksanläggningar (TMU) Sammanfattningsrapport, Swe)*; SP Technical Research Institute of Sweden: Borås, Sweden, 2015.
7. Lehnen, F.; Martens, P.N.; Rattman, L. Challenges in deep mine rescue within the European I2 Mine project. In Proceedings of the 6th International Conference on Sustainable Development in the Minerals Industry, Institute of Mining Engineering I, RWTH Aachen University, Milos Island, Greece, 30 June–3 July 2013; pp. 1–6.
8. Swedish Mining Industry's Health and Safety Committee. *Fire Safety in Mines and Underground Constructions (Brandskydd i gruv- och berganläggningar: Samlade råd och anvisningar, Swe)*; Swedish Association of Mines, Metal and Mineral Producers: Stockholm, Sweden, 2016.
9. Karlsson, S.; Saveman, B.-I.; Gyllencreutz, L. The medical perspective on mining incidents: Interviews with emergency medical service (EMS) personnel. *Int. J. Emerg. Serv.* **2019**, *8*, 236–246. [CrossRef]
10. Aléx, J.; Lundin, H.; Joansson, C.; Saveman, B.-I. Preparedness of Swedish EMS Personnel for Major Incidents in Underground Mines. *J. Health Sci.* **2017**, *5*, 239–243. [CrossRef]
11. Kim, H. Learning from UK disaster exercises: Policy implications for effective emergency preparedness. *Disasters* **2014**, *38*, 846–857. [CrossRef] [PubMed]
12. Latiers, M.; Jacques, J.-M. Emergency and crisis exercises: Methodology for understanding safety dimensions. *Int. J. Emerg. Manag.* **2009**, *6*, 73–84. [CrossRef]
13. Lee, Y.-I.; Trim, P.; Upton, J.; Upton, D. Large Emergency-Response Exercises: Qualitative Characteristics—A Survey. *Simul. Gaming* **2009**, *40*, 726–751. [CrossRef]
14. Rüter, A.; Nilsson, H.; Vikström, T. *Medical Command and Control at Incidents and Disasters: From the Scene of the Incident to the Hospital Ward*; Studentlitteratur: Lund, Sweden, 2006; pp. 22–23, 29, 83–84.
15. Crichton, M.T.; Ramsay, C.G.; Kelly, T. Enhancing Organizational Resilience through Emergency Planning: Learnings from Cross-Sectoral Lessons. *J. Conting. Crisis Manag.* **2009**, *17*, 24–37. [CrossRef]
16. Borodzicz, E.; van Haperen, K. Individual and Group Learning in Crisis Simulations. *J. Conting. Crisis Manag.* **2002**, *10*, 139–147. [CrossRef]
17. Doyle, E.E.H.; Paton, D.; Johnston, D.M. Enhancing scientific response in a crisis: Evidence-based approaches from emergency management in New Zealand. *J. Appl. Volcanol.* **2015**, *4*, 1–26. [CrossRef]
18. Berlin, J.M.; Carlström, E.D. Why is collaboration minimised at the accident scene? A critical study of a hidden phenomenon. *Disaster Prev. Manag. Int. J.* **2011**, *20*, 159–171. [CrossRef]
19. Sorensen, J.L.; Carlström, E.D.; Magnussen, L.I.; Kim, T.E.; Christiansen, A.M.; Torgersen, G.E. Old dogs, new tricks? A Norwegian study on whether previous collaboration exercise experience impacted participant's perceived exercise effect. *Int. J. Emerg. Serv.* **2019**, *8*, 122–133. [CrossRef]
20. Allen, D.K.; Karanasios, S.; Norman, A. Information sharing and interoperability: The case of major incident management. *Eur. J. Inf. Syst.* **2014**, *23*, 418–432. [CrossRef]
21. Andersson, A.; Carlström, E.D.; Ahgren, B.; Berlin, J.M. Managing boundaries at the accident scene—A qualitative study of collaboration exercises. *Int. J. Emerg. Serv.* **2014**, *3*, 77–94. [CrossRef]
22. Andersson, A.; Lindström, B. Making collaboration work—developing boundary work and boundary awareness in emergency exercises. *J. Workplace Learn.* **2017**, *29*, 286–303. [CrossRef]

23. Juffermans, J.; Bierens, J.J. Recurrent Medical Response Problems during Five Recent Disasters in the Netherlands. *Prehosp. Disaster Med.* **2010**, *25*, 127–136. [CrossRef]

24. Kristiansen, E.; Håland Johansen, F.; Carlström, E. When it matters most: Collaboration between first responders in incidents and exercises. *J. Conting. Crisis Manag.* **2019**, *27*, 72–78. [CrossRef]

25. Skryabina, E.; Reedy, G.; Amlôt, R.; Jaye, P.; Riley, P. What is the value of health emergency preparedness exercises? A scoping review study. *Int. J. Disaster Risk Reduct.* **2017**, *21*, 274–283. [CrossRef]

26. Danielsson, E.; Sparf, J.; Karlsson, R.; Oscarsson, O. *Multidisciplinary collaboration during crises. (Sektorsövergripande Samverkan vid Kriser, Swe)*; Swedish Civil Contingencies Agency: Karlstad, Sweden, 2015.

27. Berlin, J.M.; Carlström, E.D. Collaboration Exercises: What Do They Contribute? –A Study of Learning and Usefulness. *J. Conting. Crisis Manag.* **2015**, *23*, 11–23. [CrossRef]

28. Engeström, Y.; Sannino, A. Studies of expansive learning: Foundations, findings and future challenges. *Educ. Res. Rev.* **2010**, *5*, 1–24. [CrossRef]

29. Engeström, Y. Expansive Learning at Work: Toward an activity theoretical reconceptualization. *J. Educ. Work* **2001**, *14*, 133–156. [CrossRef]

30. Kerosuo, H.; Engeström, Y. Boundary crossing and learning in creation of new work practice. *J. Workplace Learn.* **2003**, *15*, 345–351. [CrossRef]

31. Daniels, H.; Leadbetter, J.; Warmington, P.; Edwards, A.; Martin, D.; Popova, A.; Apostolov, A.; Middleton, D.; Brown, S. Learning in and for multi-agency working. *Oxf. Rev. Educ.* **2007**, *33*, 521–538. [CrossRef]

32. Altrichter, H.; Kemmis, S.; McTaggart, R.; Zuber-Skerritt, O. The concept of action research. *Learn. Organ.* **2002**, *9*, 125–131. [CrossRef]

33. Toiviainen, H. Inter-organizational learning across levels: An object-oriented approach. *J. Workplace Learn.* **2007**, *19*, 343–358. [CrossRef]

34. Kajamaa, A. Boundary breaking in a hospital: Expansive Learning between the Worlds of Evaluation and Frontline Work. *Learn. Organ.* **2011**, *18*, 361–377. [CrossRef]

35. Swedish Code of Statutes. *Law Concerning the Ethical Review of Research Involving Humans; (Lag (SFS 2003:460) om Etikprövning av Forskning som Avser Människor, Swe)*; The Ministry of Education and Research: Stockholm, Sweden, 2003.

36. World Medical Association. World Medical Association declaration of Helsinki—Ethical Principles for Medical Research Involving Human Subjects. 2013. Available online: https://www.wma.net/policies-post/wma-declaration-of-helsinki-ethical-principles-for-medical-research-involving-human-subjects/ (accessed on 9 June 2020).

37. Robert, B.; Lajtha, C. A New Approach to Crisis Management. *J. Conting. Crisis Manag.* **2002**, *10*, 181–191. [CrossRef]

38. Hill, B. Diagnosing co-ordination problems in the emergency management response to disasters. *Interact. Comput.* **2010**, *22*, 43–55. [CrossRef]

39. Danielsson, E. Following Routines: A Challenge in Cross-Sectorial Collaboration. *J. Conting. Crisis Manag.* **2016**, *24*, 36–45. [CrossRef]

40. Guba, E.G. Criteria for Assessing the Trustworthiness of Naturalistic Inquiries. *ECTJ* **1981**, *29*, 75–91. [CrossRef]

41. Dahlgren, L.; Emmelin, M.; Hällgren Graneheim, U.; Sahlén, K.-G.; Winqvist, A. *Qualitative Methodology for International Public Health*, 3rd ed.; Umeå University: Umeå, Sweden, 2019; pp. 42–49.

42. Collins, C.S.; Stockton, C.M. The Central Role of Theory in Qualitative Research. *Int. J. Qual. Methods* **2018**, *17*, 1–10. [CrossRef]

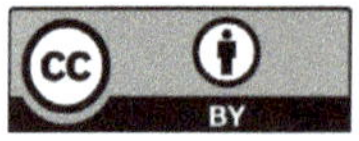

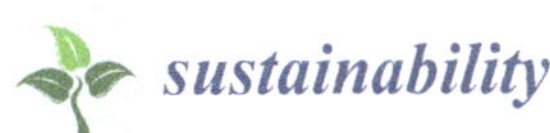 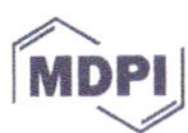

Article

"Share Your Tools"—A Utility Study of a Norwegian Wildland-Fire Collaboration Exercise

Jarle Løwe Sørensen [1,*], Carina Halvorsen [1], Jens Petter W. Aas [1] and Eric Carlström [1,2]

[1] USN School of Business, University of South-Eastern Norway, P.O. Box 235, 3603 Kongsberg, Norway; car-halv@online.no (C.H.); wergelandaas@outlook.com (J.P.W.A); eric.carlstrom@usn.no (E.C.)
[2] Sahlgrenska Academy, University of Gothenburg, 413 90 Göteborg, Sweden
[*] Correspondence: jarle.sorensen@usn.no

Received: 27 May 2020; Accepted: 10 August 2020; Published: 12 August 2020

Abstract: Based on the assumption that crisis collaboration exercises lead to better team-integration and more efficient problem solving, the aim of this study is to test whether there is a relationship between exercise participation and perceived levels of learning and utility. Online survey data was collected from participants in a 2018 two-day, full-scale, wildland-fire collaboration exercise in southeastern Norway. The instrument of choice was the collaboration, learning, and utility (CLU) scale. Findings indicate a strong covariation between participation in Norwegian wildland-fire collaboration exercises and the perceived level of learning, with a medium to small covariation between perceived learning and utility. The results indicate the importance of giving clear instructions, focus on collaboration, and sufficient forms of discussion during and after the exercise in order to gain learning. However, learning had a limited impact on utility. The study indicates joint evaluations, improvising, and testing of new and alternative strategies across sectors are important when exercises are constructed. The data was retrieved from a questionnaire, observations and interviews can add more and comprehensive insight into the studied phenomenon.

Keywords: crisis management; collaboration; exercises; learning; utility

---

1. Introduction

In 1996, Karl Weick [1] published his allegory of organizational studies "Drop your Tools." In his paper, Weick points to 10 possible reasons why 27 wildland firefighters lost their lives when they failed to follow orders to drop their tools and run when overrun by exploding fires. His study is based on values developed by James D. Thompson [2] and data collected from two main wildland fire disasters: Mann Gulch in Montana (1949) and South Canyon in Colorado (1994). Weick shows that the willingness of endangered firefighters to leave equipment behind and run was overdetermined due to deeply rooted routines and identity. An important conclusion was that fighting wildland-fires requires skills in cross-sectional collaboration to break familiar and iterative routines during extra-ordinary situations. Such skills develop through collaboration exercises. There exists an assumption in emergency preparedness that exercises lead to better team-integration and more efficient problem solving. However, though few in number, all relevant international studies indicate that the perceived effects of exercises by participants are rather limited [3–7].

As the effects of collaboration exercises and specially wildland-fire collaboration exercises are little researched, this should be considered a gap in the collaboration literature. As a contribution to closing this gap, this study focuses on the perceived effects of such exercises with an emphasis on learning and usefulness. Further, this study has a practical utility value, as it defines perceived problem areas, which can help exercise organizers and managers to further develop collaboration learning and usefulness. The following research questions were developed: (1) To what extent is there a relationship between participation in Norwegian wildland-fire collaboration exercises and perceived level of learning? (2) To what extent is there a relationship between participation in Norwegian wildland-fire collaboration exercises and perceived level of utility? A collaboration exercise is here defined as an exercise where multiple emergency stakeholders come together to develop preparedness, team-integration, and behavioral response [8]. In Norway, where this data is collected, collaboration is one out of four national emergency preparedness principles. The principle imposes on all relevant emergency stakeholders the commitment to ensure the best possible collaboration with other relevant actors across all phases of emergency preparedness [9]. The three other principles of responsibility, equality, and proximity are also formalized in the other Scandinavian countries, but thus far Norway is the only country that has adopted collaboration by law. This paper first starts out by reviewing literature on collaboration, learning, and utility. Second, it outlines the study's materials and methods, before summarizing and presenting the study's results. The discussion section then describes and interprets the findings, with the final section summarizing the answers to the stated research questions, outlining the theoretical and practical implications, and making recommendations.

1.1. Collaboration

Collaboration is here defined as a horizontal process where stakeholders, both at the organizational and individual level, share competences, unite resources, and unprestigiously work together towards a common goal. [10]. Compared with coordination and cooperation, collaboration calls for more frequent interaction, higher embeddedness, and a larger will of risk sharing [11]. There are multiple motives for engaging in collaborative processes, but possible explanations include an overall assessment of advantages vs. disadvantages [3], a desire for individual or social benefits [12], and the sharing of risks [13]. As a working form, it has over the years become popular across multiple fields and branches and received considerable attention, especially in management literature [14–17]. Well-functioning collaboration processes are often presented as a solution to task allocation and regulatory fragmentation [18], thus they represent the leading perspectives within fields such as team-development, coaching, and integration [19]. In the field of crisis management, collaboration is viewed as a key success criterion [20–22] and has been found to positively affect the overall outcome of a crisis [23]. We define a crisis as a situation or incident that outsources available resources [24] and is not confined within administrative, geographical, or physical boundaries [25]. Collaboration, or more specifically cross-sector collaboration, which is the main focus of this study, is viewed in the crisis literature as a core concern as it helps both crisis managers and societies to effectively deal with adverse consequences [23] and meet societal expectations [26]. On the contrary, if managers fail in their quest, a lack of collaboration may lead to less resilience, flexibility, and efficiency [27]. While there are examples of sudden, informal collaboration processes during major disasters such as Hurricane Katrina [28] and the 2011 terrorist attacks in Norway [29], collaboration is something that, in most cases, needs to be learned, developed, and exercised. Thus, there exists an assumption that cross-sector collaboration exercises develop, train, and test joint preparedness efforts and response [8]. The problem, however, is that recent studies have found that such exercises tend to have limited perceived levels of learning and utility [30–35]. Sources today are conflicting as to why this perceived limitation occurs, but cited reasons include a lack of focus on variation [36], lack of trust [37], and insufficient focus on collaboration learning and utility enhancing elements [3,6,7,38]. Collaborative strategies can, however, differ depending on the current situation. On a scale of less to more collaboration sequential, parallel, and synchronous types of collaboration have been identified. Sequential strategies are often used when it is optimal to go through official channels and stick to routines. Parallel routines are when tasks are carried out simultaneously, while acting "on their own". Such a subtle type of collaboration is used when members do not go in and help each other across. It is characterized by the standardization of developed roles and established procedures. Synchronous collaboration means stepping over the boundary into the unfamiliar and flexibly covering for others where needed, even if this does not lie within a specific area of competence. Synchronous collaboration is the idealized seamless form of collaboration referred to when governing bodies stress their ability to interact, but it is also a challenging and exhausting type of collaboration. These types of collaboration have been identified as useful depending on the current situation. The synchronous type of collaboration is seldom used in everyday practice, but merely when there is a lack of resources such as during mass casualty scenarios [3].

1.2. Learning and Utility

The goal of learning is to acquire new knowledge [39]. The idea of collaboration learning during exercises is, in this study rooted in, and limited to, Johan Stein's [40] and Klabber's [41] perspectives on how institutions learn, hence the differences between first- and second-order learning. First-order learning is when participants learn new things during the exercise but are unable or unwilling to transfer knowledge to practice. Second-order learning, on the other hand, is when participants manage to acquire new knowledge and apply that knowledge in real situations [31]. While the goal of obtaining new collaboration skills and understanding during exercises may seem obvious, Berlin and Carlström [3] found that while it was considered theoretically and socially correct to support collaboration engaging processes, participants, in practice, prefer their everyday, standardized working patterns, which results in a decoupling between theoretical structures and practice [42]. To increase exercise utility, planners should focus more on integrating collaboration-learning elements, hence creating new configurations of thoughts that bridge exercise learning and real life practice [43]. Bourgeois et al. [44] discovered that the promotion of collaboration enhancing factors increased the sense of team-belonging and the ability to learn, thus substantiating Borell and Eriksson's [36] later argument on how perceived crisis learning is greatly dependent on the design and applied exercise model. When designing an exercise, there are multiple ways to enhance both collaboration learning and exercise utility. Firstly, the exercise needs to have a purpose and primary objective [45], hence the exercise needs a clearly defined training content with associated learning outcomes [46]. Participants must be informed that the main goal is collaboration development, not only complex scenario solving. Secondly, the organizers need to provide clear collaborative instructions and ensure that the exercise participation feels relevant and is free from long or unnecessary waiting periods [31]. Thirdly, it is important that all participants at all times have an overview of the ongoing scenario development [45] and feel that their opinions matter. Moreover, they must be included in formative assessment and collective reflection processes throughout all stages of the exercise [39]. On that note, organizers and managers also need to take into consideration that collaboration learning processes are not always either black or white. Some professional boundaries are, and will always be non-negotiable due to e.g., jurisdiction or complexity of task [47].

2. Materials and Methods

This study reports on data collected from a 2018, two-day, full-scale, wildland-fire collaboration exercise in southeastern Norway. The main goal of the exercise was collaboration development, but included also technical, logistical and managerial elements. Participants included the Norwegian Civil Defense, County Wildland-Fire troops, local fire and rescue personnel, the Norwegian Directorate for Civil Protection, and local fire planes and helicopters. The exercise scenario ran from alarm to completion and included air- and land-based fire extinguishing, controlling of fires, and establishment of fire ditches. Logistical exercise elements included crew reception, parking, and housing/catering establishment. The exercise planning and directing staff was composed of senior representatives from the participating organizations. There were no performed joint evaluations following the exercise. The exercise was conducted in May, and data was collected in early fall. The exercise had 184 participants ($N = 184$) representing local full-time and part-time fire and rescue services, regional wildland-fire troops, civil defense, and wildland-fire planes and helicopter personnel.

The sample included both the operational and tactical level personnel. The selection of sample participants was based on an assumption that relevant personnel in need of collaboration exercise participated, and that the exercise had a relevant and clearly defined collaborative purpose and primary objective.

2.1. Data Collection and Procedures

A G*Power 3.13 analysis [48] calculated the appropriate sample size to be 82 participants. A *t*-test, linear bivariate regression—one group, two-tailed, with an alpha significance level of 0.05 [49], a statistical power of 0.80, and an effect size of 0.3—was applied. The collection of data occurred through the use of a validated online survey instrument. The collaboration, learning, and utility scale (CLU-scale) [31] became the instrument of choice as it is especially designed to measure the perceived effects of collaboration exercises, with an emphasis on learning and usefulness (Table 1). Also, as the CLU has been applied in similar studies [7,31,32], a comparison with other collaboration exercises are made possible. CLU is a Swedish developed survey tool. An expert group of five academic instrument-developing experts together with three emergency practitioners, representing blue-light response organizations, developed it. The instrument was developed in different stages based on Meyer and Rowan's 1977 decoupling theory [42], Berlin and Carlström's theories on sequential, parallel, and synchronous collaboration [50], and Stein's [40] learning theories, which have their outspring from Klabber's [41] perspectives on how institutions learn, hence the differences between first- and second-order learning. Before completion, the CLU-scale was tested in multiple pilot-studies. The final product consisted of 17 items measuring the three dimensions collaboration (C), learning (L), and utility (U). The C dimension measures the perceived collaboration characteristics, the L dimension emphasizes collaboration related lessons, and the U concerns transfer of value to real-life scenarios. The CLU-scale is based on a 5-point Likert scale with the values 1 (strongly disagree), 2 (mildly disagree), 3 (neutral), 4 (mildly agree), and 5 (strongly agree). The instrument's homogeneity was tested through a calculation of Cronbach's alpha, showing an alpha of 0.88 [51]. Analysis stems from descriptive data and bivariate and multiple regressions. Means and standard deviations were included for descriptive purposes. The instrument has earlier been applied in multiple, similar studies [7,30–33,52]. To ensure appliance with ethical research standards, the researchers sought permission from the Norwegian Center for Research Data (NSD) prior to data collection.

Table 1. The collaboration, learning, utility scale (CLU-scale).

C	The exercises were focused on collaboration
C	Sufficient forms of discussions were provided
C	There were opportunities to improvise
C	Personnel in need of exercise participated
C	I performed well-known activities
C	Collaboration was initiated immediately
C	Clear instructions of collaboration were presented
C	My points of view were regarded
L	I learned new things during the exercise
L	I learned about other's organizational aspects
L	I learned about other's communication patterns
L	I learned about other's prioritizing of activities
L	I learned other's concepts and abbreviations
U	Based on what I learned, the exercises were useful to real-life activities
U	Based on what I learned, the exercises were useful to command officers
U	Based on what I learned, the exercises were useful to ordinary operative staff
U	Based on what I learned, the experiences from the exercises impact my daily work

Dimensions: Collaboration (C), Learning (L), Usefulness (U). Source: Berlin and Carlström [31].

Prior to contacting the defined sample population, permission was sought from the participating organizations. The email contained information about the study, methods, instrument, and purpose. The letter emphasized volunteerism and assurance of anonymity. After obtaining written permissions and email addresses from the organizations, an invitation to participate was sent out to the population sample. Apart from a hyperlink to the survey designed in the online survey platform "Nettskjema" [online-form] hosted by the University in Oslo, the invitation contained information about the study, data handling, and how to contact the researchers. Volunteerism and anonymity were highlighted, as well as the option to at any time withdraw from the study without facing consequences. To ensure further anonymity, only demographical questions related to gender, age, professional experience, and professional affiliation were asked. Age and experience were divided into groupings, and affiliation was limited to public or NGO sectors. Age groupings were 1 = 18–26, 2 = 27–35, 3 = 36–44, 4 = 45–53, 5 = 54–62, and 6 = 62+. Choice of affiliation was 1 = private, 2 = public, and 3 = volunteer. Years of professional experience was divided into 1 = 0–5, 2 = 6–11, 3 = 12–15, 4 = 16–20, and 5 = 21+. Number of collaboration exercises attended over the last five years were divided into 1 = 1–3, 2 = 4–7, 3 = 8–11, and 4 = 11+. The participants were asked to complete the survey within three weeks. During this period, two reminders were sent out. After collection, all data was uploaded into Statistical Package for the Social Sciences (SPSS) and analyzed. Identifiable information in the data set was removed and replaced with a number. The scrambling key was stored on a safe drive at the University of South-Eastern Norway accessible only to the research team. The key and identifiable information were deleted after the completion of this research project.

2.2. Analysis

The analysis process commenced with the exploration of demographical information, followed by an analysis of the collaboration, learning, and usefulness (CLU) characteristics (Table 2). Here means and standard deviations were identified for describing data distribution variations [53]. The empirical relationship between the CLU variables were tested by performing two bivariate regression analyses, where the first one tested the relationship between collaboration (C) and learning (L), and the second tested the relationship between learning (L) and usefulness (U). Demographical data was collected exclusively for description purposes, thus not integrated into the regression analysis. The working assumption was that focusing on collaboration enhancing elements during a collaboration exercise leads to collaboration learning, which again leads to usefulness [50]. In this first test, collaboration was defined as an independent variable relative to learning (dependent), while in the second test, learning was the independent variable to usefulness (dependent). Pearson correlation coefficients (Pearson's r) were calculated to measure the linear dependence between the variables. Coefficients of determination ($r2$) were calculated to determine what proportions of the variance in the dependent variables could be considered predictable from the independent variables [54]. To test the difference in parameters between the observed results and the stated hypotheses, standard errors and F-values were calculated. Further, the significance level (p-value) was calculated to determine the probability of rejecting the null hypothesis. Statistical significance was set to $p < 0.05$, and all tests were two-tailed [49]. In the next step, the relevant predictor and criterion variables that were found significant were tested in multiple regression analysis [48]. Here collaboration and learning were used as integrated independent variables relative to usefulness (dependent variable). The standardized coefficient values (beta), and the differences between them, were calculated both for the bivariate and multiple regression analyses to analyze the strength of the effects of each CLU variable. Towards the end, p-values were calculated together with the performance of a Shapiro-Wilk test [55]. The last was done to ensure that the CLU variables met normal assumptions for regression analysis.

Table 2. Mean values—CLU-dimensions.

	Mean Values	**Standard Deviation**
Collaboration	4.12	0.547
Learning	3.97	0.850
Utility	3.68	0.543

Note: n = 71, sign = $p < 0.05$.

3. Results

3.1. Demographics

Seventy-one persons participated in the study; 90.1% percent were males and 9.9% were females. The overall response rate was 38.6%. Most age groups were represented, besides the 62+ group. Most respondents belonged to the 45–53 group (52.1%), while the mean age group was 36–44. Ninety-seven percent of the participants belonged to a public organization, and the number of years of professional experience ranged from the 0–5 group to the 21+ group. Most (38%) belonged to the 0–5 group. The number of collaboration exercises attended over the last five years ranged from the 1–3 group to the 11+ group. The majority (57%) had participated in 1–3 exercises during the last five years.

3.2. Collaboration

In total, 84.3% of the sample population either strongly or mildly agreed that the exercise focused on collaboration; none strongly disagreed (M = 4.43, SD = 0.791). On the question regarding whether sufficient forms of discussions were provided, 14.1% strongly agreed and 35.2% mildly agreed. Further, 15.5% mildly disagreed, while 1.4% strongly disagreed (M = 3.47, SD = 0.985). Over half of the sample population (60.6%) either strongly or mildly felt that there were opportunities to improvise, while 21.1% remained neutral (M = 3.74, SD = 1.112). When it came to perceptions of whether the collaboration had been immediately initiated, most mildly (42.3%) or strongly (36.6%) agreed. None of the participants strongly disagreed (M = 3.93, SD = 1.10). In total, 53.5% strongly agreed that they had performed well-known activities. Nobody mildly or strongly disagreed (M = 4.37, SD = 0.790). A total of 85.9% either strongly (64.8%) or mildly (21.1%) agreed that personnel in need of exercise participated, while 11.3% remained neutral (M = 4.55, SD = 0.697). Of the respondents, 77.5% either mildly or strongly agreed that instructions about collaborative practice were presented during the exercises (M = 4.28, SD = 0.922). Finally, when it came to whether the population perceived that their points of view were regarded, 42.3% strongly agreed, 16.9% mildly agreed, and 40.8% remained neutral (M = 4.01, SD = 0.918). The overall mean for the collaboration dimension was 4.12 (SD = 0.547).

3.3. Learning

Most of the respondents either strongly (69.0%) or mildly (18.3%) agreed that they had learned new things during the exercise (M = 4.51, SD = 0.980). A total of 74.6% either strongly (39.4%) or mildly (35.3%) agreed that they had learned about others' organizational aspects (M = 4.07, SD = 1.041), while more than half (71.8%) had learned about others' communication patterns. Here, 19.7% remained neutral (M = 4.03, SD = 1.021). As to whether the exercise participants felt that they had learned about how collaborating organizations prioritized their activities, 7.0% mildly disagreed while 2.8% strongly disagreed (M = 3.77, SD = 1.002). Some 45.1% agreed that they had either strongly (16.9%) or mildly (28.2%) learned new concepts and abbreviations (M = 3.43, SD = 1.050). The overall mean for the learning dimension was 3.97 (SD = 0.850).

3.4. Utility

Most of the sampled population (94.4%) found the exercise useful for real-life activities (M = 4.69, SD = 0.623). While 18.3% strongly and 19.7% mildly agreed that the exercise was useful for commanding officers, 29.6% remained neutral (M = 3.17, SD = 1.248). Some 42.3% either mildly or strongly agreed that the exercises were useful for ordinary operative staff. Here, 42.3% remained neutral (M = 3.40, SD = 0.900). Finally, under half (45.1%) agreed that their experiences of the exercises would affect their daily work, while 33.8% remained neutral (M = 3.40, SD = 1.102). The overall mean for the utility dimension was 3.68 (SD = 0.543).

3.5. Bivariate and Multivariate Regression Analysis.

RQ 1: *To what extent is there a relationship between participation in Norwegian wildland-fire collaboration exercises and perceived level of learning?*

Bivariate analysis. The most pronounced significance was found between learning and the item "Clear instructions of collaboration were presented" (r = 0.501, r2 = 0.239, F = 20,761, $p \leq 0.000$). The item "The exercises were focused on collaboration" had the second highest pronounced significance (r = 0.451, r2 = 0.191, F = 16.349, $p \leq 0.000$), followed by "Sufficient forms of discussions were provided" (r = 0.421, r2 = 0.164, F = 13.564, $p \leq 0.000$). "My points of view were regarded" had an R-value of 0.398 (r2 = 0.145, F = 12.034, $p \leq 0.001$), while "there were opportunities to improvise" had an R-value of 0.282 (r2 = 0.65, F = 5.508, $p \leq 0.022$). "Collaboration was initiated immediately" had somewhat lower significance level (r = 0.255, r2 = 0.050, F = 4.439, $p \leq 0.039$). The final item with a pronounced significant was "Personnel in need of exercise participated" with an R-value of 0.253 (r2 = 0.049, F = 4.291, $p \leq 0.042$). The item "I performed well-known activities" was found insignificant (r = 0.06, r2 = −0.01, F = 0.30, $p = 0.58$) and was therefore excluded from the multiple regression analysis (Table 3).

Table 3. Bivariate regression of the collaboration dimensions of learning.

Dependent Variable: Learning. Independent Variables: Collaborative Characteristics of Exercises	R	R2	F	Sign (*p*)
The exercises were focused on collaboration	0.451	0.191	16.349	0.000
Sufficient forms of discussions were provided	0.421	0.164	13.564	0.000
There were opportunities to improvise	0.282	0.065	5.508	0.022
Personnel in need of exercise participated	0.255	0.050	4.439	0.039
I performed well-known activities	0.045	−0.014	0.124	0.726
Collaboration was initiated immediately	0.253	0.049	4.291	0.042
Clear instructions of collaboration were presented	0.501	0.239	20.761	0.000
My points of view were regarded	0.398	0.145	12.034	0.001

Note: N = 71, sig = $p \leq 0.05$.

Multivariate analysis. The joint collaborative characteristics predicted 29.3% (r2 = 0.293) of the learning variance, meaning that the remaining 70.7% of the predicted variance was unaccounted for. Still, the variables "There were opportunities to improvise," "Collaboration was initiated immediately," and "Personnel in need of exercise participated" were found to be significant (Table 4). The regression analysis indicated a 61% (r = 0.61) covariation between collaboration and learning, which is considered strong [49].

Table 4. Multiple regression of the collaboration dimensions of learning.

Dependent Variable: Learning Independent Variables: Collaboration Characteristics	Biv. reg. Stand.Beta	Mult.regr. Stand. Beta	Sign. (*p*)
The exercises were focused on collaboration	0.451	0.286	0.056
Sufficient forms of discussions were provided	0.428	0.203	0.129
There were opportunities to improvise	0.282	−0.049	0.722
Personnel in need of exercise participated	0.255	−0.064	0.641
Collaboration was initiated immediately	0.253	−0.025	0.839
Clear instructions of collaboration were presented	0.501	0.308	0.023
My points of view were regarded	0.398	0.101	0.469

Note: N = 71, R = 0.611, r2 = 29.3 sig = $p \leq 0.05$

RQ 2: (2) *To what extent is there a relationship between participation in Norwegian wildland-fire collaboration exercises and perceived level of usefulness?*

Bivariate analysis (Table 5). The most pronounced significance was found between usefulness and "I learned other's concepts and abbreviations" (r = 0.436, r2 = 0.177, F = 14.755, $p \leq 0.000$). This was followed by "I learned about other's organizational aspects" (r = 0.388, r2 = 0.137, F = 10,998, $p \leq 0.002$) and "I learned new things during the exercise" (r = 0.343, r2 = 0.103, F = 8.259, $p \leq 0.006$). The item "I learned about other's prioritizing of activities" received a R-value of 0.324 (r2 = 0.091, F = 7.290, $p \leq 0.009$), and "I learned about other's communication patterns" a R-value of 0.323 (r2 = 0.090, F = 7.358, $p \leq 0.009$).

Table 5. Bivariate regression of the learning dimension of usefulness.

Dependent Variable: Utility Independent Variables: Learning Characteristics of Exercises	R	R2	F	Sign (*p*)
I learned new things during the exercise	0.343	0.103	2.874	0.006
I learned about other's organizational aspects	0.388	0.137	3.316	0.002
I learned about other's communication patterns	0.323	0.090	2.713	0.009
I learned about other's prioritizing of activities	0.324	0.091	2.700	0.009
I learned other's concepts and abbreviations	0.436	0.177	3.841	0.000

Note: N = 71, sig = $p \leq 0.05$.

Multivariate analysis (Table 6.). The perceived learning items predicted 17% (r2 = 0.170) of the usefulness variance, meaning that the remaining 83% of the predicted variance was unaccounted for. The only item that was found significant was "I learned about other's prioritizing of activities" (p = −0.049). Thus, these results indicate a medium to small [49] covariation between learning and utility.

Table 6. Multiple regression of the learning dimensions of usefulness.

Dependent Variable: Utility Independent Variables: Learning Characteristics	Biv. reg. Stand.Beta	Mult.regr. Stand. Beta	Sign. (*p*)
I learned new things during the exercise	0.343	−0.072	0.743
I learned about other's organizational aspects	0.388	0.256	0.277
I learned about other's communication patterns	0.323	−0.049	0.826
I learned about other's prioritizing of activities	0.324	0.078	0.649
I learned other's concepts and abbreviations	0.436	0.345	0.022

Note: N = 71, R = 0.488, r2 = 0.170, sig $p \leq 0.05$

4. Discussion

The results from this study indicate a strong covariation between participation in Norwegian wildland-fire collaboration exercises and perceived level of learning, and a medium to small covariation between perceived learning and utility. Thus, our results support findings in past international studies, all of which indicate that participants' perceived effects of exercises are rather limited [3–7]. Initially, a significant majority of the sample population in this study (84.3%) agreed that the exercise focused on collaboration. This supports the assumption that it is considered rhetorically correct to be in support of collaboration-enhancing initiatives and exercises [3], hence contributing to maintaining the crisis management assumption that collaboration is viewed as a core concern, as it helps managers and societies to effectively deal with the adverse consequences of a crisis [22]. The results indicate the importance of giving clear instructions and sufficient forms of discussion during and after the exercise in order to gain learning. The study indicates joint evaluations, improvising and testing of new and alternative strategies across sectors as successful. An extensive crisis sometimes requires more focus on flexibility, e.g., synchronous collaboration compared to an everyday emergency, e.g., sequential and parallel collaboration. Exercises are opportunities to train horizontal and vertical working processes, either mechanistic or a more organic approach. Even non-collaborative decisions when a situation requires acts of demarcation or exclusion can be tested and evaluated [56]. The skill of choosing alternative strategies and approaches can be of special value during catastrophes and disasters [45].

Over half (53.3%) strongly agreed to whether they had performed well-known activities, while the rest mildly agreed or remained neutral. This suggests that the exercises contained elements of drilling, which have a focus on developing and repeating discipline-specific key procedures [4]. It should here be taken into consideration that putting out wildland-fires, together with flying planes and helicopters, requires specific skills and training and is thus difficult to entrust to others, something that may explain the finding that 85.9% agreed that personnel in need of exercise participated. This assumption is further supported by the fact that 97% of the participants belonged to a public organization, suggesting that these exercise participants were by and large specialists within their own fields.

A clear majority of participants (87.3%) agreed that they had learned new things. Over half agreed that they had learned about others' organizational aspects (74.6%) and communication patterns (71.8%). While these are high numbers, we argue for the need to see them in a context involving exercise participants that are highly trained, specialist professionals who already perform well-known activities. It may thus be assumed that the participants, as fire professionals, through everyday interaction and common training, already had a basic knowledge of each other's way of organizing. That under half (45.1%) agreed that they had learned new concepts and abbreviations suggests, however, that there were organizational differences and a slight lack of focus regarding cross-organizational communication development during the exercise. This, together with the high degree of familiar task performance, indicates that the exercise was dominated by sequential or parallel working patterns [19], where participants either perform their task in a defined order, similar to an assembly-line approach, or work side by side, while maintaining focus on an individual sector specific task. Even if all levels of collaboration are necessary to practice depending on the current situation, there is, according to past studies, a tendency to avoid synchronous collaboration during exercises. The reason can be a desire to avoid challenges associated with having to understand the collaborating organization's way of working or communicating [3], or as a means to reach individual professional goals [35]. However, in this study, it may also be a result of the practical need to perform tasks in a certain order, such as when to apply air vs. ground resources.

While most of the sample population (94.4%) initially found the exercise useful for real-life activities, the analysis of the other utility items suggests that there was some uncertainty related to who the exercise was for and which organizational level found it most useful. While 38% agreed that the exercise was useful for commanding officers, 42.3% agreed it was useful for ordinary operative staff. However, an interesting observation was that 29.6% and 42.3% chose to respond neutrally to the same questions. This suggests that the exercise lacked a clearly defined purpose, joint discussions, and the presentation of clear instructions. These assumptions are also supported by the fact that barely half (49.3%) agreed that sufficient forms of discussion were provided, and just above half (59.2%) perceived that their points of view were regarded. Overall, under half (45.1%) agreed that their experiences of the exercises would affect their daily work, while 33.8% remained neutral. From a learning point of view, these numbers suggest a potential of improvement. The results can be explained by the discovery that exercise participants have a tendency to distinguish between exercise and real-life behavior [57].

Limitations

First, this study was limited in scope as data was collected from a limited number of exercise participants during a short period. Second, the achieved population sample of 71 resulted in a statistical power of 0.86. Nevertheless, due to the relatively few wildland-fire collaboration exercises involving a large number of participants, data from this exercise gave good indications of the perceived levels of collaboration, learning, and utility. Also, the achieved power is, according to Cohen [49], still to be considered strong. Thirdly, the possible occurrence of a somewhat low term-validity needs to be taken into consideration, as the researchers did not pre-define the meaning of the CLU variables for the exercise participants. Fourth, the time passed between participants' participation in the exercise and time answering the survey may have led to lower response rate, as well as possible lower response validity. The data was retrieved from a questionnaire, observations and interviews can add more and comprehensive insight into the studied phenomenon.

5. Conclusions

As Karl Weick [1] found in his study, wildland-fire fighters have a strong identity and prefer keeping "their familiar tools in a frightening situation" (p. 7). Weick assumed that this was because they considered the unfamiliar alternative even more frightening. As such, the results from our study may be seen as supportive of Weick's supposition, as they indicate that the exercise population prefers working in familiar patterns. While this study found a strong covariation between participation in Norwegian wildland-fire collaboration exercises and perceived level of learning, it also found a medium-to-small covariation between perceived learning and utility. The results show that the exercise contributed positively to adding new learning. However, on the basis that the goal was to strengthen collaboration utility value, the study indicates the need to focus more on collaboration building and enhancing elements throughout all phases of the exercise. To ensure an effective and optimized use of available resources in crisis, cross-boundary tasks need to be integrated into the exercise; more room for improvising and testing of unfamiliar and alternative strategies are suggested. As this study was limited in scope and population, we recommend conducting similar studies, preferably through the use of the same instrument.

Author Contributions: Conceptualization, C.H., J.P.W.A., and J.L.S.; methodology, C.H., J.P.W.A., E.C., and J.L.S.; validation, E.C. and J.L.S.; formal analysis, C.H. and J.P.W.A.; investigation, C.H. and J.P.W.A.; writing—original draft preparation, C.H. and J.P.W.A.; writing—review and editing, C.H., J.P.W.A., E.C., and J.L.S.; visualization, C.H. and J.P.W.A.; supervision, J.L.S. All authors have read and agreed to the published version of the manuscript.

Funding: This research received no external funding.

Acknowledgments: Reported data were first were first published in Halvorsen, C., & Aas, J.P.W. (2019). [Samvirke–Går vi mot felles mål? Subjektiv opplevelse av læring og nytte i en skogbrannkontekst (Master's thesis, University of South-Eastern Norway).

Conflicts of Interest: The authors declare no conflict of interest.

References

1. Weick, K.E. Drop your tools: An allegory for organizational studies. *Adm. Sci. Q.* **1996**, *41*, 301–313. [CrossRef]
2. Thompson, J.D. On building an administrative science. *Adm. Sci. Quart.* **1956**, *1*, 102–111. [CrossRef]
3. Berlin, J.M.; Carlström, E.D. Why is collaboration minimised at the accident scene? *Disaster Prev. Manag. Int. J.* **2011**, *20*, 159–171. [CrossRef]
4. Berlin, J.M.; Carlström, E.D. The three-level collaboration exercise–impact of learning and usefulness. *J. Conting. Crisis Manag.* **2015**, *23*, 257–265. [CrossRef]
5. Perry, R.W. Disaster exercise outcomes for professional emergency personnel and citizen volunteers. *J. Conting. Crisis Manag.* **2004**, *12*, 64–75. [CrossRef]
6. Magnussen, L.I.; Carlstrøm, E.; Sørensen, J.L.; Torgersen, G.-E.; Hagenes, E.F.; Kristiansen, E. Learning and usefulness stemming from collaboration in a maritime crisis management exercise in Northern Norway. *Disaster Prev. Manag.* **2018**, *27*, 129–140. [CrossRef]
7. Sørensen, J.L.; Magnussen, L.I.; Torgesen, G.-E.; Christiansen, A.M.; Carlstrom, E. Perceived usefulness of maritime cross-border collaboration exercises. *Arts Social. Sci. J.* **2018**, *9*, 1–5.

8. Rutty, G.N.; Rutty, J.E. Did the participants of the mass fatality exercise Operation Torch learn anything? *Forensic Sci. Med. Pathol.* **2012**, *8*, 88–93. [CrossRef] [PubMed]

9. Norwegian Ministry of Justice and Public Security. National Emergency Preparedness Principles 2019. Available online: https://www.regjeringen.no/no/tema/samfunnssikkerhet-og-beredskap/innsikt/hovedprinsipper-i-beredskapsarbeidet/id2339996/ (accessed on 20 May 2020).

10. Murphy, M.; Arenas, D.; Batista, J.M. Value creation in cross-sector collaborations: The roles of experience and alignment. *J. Bus. Eth.* **2015**, *130*, 145–162. [CrossRef]

11. Martin, E.; Nolte, I.; Vitolo, E. The Four Cs of disaster partnering: Communication, cooperation, coordination and collaboration. *Disasters* **2016**, *40*, 621–643. [CrossRef] [PubMed]

12. Mill, J.S. On liberty. In *A Selection of His Works*; Springer: New York, NY, USA, 1966; pp. 1–147.

13. Elkington, N.E.; Massie, D. The changing nature of international resource sharing: Risks and benefits of collaboration. *Interlend. Doc. Supply* **1999**, *2*, 95–103. [CrossRef]

14. Austin, J.E. Strategic collaboration between nonprofits and businesses. *Nonprofit Volunt. Sect. Q.* **2000**, *29*, 69–97. [CrossRef]

15. Gray, B. Collaborating: Finding common ground for multiparty problems. *Acad. Manag. Rev.* **1989**, *15*, 545–547.

16. Kourula, A.; Laasonen, S. Nongovernmental organizations in business and society, management, and international business research: Review and implications from 1998 to 2007. *Bus. Soc.* **2010**, *49*, 35–67. [CrossRef]

17. Richter, J. Public–private Partnerships for Health: A trend with no alternatives? *Development* **2004**, *47*, 43–48. [CrossRef]

18. Drucker, P.F. *Management Challenges for the 21st Century*; Routledge: Abingdon-on-Thames, UK, 2007.

19. Berlin, J.M.; Carlström, E.D. The 20-minute team—A critical case study from the emergency room. *J. Eval. Clin. Pract.* **2008**, *14*, 569–576. [CrossRef] [PubMed]

20. Brattberg, E. Coordinating for contingencies: Taking stock of post-9/11 homeland security reforms. *J. Conting. Crisis Manag.* **2012**, *20*, 77–89. [CrossRef]

21. Kapucu, N. Collaborative emergency management: Better community organising, better public preparedness and response. *Disasters* **2008**, *32*, 239–262. [CrossRef]

22. Powley, E.H.; Nissen, M.E. If you can't trust, stick to hierarchy: Structure and trust as contingency factors in threat assessment contexts. *J. Homel. Secur. Emerg. Manag.* **2012**, *9*, 1–9. [CrossRef]

23. Sawalha, I.H.S. Collaboration in crisis and emergency management: Identifying the gaps in the case of storm "Alexa". *J. Bus. Contin. Emerg. Plan.* **2014**, *7*, 312–323.

24. Van Wart, M.; Kapucu, N. Crisis management competencies: The case of emergency managers in the USA. *Public Manag. Rev.* **2011**, *13*, 489–511. [CrossRef]

25. Ansell, C.; Boin, A.; Keller, A. Managing transboundary crises: Identifying the building blocks of an effective response system. *J. Conting. Crisis Manag.* **2010**, *18*, 195–207. [CrossRef]

26. Boin, A.; Bynander, F. Explaining success and failure in crisis coordination. *Geografiska Annaler A Phys. Geogr.* **2015**, *97*, 123–135. [CrossRef]

27. Jung, K.; Song, M. Linking emergency management networks to disaster resilience: Bonding and bridging strategy in hierarchical or horizontal collaboration networks. *Qual Quant.* **2015**, *49*, 1465–1483. [CrossRef]

28. U.S. Centers for Disease Control and Prevention. *Health hazard evaluation of police officers and firefighters after Hurricane Katrina–New Orleans, Louisiana, -28 and November 30-December 5, 2005*, MMWR: Morbidity and mortality weekly report. 2006; pp. 456–458.

29. Norwegian Official Report 2012:14. Rapport fra 22. juli-kommisjonen: Oppnevnt ved kongelig resolusjon 12. august 2011 for å gjennomgå og trekke lærdom fra angrepene på regjeringskvartalet og Utøya 22. juli 2011; avgitt til statsministeren 13. august 2012. Available online: https://www.regjeringen.no/contentassets/bb3dc76229c64735b4f6eb4dbfcdbfe8/no/pdfs/nou201220120014000dddpdfs.pdf (accessed on 20 May 2020).

30. Carlström, E.; Berlin, J. Var och en på sin kant om avsaknaden av synkron samverkan på olycksplatsen. *Kommunal Ekonomi och Politik* **2009**, *13*, 3.

31. Berlin, J.M.; Carlström, E.D. Collaboration exercises: What do they contribute? *—A study of learning and usefulness*. *J. Conting. Crisis Manag.* **2015**, *23*, 11–23. [CrossRef]

32. Sørensen, J.L. Norwegian Maritime Crisis Collaboration Exercises: Are They Useful? Ph.D. Thesis, Northcentral University, San Diego, CA, USA, May 2017.

33. Carlström, E.; Berlin, J.; Sørensen, J.L. Collaboration exercises in emergency work: Outcomes in terms of learning and usefulness. *Disaster Divers. Emerg. Prep.* **2019**, *146*, 147.

34. Sorensen, J.L.; Kim, T.-E.; Christiansen, A.; Torgensen, G.-E. Old dogs, new tricks? A Norwegian study on whether previous collaboration exercise experience impacted participant's perceived exercise effect. *Int. J. Emerg. Serv.* **2018**, *8*, 122–136. [CrossRef]

35. Kristiansen, E.; Sorensen, J.L.; Magnussen, L.I.; Carlstrøm, E. Time to rethink Norwegian maritime collaboration exercises. *Int. J. Emerg. Serv.* **2017**, *6*, 14–28. [CrossRef]

36. Borell, J.; Eriksson, K. Learning effectiveness of discussion-based crisis management exercises. *Int. J. Disaster Risk Reduct.* **2013**, *5*, 28–37. [CrossRef]

37. Curnin, S.; Owen, C.; Paton, D.; Trist, C.; Parsons, D. Role clarity, swift trust and multi-agency coordination. *J. Conting. Crisis Manag.* **2015**, *23*, 29–35. [CrossRef]

38. Berlin, J.M.; Carlström, E.D. Collaboration exercises—The lack of collaborative benefits. *Int. J. Disaster Risk Sci.* **2014**, *5*, 192–205. [CrossRef]

39. Sommer, M.; Njå, O. Dominant Learning Processes in Emergency Response Organizations: A Case Study of a Joint Rescue Coordination Centre. *J. Conting. Crisis Manag.* **2012**, *20*, 219–230. [CrossRef]

40. Stein, J. How institutions learn: A socio-cognitive perspective. *J. Econ. Issues* **1997**, *31*, 729–740. [CrossRef]

41. Klabbers, J. *The Exercises Planners Guide*; HMSO: London, UK, 1999.

42. Meyer, J.W.; Rowan, B. Institutionalized organizations: Formal structure as myth and ceremony. *Am. J. Sociol.* **1977**, *83*, 340–363. [CrossRef]

43. Gredler, M.E. *Learning and Instruction: Theory into Practice*; Macmillan: New York, NY, USA, 1992.

44. Bourgeois, S.; Drayton, N.; Brown, A.-M. An inovative model of supportive clinical teaching and learning for undergraduate nursing students: The cluster model. *Nurse Educ. Pract.* **2011**, *11*, 114–118. [CrossRef]

45. Andersson, A.E.C.; Berlin, J. Organizing a simulated reality: On exercises with public safety organizations. *Nord. Organ. Stud.* **2013**, *15*, 34–64.

46. van Laere, J.; Lindblom, J. Cultivating a longitudinal learning process through recurring crisis management training exercises in twelve Swedish municipalities. *J. Conting. Crisis Manag.* **2019**, *27*, 38–49. [CrossRef]

47. Andersson, A. Boundaries as mechanisms for learning in emergency exercises with students from emergency service organisations. *J. Vocat. Educ. Train.* **2016**, *68*, 245–262. [CrossRef]

48. Faul, F.; Erdfelder, E.; Buchner, A.; Lang, A.-G. Statistical power analyses using G* Power 3.1: Tests for correlation and regression analyses. *Behav. Res. Methods* **2009**, *41*, 1149–1160. [CrossRef]

49. Cohen, J. *Statistical Power Analysis for the Behavioral Sciences*; Academic press: Cambridge, MA, USA, 2013.

50. Berlin, J.; Carlström, E. *Samverkan På Olycksplatsen: Om Organisatoriska Barriäreffekter*; University West: Trollhattan, Sweden, 2009.

51. Altman, D.G. *Practical Statistics for Medical Research*; CRC Press: Boca Raton, FL, USA, 1990.

52. Sørensen, J.L.; Carlström, E.; Torgensen, G.-E.; Christiansen, A.; Kim, T.-E.; Wahlstrøm, S.; Magnussen, L.I. The organizer dilemma: Outcomes from a collaboration exercise. *Int. J. Disaster Risk Sci.* **2019**, *10*, 261–269.

53. Bennett, J.; Briggs, W.; Triola, M. *Statistical Reasoning for Everyday Life*; Pearson: London, UK, 2009.

54. Trochim, W.; Donnelly, J.P. *The Research Methods Knowledge Base Mason*; Atomic Dog: Cincinnati, OH, USA, 2008.

55. Shapiro, S.S.; Wilk, M.B. An analysis of variance test for normality (complete samples). *Biometrika* **1965**, *52*, 591–611. [CrossRef]

56. Burns, T.; Stalker, G. Mechanistic and organic systems. *Organ. Behav.* **2005**, *2*, 214–225.

57. Berlin, J.M.; Carlström, E.D. The 90-second collaboration: A critical study of collaboration exercises at extensive accident sites. *J. Conting. Crisis Manag.* **2008**, *16*, 177–185. [CrossRef]

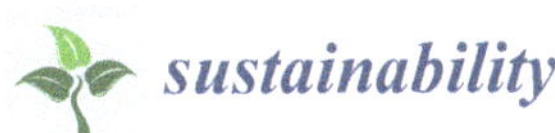 *sustainability*

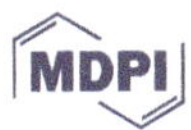

Article

Preparedness and Multiagency Collaboration—Lessons Learned from a Case Study in the Norwegian Armed Forces

Trygve J. Steiro [1],* and Glenn-Egil Torgersen [2]

[1]   Department of Teacher Education, Norwegian University of Science and Technology,
      7012 Trondheim, Norway
[2]   Department of Business, History and Social Sciences, USN School of Business, University of South-Eastern
      Norway, Campus Vestfold, 3184 Borre, Norway; Glenn-Egil.Torgersen@usn.no
*   Correspondence: trygve.j.steiro@ntnu.no

Received: 10 August 2020; Accepted: 1 September 2020; Published: 4 September 2020

Abstract: The objective of this study is to investigate the structure for learning and the learning outcomes from a paper exercise based on multiagency collaboration, and point to potential benefits for crisis leadership and management in civil organizations. The current study was conducted by participant observation in one exercise and a questionnaire was handed out in the following exercise to measure outcomes. Social interaction and concurrent learning are used as the theoretical foundation in the current study. The exercise can be used as an input for multiagency collaboration when linked to the strategic and operative context. The Norwegian Armed Forces operate from a leadership perspective of intention-based leadership. The organization has also developed a pedagogical platform that guides learning activities. In a complex world, we aim at finding training areas that can prepare the cadets for scenarios that also heavily involve the unforeseen. Improvisation is seen as important for military leaders and the exercise provides a sound arena for this purpose. We have seen that even for a table exercise, important lessons can be learned. The current study makes suggestions as well as improvements that could be performed based on the lessons learned for both the Norwegian Armed Forces as well as for other organizations that find the experiences interesting. The article identified five management principles for interaction under unforeseen conditions: (1) develop a pedagogical view for the organization, (2) facilitate and train using processes for complementary process development, (3) develop precise and common language, (4) train the organization in concurrent learning, (5) develop tolerance and mutual respect.

Keywords: interaction; concurrent learning; exercise; unforeseen

1. Introduction

An air force is termed as a high-risk organization within the taxonomy of Charles Perrow [1]. It has been argued that military operations and especially sharp operations can be described as dynamic, turbulent and competitive [2]. Norway, like many other nations, has applied "mission command" that aims to reduce the gap between plans and the actual chaos of war. Today's officers must be capable of autonomous decision-making in both rapidly changing and ambiguous situations. Officers will even, early in their career, need a capacity for divergent thinking and problem-solving skills. Military officers can be put in command and control situations depending on their skills and experience, but also ones demanding improvisation [3]. Clausewitz (1832/1976, p. 119) [4] termed "friction" as a discrepancy between the plan and what was occurring on the battlefield [5,6]. Considering this, the United Nations Air Power Operation (UNAPO) is a fictional operation run as a paper exercise. The end of the exercise does not seek a "fixed" solution or "the school's solution" as it is pointed out in the start of the exercise.

The cadets are presented with a mission and the intention of the commander. The commander is typically an operative officer. Then the cadets representing the different nations pull back to develop a plan and present it in a plenary. The following tasks are performed in the exercise:

-   Setting up an air defence involving different nations
-   A planned air assault on a strategic target with the presentation of different solutions by the different nations with suggested efforts from the other nations
-   An opportunity to strike an enemy target that is time-sensitive
-   A combat search and rescue operation of a fighter pilot who has been forced to bail out over enemy territory
-   Moving a large number of refugees from an insecure to a safe location.

The Royal Norwegian Air Force Academy (RNoAFA) is a branch of the Norwegian Defence College responsible for educating officers for the different branches of the Royal Norwegian Air Force. One of the key aspects is mission command and to be educated in, understand, and know how to use air power with its strengths and limitations. The cadets come from different branches of the Air Force and understanding the different concepts of the Air Force is important. It is also important to understand the interplay with other air forces as well for the understanding of air power. The cadets will serve as officers in positions both nationally and internationally as officers operating on the line or as staff officers. In 2011, the Royal Norwegian Air Force participated in the air campaign over Libya and played a very active role in the operation. This has called for a focus on the use of air power in an international context and for the scaffolding of the experiences obtained in the operation.

The objective of this study is to investigate the structure for learning and the learning outcomes of such an exercise, report on experiences, and point to factors that might be relevant for crisis management. The theoretical foundation the article is based on is learning leadership, mission-based leadership, social interaction and concurrent learning. The current study might be a case example for contributing to the fight against pandemics, in particular COVID-19.

2. Theoretical Framework

The theoretical section is divided into five sections:

-   The leadership context
-   Learning leadership
-   Mission-based leadership
-   Social interaction ("samhandling")
-   Concurrent learning.

2.1. The Leadership Context

Northouse [7] writes that leadership must be understood in the context in which one operates. Northouse [7] divides leadership competence into three parts:

1. Substantial competence such as production and technology and industry
2. Competence in people and social relationships
3. The ability for abstraction.

A central aspect of leadership in the Armed Forces of Norway and allied nations is mission command. Mission command or "intention-based" leadership as it is termed in Norway is based on the commander given the objective or intent and the "why". The operative level must within the framework find out the "how". This implies decentralized decisions and task solving is based on the practical judgement of the commanding officer at the sharp end [8]. Information regarding the why is very important to determine [9,10]. Hence, the commander would form the "intent" of the mission, thus providing a framework and guidance. Within the framework the operative level is also able to improvise on the battlefield to fulfil the mission, but in addition also exploit opportunities that occur from the friction in the war [11,12].

2.2. Learning Leadership

A central aspect of the RNoAFA is educating leaders that will operate within the context of air power. Learning leadership means that working and learning is as much a way of life at the RNoAFA for educating leaders, as it is among the staff [13]. The RNoAFA operates as a community of interdisciplinary practitioners with diverse expertise that must be aligned, and therefore a key characteristic is that each is valued for their contribution irrespective of rank and seniority. There is a focus on embracing diversity and celebrating heterogeneity [13]. This in everyday practice means that critiquing is a way of living and working. The staff at RNoAFA reinforce ongoing learning individually and collectively [13]. In "Global Competence in an Inclusive World" [14], the OECD writes: "Global competence includes the acquisition of in-depth knowledge and understanding of global and intercultural issues, the ability to learn from and live with people from different backgrounds, and the attitudes and values necessary to interact respectfully with others" (OECD, 2016: 1) [14].

2.3. Mission-Based Leadership

The purpose of developing "mission-based leadership" in the Armed Forces is to better deal with uncertainty and to meet an unknown future with greater agility. This implies that education must include creating solutions; maintaining self-awareness and situational awareness and forming a comprehensive understanding, as well as exercising independent decisions and translating plans and intentions into action. With this, the Armed Forces have chosen a decentralized command system, where the operative level will be able to act independently and flexibly and independently within the commander's intention [9,10]. This requires leadership that emphasizes cooperative and relational skills to create common understanding as to why it should be done (commitment) and how to do it (interaction) [13]. The benefits of the UNAPO exercise should therefore be seen in light of mission command.

2.4. Social Interaction (Samhandling)

Herberg, Torgersen and Rundmo (2019) have identified social interaction and concurrent learning (CL) as key factors for meeting the unforeseen in a study conducted among military personnel [15]. Torgersen and Steiro defined "samhandling" as: "Samhandling is an open and mutual communication and development between participants, who develop skills and complement each other in terms of expertise, either directly, face-to-face, or mediated by technology or by hand power. It involves working towards common goals. The relationship between participants at any given time relies on trust, involvement, rationality and industry knowledge" [16]. Samhandling is not only reserved for senior management and it typically takes place in production and common processes in which people work and act together. This action is based on shared and exchanged expertise which is often extensive, specialized, and used in a complementary manner [16,17]. Miles and Watkins [18] support the notion that interaction is more than the sum of its parts and focus on complementary competencies.

2.5. Concurrent Learning

As we saw, Herberg, Torgersen and Rundmo (2019) have highlighted CL in military organizations. CL can be defined as: "A deliberate and continuously functional and interacting learning process among actors that occurs simultaneously with the interaction" [17] (p. 335). Learning in this form does not merely take place by chance. CL is both intentional and purposeful. Stakeholders or participants need to be aware of this process and focus on the relationship between one's own and others' expertise and diversity and focus on the complementary. Samhandling and CL represent a mindset to tackle the challenges of flexible organizations [16]. Therefore, the utilization of complementary expertise and CL are important strategic measures for the efficient development of flexible features for organizations [17].

This is also highlighted in Torgersen and Steiro [19]. The distinction between interaction, collaboration and teamwork is that interaction is an extra emphasis and awareness of the complementary:

- with arrangements for the exchange and utilization of the participants' different competence, experience, background and culture,
- and channeling (coordination) of this into the work towards a common goal in a work or meeting process.
- In collaboration, common understanding is built and developed with different competence and understanding through concurrent learning [19].

They refer to the corresponding exchange of a number of knowledge structures combined with developing the ability to interact, and teach as an event occurs, as CL, and which is defined as: "A deliberate and continuously functional and interacting learning process among actors that occurs simultaneously with the interaction" [18] (p. 253).

In military contexts, CL can be compared to the principle of "train as you fight" [20,21] as we see it, but CL has a more systematic and combined learning content, which also includes the debrief phase. Therefore, CL competence will be important to develop in all types of emergency environments, both civilian and military. Heifetz, Grashow and Linsky [22] think of leadership in terms of "putting a hand on a thermostat". They argue that if the heat is too low, people will not make a decision. If the heat is too high, people might panic. This implies, as we see it, the need for CL. This could be assured by, for instance, the extensive use of debriefing [23].

3. The Context of the Exercise

The Air Force Academy of Norway has invested a great deal of resources in the education of cadets. The curricula are based on a blend of theory, practice and reflection [24]. The challenge is to ensure an appropriate mix of these factors and set them in a relevant context. The exercise is inspired by a human rights concept of the Air Force Academy in Italy, where an air operation is simulated and cadets from different nations are challenged in San Remo to provide human rights answers to commanders in an air operation. The RNoAFA was inspired by the concept and has created its own exercise for cadets in Norway. The Norwegian version is based on a joint international air operation to protect a group of people from attack in one nation. The exercise is played out under a United Nations umbrella. However, points made in the exercise and expressed in this article must not be seen as the opinion of the United Nations. It is an exercise played out where the nations are labeled "Blue", "Black", and "Green" etc. Each nation is assigned air power capacities with individual descriptions. The first author played the role of nation "Green" with eight F-16 fighters, one Hercules air transport and a platoon of Special Operation Forces (SOF), meaning a medium-large player in the field. In addition, they were given a mandate of being offensive and were known to follow the line of the lead nation "Blue". Both "Green" and "Blue" nations had few caveats (restrictions mandated by the respectively politicians). The exercise demanded the cadets operate on a table (or paper-based exercise) in a complex environment, demanding heterogeneous competence and involving ethical consideration. The exercise can therefore be perceived as an example of Bennis and O'Toole's [25] suggestion for management training. The airpower exercise lasts for five full days and ends in with a wrap-up and lessons learned in a session on day five. Antonacopoulou and Sheaffer's [26] account for why organizations and individuals fail to learn from failure and repeat the same mistakes again by embedding crisis in learning is a mode of learning they define as "learning in crisis" [26] (p. 4). This means that the UNAPO exercises should not be about finding the right solutions, but rather learning from experience and from mistakes.

4. Methods and Materials

The method applied was participant observation of the exercise. The first author participated in the exercise in 2015 as a participant playing the Green nation, as mentioned earlier. At that time research was not thought of as just being part of a learning area with the staff and cadets. The first author was working as an associate professor at RNoAFA, but with no participation in the planning and the execution of the exercise, only as a participant. After participating in the exercise, the first author discussed the experience with the second author and both agreed that the exercise would be of interest to explore in greater detail. The idea of conducting research was further discussed with the officer responsible for the exercise. He was positive and allowed us to conduct research. Having been part of the exercise was a major advantage for developing a questionnaire for conducting research the next time the exercise was performed with a new group of cadets in December 2015. It was decided to hand out the questionnaire to the cadets on the morning of day five (the last day of the exercise) before the "hot wash-up" and debrief of the exercise. "Hot wash-up" involves the immediate responses from the participants taking part in the exercise. This is unfiltered and can be seen as a "brainstorming" session. Next, a structural debrief is performed. By providing the questionnaire before these processes, the research material was not influenced by the processes. All 25 cadets were asked to fill out the questionnaire and all 25 gave their consent for the second exercise in 2015. Of the 25 cadets, there were five women and 20 men ranging from 22 to 32 years with a mean of 25 years. The questionnaire was taken directly from Berlin and Carlström [27] (p. 32), focusing on themes regarding:

-   Collaboration
-   Learning
-   Usefulness

In addition, some questions (items) from Torgersen and Steiros's 10-factor questionnaire for relational indicators for effective social interaction in organizations [16] were also included. The questions asked were:

-   Are all actors in the exercise treated with the same respect?
-   Involvement awareness. Are all actors in the exercise equally willing to contribute actively?
-   Complementary competence (complement each other with unique competence). Did all actors contribute with their industry-specific expertise?
-   Did the exercise help to develop a common understanding of language?
-   Through the exercise, have I gained more confidence in the other actors?

All questions in the battery ($n = 23$) were based on a 5-point Likert scale from strongly disagree to strongly agree. In addition, we added a category "I do not know/no view" because we wanted this as a further option. No cadets used this category for any questions, implying that all questions could be seen as relevant.

The study will present the exercise in detail and assess the learning outcome. It will link the learning outcome to relevant operations. It will also argue that such an exercise plays a valuable role in meeting demands for training managers for performing of complex assignments in organizations [25]. The study will not only document responses but also investigate means for the improvement of the structure of the exercise and the learning output and potential benefits for other organizations.

5. Results

The questionnaire revealed several interesting findings. Based on the response, the following table can be presented. The questionnaire was based on a 5-item Likert scale. However, we have merged disagree/strongly disagree and agree/strongly agree in order to make it more readable and to ensure a better overview. The results are presented in Table 1.

Table 1. Participants' report on outcome of the exercise. (n = 25).

Questions	Disagree/Strongly Disagree	Middle Value	Agree/Strongly Agree
Opportunities to improvise between organizations	8%	8%	84%
My points of view were acknowledged	4%	12%	84%
I learned new things during the exercise	-	4%	96%
It is useful for real-life activities	4%	28%	64%
Impact on my daily work	16%	40%	44%
All actors treated with the same respect	16%	20%	64%
Complementary competence was used	12%	16%	72%
More trust during the exercise	16%	40%	44%

The questionnaire reveals that the exercise produces several important outcomes. However, the number of respondents was low, so we have used it for creating an overall impression. It can be argued based on the response to the questionnaire that the exercise strengthens the collaboration within the group. However, this is reported and is not viewed in practice. Therefore, it is fair that the respondents expect a strengthening rather than actually experiencing a strengthening. It was also reported that room for discussions during and after the exercise is needed and might be structured for CL and social interaction. This has been stressed as very important in order to strengthen collaboration [16]. Debriefing is important in order to strengthen CL. The exercise, as noted earlier, consisted of different types of operations which were concluded before moving to the next operation. We also found support from the cadets' point of view that the exercise provides opportunities for improvisation and trying out different strategies regarding collaboration among the participating organizations. In this regard, the different nations [3] focused on the importance of military leaders' ability to improvise. Another finding is that they reported that they learned about collaborating organizations' priorities. This is a reported outcome but still might assume strengthening the knowledge regarding what decisions are made, but to a lesser degree on how the actual priorities are decided or negotiated in real life. Regarding elements that are not so positive, there are some aspects that stand out, despite an overall positive impression. The cadets were divided down the middle on whether they perceived the exercise as useful in their daily life. This might imply that different cadets or branches of the Royal Norwegian Air Force are better covered. Air operations are complex and covering several scenarios in just four days could be too ambitious. One must ask, how much did they learn in detail from such an exercise? More instructions regarding collaboration could be provided. Having said that, the exercise seems to be most heavily focused on air power planning and decision making. At the same time, it is hard to put too many expectations into an exercise. But there is a potential as we see it to strengthen this part. This could be achieved by having a "time out" focusing on this issue and asking the cadets to write down their reflections regarding collaboration issues given the use of a "Blue Book". The academy uses a so-called Blue Book in which to write down reflections [16]. We did not observe the use of this Blue Book when the first author was part of the exercise. In the exercise, an air raid resulted in severe collateral damage so the success of the mission was, to say the least, very questionable. However, no further discussion was raised. There could have been a possibility to raise questions. But the participants, including the first author, did not raise any questions, nor was it encouraged. We think that what you focus upon is important for addressing different issues. We also observed that the cadets did not report increased trust in each other. This might, however, imply that trust was high before the start of the exercise. An alternative might be that the content of the exercise does not go into any real depth. The case of collateral damage was one where participants were vulnerable. Who is to blame? What should be done to mitigate the damage? A third assumption might be that this was a paper exercise and that, by playing different nations, the cadets were playing roles, rather than truly giving themselves. Being in a more naturalistic and hostile environment, say crossing the mountains as a team in the winter, combating stormy weather, fatigue, and stress would be better suited for building trust. This curriculum was also covered earlier at the RNoAFA. This can be viewed as a negative aspect. In addition, the cadets were together almost every day following a tight schedule and curricula and at the time of the exercise half the class had been together for 1.5 years. All of them were together for half a year (the last ones to enter were experienced officers that had earlier gone through the the first year, which is mandatory before going for pilot training in the USA). It can be argued that, for this group, trust was not strengthened. It might already have been at a very high level [27]. The exercise focuses on a strategic planning team that bring to getter personnel from different organizations or different departments in large organizations. So, the question is also relevant for the cadets. They also reported less relevance to daily activity. That could be interpreted as meaning that this exercise is on a high level that is said to be relevant. There might be a greater complexity demanding interdisciplinary collaboration and involving ethical dilemmas that might be less visible in the day-to-day activities at the academy [27]. It stresses the importance of training students in complex scenarios demanding interdisciplinary collaboration and ethical dilemmas. Perhaps it could be argued that more of the curricula at the academy should be linked to the exercise? This means that more resources should be used in order to foster more learning from the exercise and that teachers and facilitators should be used to scaffold the exercise and later use it as examples in the curricula. A natural development from the UNAPO exercise is that the cadets are put in the role of the commander and writing the intention of missions. In the UNAPO exercise, all cadets play the same role as executors, not the mission commander. Having one group acting as the mission command team could challenge the cadets even more.

6. The Norwegian Defence Pedagogical View (FPG)

The Norwegian Armed Forces has a comprehensive strategic curriculum with regards to the pedagogical approach and overall learning objectives for learning activity. This is the Armed Forces' pedagogical basic view [27]. This plan focuses consistently on collaboration, development of creativity and problem solving. In addition, emphasis is placed on teaching and exercise methods, where no work is performed towards a defined conclusion, but instead situation-oriented solutions adapted to the challenges and conditions that exist. Competence is important for dealing with unforeseen events. In the preface of the document, it is stated, among other things:

> " ... *The military profession presupposes the ability to mobilize knowledge, attitudes and skills in both familiar, new and unexpected circumstances in relation to persons with different backgrounds, to equipment and new technology. This makes great demands on the learning activity that is taking place in the Armed Forces in relation to education and training. There are also demands on the individual's ability learn, cooperate, evaluate and adapt to different situations.*
>
> *The changes in the organization and the tasks of the Defense demand inspection of and development of the pedagogical activity. The pedagogical execution of the Defense's branches of education and courses will be an important success criterion to succeed in developing a quality oriented, effective, flexible and alteration willing Defense.*
>
> *The Defense already has a good and well-developed educational system, but there may be aspects that have to be improved to meet new challenges. The basic pedagogical view (FPG) of the Defense shall make sure of a common platform for teaching, both internally and what is bought externally. FPG shall be the guideline for all pedagogical activities within the Defense. FPG is based upon the basic values of the Defense, and must also be seen in relation to basic military leadership (GML) the common operative doctrine (FFOD) of the Defense and the personnel manual (FPH). These together are an important force to produce effective learning ... "* ([27], preface).

Of course, training is also based on basic fixed procedures and solutions, but the concept of learning and pedagogy has several dimensions and is more holistic than that which has traditionally been seen in military organizations (before FPG was introduced). In itself, the development and implementation of an organization's pedagogical philosophy will be a feature to be determined for the competence development in an organization. Therefore, it is somewhat surprising that several large civilian companies and institutions, and other countries' military organizational zones, do not already have this. This is an important lesson, and we believe that we can strongly state that a well-functioning FPG in the organization is crucial for successful competence development. Without FPG, strategic management and training are built without a foundation.

7. The Lessons Learned: Overall Discussions and Implications

The cadets reported overall positive experiences regarding collaboration and learning. They reported less favorable ones regarding the usefulness in daily activities and trust. However, the number of reports was small, which should also be a consideration. Further distribution of the questionnaire is recommended in order to gather more data and compare the different classes of cadets and thereby create CL in order to strengthen the pedagogical outcome, as pointed out in FPG [27]. We will also advise distributing the questionnaire during the exercise to facilitate more CL. If teamwork was essential and the cadets reported low scores on this issue, more emphasis on this could be introduced during the exercise. In a complex world we aim to find training areas that can prepare the cadets for scenarios that also heavily involve the unforeseen. Improvisation is seen as important for military leaders and the exercise provides a sound arena for this purpose. However, again, it is necessary to ask how they will use improvisation after the exercise. We have seen that, even for a table exercise, important lessons can be learned. The point is not having live planes, but rather solving tasks and garnering feedback and learning. The overall experience is reported to be very positive. In the current study, only the cadets filled out the questionnaire. For further exercises, the instructors might also fill out a questionnaire for creating a more dynamic learning environment and enabling more CL, thereby fostering CL between teachers/facilitators and cadets. It can also be supported by semi-structured interviews by researchers not playing a part of the planning and execution of the exercise. Another point to address is that, in another study [28], it was pointed out that some instructors focus only on the product and not on the process. The students, however, favored instructors focusing on both the process and product [28]. Further development of the UNAPO exercise would benefit from addressing both the product and the processes. Another factor is that CL will demand that instructors and cadets need to stop, reflect and adjust when under way, as [22] when thinking of leadership as putting a hand on the thermostat. The idea of the hand on the thermostat, which either speeds up the pace of the exercise or pauses it to reflect on something emergent, could be a fruitful path to take. If the exercise is perceived either by cadets or teachers/ facilitators as going slow, the "heat" could be turned up to create more stress, or strengthen the complexity, or to reveal an ethical dilemma that could be further explored [25]. In addition, it will be necessary for the organization to have developed a unified pedagogical philosophy, which can form the foundation for strategic management, training and renewal. Not least, this applies to building the right skills and a flexible and adaptable mindset to deal with unforeseen events during situations, including pandemics. The UNAPO exercise is developed within an air power context. We have seen that context is important for the leadership of organizations [7], but we think there are some generic lessons that could be addressed. A paper exercise allows for complex scenarios to be played out. We also know from scenario planning that it contributes to strengthening the relations between the participating actors [29]. In this respect the current study provides an example of the seminal work of De Geus (1988) [29]. Regarding more recent research, we think the current study should be seen in light of the work of Herberg et al. (2019) [15], understanding CL and social interaction. The current study might provide a concrete example to facilitate such processes. The current study might be a case example for contributing to the fight against pandemics, in particular COVID-19, especially in relation to extracting experiences and research finding from military pedagogy and psychology, with implications for handling competence and knowledge strategies to provide infection control [22].

8. Conclusions: Five Crisis Management Principles

All in all, in this study we have identified five crisis management principles for developing competence for interaction under unforeseen conditions and these principles are identified as:

(1)   Develop a pedagogical view for the organization
(2)   Facilitate and train for complementary competence process development
(3)   Develop precise and common language
(4)   Train the organization in concurrent learning
(5)   Develop tolerance and mutual respect

These principles should permeate strategic contingency plans and practical crisis management, to ensure the development of the necessary expertise for interaction under risk and unpredictable conditions. The principles can also serve as quality indicators in evaluation and improvement processes in the organization. However, it is necessary for the individual organization to adapt and concretize the principles to its specific activities and tasks.

Author Contributions: The first author (T.J.S.) has planned, executed the data collection and analysed the results. The second author (G.-E.T.) contributed in the planning of the study, analysed the results, deduced conclusions, and contributed in the writing process. All authors have read and agreed to the published version of the manuscript.

Funding: This research received no external funding.

Conflicts of Interest: The authors declare no conflict of interest.

References

1.   Perrow, C. *Normal Accidents: Living with High-Risk Technologies*; Basic Books: New York, NY, USA, 1999.
2.   Visser, M. Teaching giants to learn: Lessons from army learning in World War II. *Learn. Organ.* **2017**, *24*, 159–168. [CrossRef]
3.   Brady, M. Improvisation versus rigid command and control at Stalingrad. *J. Manag. Hist.* **2011**, *17*, 27–49. [CrossRef]
4.   Clausewitz, C.V. *On War*; The Complete Edition; Princeton University Press: Princeton, NJ, USA, 1976; Originally published in 1832.
5.   Gross, G.P. *The Myth and Reality of German Warfare: Operational Thinking from Moltke the Elder to Heusinger*; University Press of KY: Lexington, KY, USA, 2016.
6.   Vandergriff, D.E. From Swift to Swiss: Tactical decision games and their place in military education and performance improvement. *Perform. Improv.* **2006**, *45*, 30–39. [CrossRef]
7.   Northouse, P.G. *Leadership: Theory and Practice*; Sage Publication: Thousand Oaks, CA, USA, 2018.
8.   Antonacopoulou, E.P.; Moldjord, C.; Steiro, T.J.; Stokkeland, C. The New Learning Organisation: PART I–Institutional Reflexivity, High Agility Organising and Learning Leadership. *Learn. Organ.* **2019**, *26*, 304–318. [CrossRef]
9.   Chief of Defense. *Chief of Defense Basic View on Leadership*; Forsvarsstaben: Oslo, Norway, 2012; pp. 6–7.
10.   Norwegian Defense University College. *Armed Forces Joint Doctrine*; Forsvarssjefen: Oslo, Norway, 2014; p. 166.
11.   Murray, W. *Military Adaptation in War: With Fear of Change*; Cambridge University Press: New York, NY, USA, 2011.
12.   Shamir, E. *Transforming Command: The Pursuit of Mission Command in the US, British and Israeli Armies*; Stanford University Press: Stanford, CA, USA, 2011.
13.   Antonacopoulou, E.P.; Moldjord, C.; Steiro, T.J.; Stokkeland, C. The New Learning Organisation: PART II–Lessons from the Royal Norwegian Air Force Academy. *Learn. Organ.* **2019**, *27*, 117–131. [CrossRef]
14.   OECD. *Global Competency for an Inclusive World*; OECD: Paris, France, 2016.
15.   Herberg, M.; Torgersen, G.-E.; Rundmo, T. Competence for the Unforeseen: Social Support and Concurrent Learning as Basic Components of Interaction under Risk. *Front. Commun.* **2019**, *4*, 19. [CrossRef]

16. Torgersen, G.E.; Steiro, T.J. *Ledelse, Opplæring og Samhandling i Fleksible Organisasjoner. Om Menneskeliggjøring av Styringssystemer. [Leadership, Training and Collaboration in Flexible Organisations. On the Humanization of Management Systems]*; Læringsforlaget: Stjørdal, Trøndelag, 2009.

17. Steiro, T.J.; Torgersen, G.-E. The Terms of Interaction and Concurrent Learning in the Definition of Integrated Operations. In *Handbook of Research on Multidisciplinary Approaches to Entrepreneurship, Innovation, and ICTs*; Rosendahl, T., Hepsø, V., Eds.; IGI Global: Hershey, PA, USA, 2013; pp. 328–340.

18. Miles, S.A.; Watkins, M.D. The leadership team: Complementary strengths or conflicting agendas? *Harv. Bus. Rev.* **2007**, *85*, 186.

19. Torgersen, G.-E.; Steiro, T.J. Defining the Term Samhandling. In *Interaction: 'Samhandling' Under Risk. A Step Ahead of the Unforeseen*; Torgersen, G.-E., Ed.; Cappelen Damm Akademisk: Oslo, Norway, 2018; pp. 39–54. [CrossRef]

20. Heifetz, R.; Grashow, A.; Linsky, M. Leadership in a (permanent) crisis. *Harv. Bus. Rev.* **2009**, *87*, 62–69. [PubMed]

21. Torgersen, G.E. The Idea of a Military Pedagogical Doctrine. In *Military Pedagogies. And Why They Matter*; Kvernbekk, T., Simpson, H., Peters, M.A., Eds.; Educational Futures Series—Rethinking Theory and Practice; Sense Publishers: Rotterdam, The Netherlands, 2008.

22. Torgersen, G.E.; Firing, K.; Steiro, T. Make the Invisible Enemy Visible: Military Debriefing in the Time of Unforeseen. In *Military Psychology Response to Post Pandemic Reconstruction*; Rawat, S., Boe, O., Piotrowski, A., Eds.; Rawat Publications: Jaipur, India, 2020; forthcoming.

23. Steiro, T.J.; Firing, K. Coaching and Mentoring in Military Training: An Educational Perspective. In *Mentoring og Coaching i et Læringsperspektiv*; Karlsdottir, R., Kvalsund, R., Eds.; Tapir Akademisk Forlag: Trondheim, Norway, 2009.

24. Bennis, W.G.; O'Toole, J. How business schools lost their way. *Harv. Bus. Rev.* **2005**, *83*, 96. [PubMed]

25. Antonacopoulou, E.P.; Sheaffer, Z. Learning in crisis: Rethinking the relationship between organizational learning and crisis management. *J. Manag. Inq.* **2014**, *23*, 5–21. [CrossRef]

26. Berlin, J.H.; Carlström, E.D. Collaboration Exercises: What Do They Contribute?—A Study of Learning and Usefulness. *J. Contingencies Crisis Manag.* **2015**, *23*, 11–23. [CrossRef]

27. Torgersen, G.E.; Bergh, J. *Forsvarets Pedagogiske Grunnsyn. Med fokus på læring*; Forsvarets Skolesenter: Oslo, Norway, 2006.

28. Nyhus, I.; Steiro, T.J.; Torgersen, G.-E. Apprenticeship Learning in Preparation for Meeting the Unforeseen. In *Interaction: 'Samhandling' Under Risk. A Step Ahead of the Unforeseen*; Torgersen, G.-E., Ed.; Cappelen Damm Akademisk: Oslo, Norway, 2018; pp. 107–126.

29. De Geus, A.P. Planning as Learning. *March/April Harv. Bus. Rev.* **1988**, *88*, 70–74.

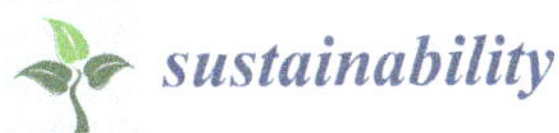 *sustainability*

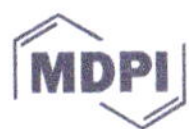

Article

Regional Flexible Surge Capacity—A Flexible Response System

Viktor Glantz [1], **Phatthranit Phattharapornjaroen** [1,2], **Eric Carlström** [3,4] **and Amir Khorram-Manesh** [1,5,*]

[1] Institute of Clinical Sciences, Department of Surgery, Sahlgrenska Academy, Gothenburg University, 40010 Gothenburg, Sweden; viktor.glantz@vgregion.se (V.G.); phatthranit.pha@mahidol.edu (P.P.)

[2] Department of Emergency Medicine, Ramathibodi Hospital, Mahidol University, Bangkok 10400, Thailand

[3] Institute of Healthcare Sciences, Sahlgrenska Academy, Gothenburg University, 40010 Gothenburg, Sweden; eric.carlstrom@gu.se

[4] USN School of Business, University of South-Eastern Norway, P.O. Box 235, 3603 Kongsberg, Norway

[5] Department of Research and Development, The Swedish Armed Forces Center for Defense Medicine, 40010 Gothenburg, Sweden

* Correspondence: amir.khorram-manesh@surgery.gu.se

Received: 1 July 2020; Accepted: 22 July 2020; Published: 24 July 2020

Abstract: Surge capacity is the ability to manage the increased influx of critically ill or injured patients during a sudden onset crisis. During such an event, all ordinary resources are activated and used in a systematic, structured, and planned way to cope with the situation. There are, however, occasions where conventional healthcare means are insufficient, and additional resources must be summoned. In such an event, the activation of existing capabilities within community resources can increase regional surge capacity in a flexible manner. These additional resources together represent the concept of Flexible Surge Capacity. This study aims to investigate the possibility of establishing a Flexible Surge Capacity response system to emergencies by examining the main components of surge capacity (Staff, Stuff, Structure, System) within facilities of interest present in the Western Region of Sweden. Through a mixed-method and use of (A) questionnaires and (B) semi-structured key-informant interviews, data was collected from potential alternative care facilities to determine capacities and capabilities and barriers and limitations as well as interest to be included in a flexible surge capacity response system. Both interest and ability were found in the investigated primary healthcare centers, veterinary and dental clinics, schools, and sports and hotel facilities to participate in such a system, either by receiving resources and/or drills and exercises. Barriers limiting the potential participation in this response system consisted of a varying lack of space, beds, healthcare materials, and competencies along with a need for clear organizational structure and medical responsibility. These results indicate that the concept of flexible surge capacity is a feasible approach to emergency management. Educational initiatives, drills and exercises, layperson empowerment, organizational and legal changes and sufficient funding are needed to realize the concept.

Keywords: capacity; community; crisis; disaster; flexible; major incident; surge; management

---

1. Introduction

Adequate preparedness efforts and proper contingency planning can mitigate and minimize the impact of major incidents and disasters (MID) in societies [1]. Contingency plans are the organized and coordinated courses of action that present institutional roles and resources, information processes, and operational arrangements based on scenarios of potential crises and hazard analyses [2]. Strategies for disaster management include establishing command and control, reliable and efficient communication, information, organization, warning systems, stockpiling of resources, and response plans for the mobilization and management of resources such as personnel, equipment, volunteers, and emergency facilities. The efficiency of the organizational structure is paramount for the outcome of the event [3,4]. Disaster preparedness and contingency planning involve all actors in society. However, in particular, the healthcare sector is designated to respond in a planned and efficient manner to prevent mortality and morbidity, resulting from an increasing number of global and local threats, at the lowest possible cost to society [3–5].

The initial approach to proper management of MID is to increase the management system's capacity, i.e., Surge Capacity (SC). Three broad areas of healthcare demand SC in response to a MID [6]: Firstly, Public health Surge capacity (the ability of the public health system to increase capacity for patient care, epidemiological investigation, laboratory services, mass fatality management, etc.); secondly, Healthcare Facility-Based Surge Capacity (augments the response within the healthcare facility structure, e.g., triage-tent on hospital grounds); and finally, Community-based Surge Capacity (the public effort to support and augment the healthcare system). The four essential elements of SC, i.e., Staff, Stuff, Structure, and System (4S), should rapidly and effectively be surged in the affected areas. Staff refers to available/alternative personnel, Stuff refers to available/alternative equipment, Structures refer to hospitals, clinics and Alternate Care Facilities (ACF), and systems are procedures and guidelines that govern the emergency management process [7,8].

The expansion of MID necessitates a new surge capacity (secondary SC), which underlines the need for increased effort to obtain additional resources still available within the management system [9–11]. A further expansion of incidences demands new approaches, policies, and adjustable preparedness within the community to scale up and down resources in a quick and seamless manner, i.e., "flexible surge capacity" (FSC) [12]. The concept of FSC is concordant with the new paradigm of proactivity in disaster management and emphasizes risk reduction rather than focusing on pure relief operations to reduce vulnerability and increase resilience within communities [13]. Therefore, risk assessment and focus on all four elements of SC is necessary for achieving a FSC. The disaster management cycle should incorporate, recognize, and value the participation of affected communities [14], and it is therefore necessary that adequate infrastructure is in place to ensure access to emergency services [15]. In this perspective, the readiness of community-owned resources is essential and includes alternative facilities to take care of victims or to unburden hospitals [16–18].

Focus on all four elements of SC is necessary for achieving a FSC. Staff pools may be needed, and new staff categories should be considered to replace the regular staffing structure. Equipment and devices placed in different parts of a community should be registered and available for use. Buildings of opportunity, i.e., facilities with the capacity to hold a high number of people that can act as an ACF should be identified [4,6,18]. Finally, relevant systems and guidelines should be produced to link all these measures. The focus of this paper, however, is on ACFs at predesignated, strategic buildings. These untapped resources available within a community can be lifesaving and deserve recognition and support from all agencies within the emergency management network [12,16]. A more comprehensive view of the Structure component of SC includes *buildings of opportunity* and *facilities of interest* that can be designated and converted to act as an ACF. Such buildings can consist of, but are not restricted to, outpatient clinics, dental and veterinary clinics, schools, hotels, convention centers, and sports facilities [6,10,12,17,18].

In the Swedish crisis and emergency management system, the responsibility for crisis and disaster management resides at national, regional, and local levels based on the principles of Responsibility, Parity, and Proximity [19]. According to these principles, all actors retain their responsibilities during MID management while the methods and structures should be kept as similar as possible to those used in normal circumstances. The geographical responsibility to manage an event lies with those parties affected at the local level, i.e., close to the incident [19]. The Region Västra Götaland (VGR) in Sweden has about 1.6 million inhabitants in 49 municipalities in its 300 km long and 250 km wide area. VGR is responsible for healthcare, growth, and development within the region and is one of the largest employers in Sweden with over 50,000 employees. According to current legislation, the preparedness of Swedish healthcare should be formed in close collaboration and cooperation between primary healthcare, hospitals, municipalities, county administrative boards (CAB), ambulance dispatch centers, and medical officers [19].

2. Aim

This study aims to investigate the possibility of implementing a FSC response system to MIDs by examining the feasibility and the potential need for additional resources and barriers in ACFs within VGR of Sweden.

3. Method

This study uses mixed methods, has an explanatory sequential design, and is partitioned into four phases of data collection and analysis [20–22].

3.1. Sample

The potential for FSC planning regarding ACFs was investigated in five VGR cities with a population ranging from 40,000 to over 600,000 inhabitants [23]. The cities were chosen because they all have essential healthcare infrastructure. Due to limited previous research in this field, a pilot study was planned with an approximate sample size of 99 facilities (around 20 facilities in each city) to receive questionnaires and supplementary informant interviews to a point of saturation [22,24]. Sampling was performed mainly using online search engines with map services to identify facilities of interest in each city. Each facility of interest/potential ACF, defined as veterinary and dental clinics, schools, sports clubs, and hotels, was checked for suitability by using information from the actors' websites and by Google Street View© to assess the location, accessibility, size, and proximity to hospitals. The final sample was relatively well distributed across the ACF categories in the investigated cities.

3.2. Questionnaire

The questionnaire (Appendix A) was developed by using the Nominal Group Technique [25]. Three academically skilled experts with extensive experience in instrument development and disaster and emergency management (one physician, one prehospital nurse, and one hospital nurse) developed the tool and tested it for face validity based on logic, relevance, comprehension, legibility, clarity, usability, and consensus. The questionnaires contained a vignette where the facility of interest faces a fictitious scenario of a mass casualty incident and is asked to help the healthcare sector to respond. It included both open-ended and close-ended questions to capture and generate relevant data [26,27]. Questionnaires were sent out January–March 2020 to 99 primary healthcare centers, dental and veterinary clinics, schools, sports facilities, and hotels during the first phase of this study.

3.3. Interviews

Qualitative data collection was performed through semi-structured interviews with 12 key informants [26,27]. The interview framework was constructed from the same general questions as the ones used in the questionnaire, but more in-depth. Before each interview, the actor's previous answers from the questionnaire were reviewed for content. The questionnaire and review notes were brought to the interview to allow for follow-up questions to written answers and comments. The interview framework contained open-ended questions to enable the conversation to capture all content of interest. The interviewees were allowed to diverge from the interview guide and explore other areas related to the subject. No more interviews were held after reaching the point of data saturation [22,26,27].

3.4. Data Processing

The data was analyzed for results, discussion, and conclusion. Sequential analysis was performed [21,27] to determine what the qualitative data added to the questionnaire data. The qualitative analysis consisted of coding for thematic content to identify capabilities, barriers, and interest to partake in a FSC-response system.

3.5. Statistical Analysis

Cronbach's alpha was measured on the finalized tool and showed internal consistency of 0.739 [28].

4. Results

The results are presented in four sections. All conclusions about capabilities and barriers that pertain to a specific category of facilities of interest are presented in Section 4.4.

4.1. Central Measurements, Phase One

Roughly 42% of respondents answered the questionnaire (41/97). The response rate was higher in a smaller city than in a larger city (86% vs. 34%, respectively). Reliability analysis was performed on the 14 items of questionnaire data. The value for Cronbach's alpha was acceptable at 0.739 [28], and the questionnaire could be deemed a valid instrument. All returned questionnaires had comments and notes written on them. About half of the respondents answered several questions in the comment section. Some respondents did not answer all the items in the questionnaire. Two questionnaires, both belonging to sports facilities, were not returned due to absent mailboxes.

4.2. Central Measurements, Phase Two

Several interviews had to be rescheduled due to the social distancing strategy implemented to counter the COVID-19 outbreak. Three face-to-face interviews were conducted with one Primary Health Care Center (PHCC) physician, two school nurses (from one school), and one chief veterinary surgeon from a major veterinary clinic. Nine more interviews were conducted via telephone: with one PHCC physician, three chief dentists, one manager for dental care development in the regional council for dental care, two more chief veterinary surgeons, one school nurse, one sports facility administrator, and two hotel managers. The average duration of an interview was approximately 28 min. The face-to-face interviews were notably longer than telephone interviews. They were more beneficial to this study because the meetings took place at the potential ACFs, allowing for visual inspection of facilities.

4.3. General Results

The majority of interview respondents from investigated facilities of interest indicated that their workplace could be converted into an ACF to care for affected persons from a MID. Some could also accept patients not affected by the emergency to alleviate pressure on the nearest hospitals. Many respondents had materials in limited amounts for minor surgery, while some facilities only had small first aid kits. Many respondents indicated that additional resources were needed for a further developed capacity and preparedness. The most common materials missing for an increased capability were suture kits and first aid packages (basic and advanced). Many potential ACFs would accept a package or cache with more advanced medical equipment (e.g., tracheal tube, thoracic drainage system, etc.) if proper education was provided and the FSC-response system managed maintenance of the cache. Many respondents and interviewees expressed enthusiasm for the ACF concept; however, they also mentioned a need for an overarching organization governing the planning processes for the FSC response system and a need for educational exercises and drills to further develop their capabilities as well as a clear legal definition of the role they may have during a MID response [29]. The suggested educational initiatives were CPR, first aid, advanced first aid, basic trauma care, ATLS-based courses, disaster management, scene management and task-specific training (e.g., cast appliances, intubation techniques). Most respondents indicated a need for financial support and reimbursement for any invested time and effort into the FSC-response system.

4.4. ACF Specific Results

The following section presents a summary of ACF-specific results. The triage colors mentioned in the text are standard triage models used in MID and are widely used in many countries. The colors define the type of injury and the acuity of medical management. Red stands for immediate management (life-threatening injuries), yellow for delayed management (non-life-threatening injuries) and green for minimal supervision (minor injuries) [30].

4.4.1. Primary Healthcare Centers (PHCCs)

Eight out of 11 sampled PHCCs answered the questionnaire, and two key informant physicians were interviewed before the point of saturation. One interview was conducted in person and another over telephone. All eight clinics indicated an interest in taking part in a FSC-response system, and various levels of involvement were suggested in both questionnaire comments and notes and interviews. All clinics reported capability to receive green patients, and one clinic indicated the ability to stabilize yellow patients before transport to a major hospital. Three clinics stated that they could receive patients from a hospital, unrelated to the type of MID, to alleviate emergency departments. Half of the PHCCs could offer psychosocial support to people affected by a major incident.

4.4.2. Dental Clinics

Ten out of 12 questionnaires were returned with answers outlining capabilities useful to SC planning. Two interviews were conducted with chief dental officers at two clinics before the point of saturation was reached. All responding dental clinics reported both interest and a type of ability to participate in a FSC-response system. Nonetheless, some significant barriers were also reported regarding missing competence to care for injuries other than dental. Three clinics indicated that they could care for green patients from a major incident to alleviate hospital emergency wards. One clinic did not want to fully answer the questionnaire because it was perceived to obligate competency that was absent at the clinic and instead referred the issue to the regional level. At the regional level, one key informant was identified and interviewed. This key informant confirmed the data from both questionnaires and interviews but also shed new light on possible implementation procedures to involve the public dental care resources in a FSC-response system. The results from the interview with the regional informant contextualized and corroborated findings from both phases one and two of this study that pertain to all components of SC.

4.4.3. Veterinary Clinics

All responding veterinary clinics reported interest in participating to some extent in a FSC-response system. All clinics offered to make equipment and facilities available to the FSC-response system, and five out of six indicated capability to receive green patients from a MID. Two clinics also reported the ability to receive yellow patients and other patients from hospitals, unrelated to the type of emergency. Most clinics indicated the ability to treat minor surgical injuries, clean and suture wounds, administer intravenous fluids, and diagnose acute conditions. Many clinics reported to house diagnostic resources that can be useful during a disaster or major incident, such as ultrasonography and radiology, and capabilities to monitor patients for respiratory distress or other somatic deterioration. One clinic indicated that they could not provide healthcare to humans without having to close their veterinary operations. Barriers for veterinary clinics to partake in a FSC-response include the lack of competence to care for humans, legal hindrances for providing healthcare to humans, and the degree of difference between human and veterinary medicine in terms of beds, materials, and equipment. Some veterinarians had different views on how they can be involved in a FSC-response system. One interviewee expressed the belief that similar anatomy amongst all mammals makes trauma surgery similar for both human and veterinary medicine.

Another veterinarian expressed his concerns about the legal aspects and emphasized the need for clear and transparent legislation to enable their participation in a FSC-response system.

4.4.4. Schools

Nine out of 14 questionnaires were returned answered by a school dean, principal, or nurse. All responding schools reported capabilities and interests to be included in a FSC-response system, and all but one school indicated the ability to receive green patients from a MID. Some schools reported limited healthcare resources as school nurses have many students to care for during often limited office hours. One school reported hesitance to receive injured persons for care and treatment and preferred to distribute food and water and administer psychosocial support exclusively. One interviewee questioned having injured persons at the school at all. The reported barriers to partaking in a FSC-response system included the lack of personnel and medical expertise, lack of beds and healthcare materials, and the priority of keeping the school open.

4.4.5. Hotels

Five out of the ten questionnaires were returned answered, and all respondents indicated interest and ability to partake in a FSC-response system. One hotel reported the capacity to receive green patients from a major incident, and the remaining four reported the ability to prepare food, water, and shelter for over 40 persons. All responding hotels indicated that they could house evacuees or injured for treatment by healthcare professionals. Both interviewees expressed an enthusiastic interest in partaking in the proposed FSC-response system. A lack of competency and material were reported as barriers.

4.4.6. Sports Facilities

It was difficult to establish contact with sports facilities. From the twelve distributed questionnaires, two envelopes were returned due to missing mailboxes and only three questionnaires were answered. Two sports facilities indicated a capacity to participate in a FSC-response system. One facility did not answer the questions in the questionnaire but informed that they have no beds, no material, and no regular staff to contribute. Another informant responded that they could help, but they were limited in terms of what they could do. Multiple sites were contacted for interviews, but neither the owners nor managers were available for discussion or interested in being interviewed because nobody could answer for the whole facility. One sports facility administrator was briefly interviewed via telephone. The sports facilities that did report a capability to be included in a FSC-response system indicated that they could provide shelter and water for many people and distribute food. An important caveat regarding the mapping of sports facilities' capabilities is that they are often owned by the public and are managed by a municipal sport and association board. The power of decision making over daily operations often lies in municipal political councils that are disconnected from the day-to-day work at the facility.

5. Discussion

The study's results emphasize the importance of inter-organizational collaboration and the willingness of other stakeholders to participate in the management of MIDs. These findings also demonstrate the feasibility of the FSC-concept and enable all contingency planners to approach this concept fairly. A FSC-plan may offer the crisis management system another tier of resources, resulting in a regionally increased capacity to safely treat many victims. However, before any attempts to retrofit facilities of interest into functional ACFs are undertaken, a range of issues must be considered carefully. The following sections discuss the proposed FSC-concept concerning the four main components of surge capacity.

5.1. Staff

The required staffing of a FSC-response system is crucial. Those who are supposed to operate the ACFs must have both the necessary competencies and be readily available when the need arises. Some facilities of interest, such as PHCCs and veterinary clinics, have the capacity and ability to care for a few patients with minor injuries from a MID. Nonetheless, if they are to care for a group of patients or to deliver a higher level of care, they must be reinforced with additional staff. Other facilities, such as dental and veterinary clinics, lack competent staff to care for injured patients. Hotels and sports arenas may not have staff resources that are appropriately trained to care for even patients with minor injuries [12]. Establishing a dynamic personnel base between competencies and across disciplines could solve some issues of staffing. Staff can, to some extent, be reassigned from ambulatory or home-service care and from hospital wards not under severe pressure from the MID. Emergency staff, including physicians, will likely have a prominent role in managing the care at ACFs, as their competency is required at the center of all responses to MIDs [31]. Volunteers with appropriate skills and competencies (e.g., from the Red Cross or other volunteer civil defense organizations) can also report to an established ACF and help healthcare professionals to deliver appropriate care. There have been exciting developments regarding the use of immediate responders and initiatives such as CITIZENAID and Stop the bleed that educate the public in simple and lifesaving techniques that can be used in a MID [32]. A recent publication from Sweden indicated a high willingness among civilians to participate in the management of MIDs [32]. Civilian defense conscription can be activated by the government without declaring heightened alert and can potentially contribute (at least in part) to staffing ACFs [33–36].

5.2. Stuff (Healthcare Equipment and Materials)

Ensuring the adequate distribution of sufficient critical equipment is a significant task for the proposed FSC-response system. Many respondents indicated that the amount of material and equipment present at their facilities are among the most constricting factors on their capability and capacity. Distributing a material cache to potential ACFs appears to be an efficient and viable way of stocking and equipping a functional FSC response system [18]. The content of the proposed material cache should be adapted to the size and assigned task. Stockpiling used to be a convenient method to secure the provision of essential goods, but the contemporary strategy is generally built on "just-in-time delivery" and access to international markets and imports [34,35]. Altogether, the purveyance of healthcare goods and materials to countries such as Sweden has become more vulnerable than previously recognized [34–37]. To compensate for resource scarcity, many county administrative boards have developed and should develop creative solutions for supplemental reinforcement, including networking with other committees for shared resource pools and infrastructure for improved response.

5.3. Structure

Many of the investigated facilities (PHCC, veterinary, and dental clinics) are suitable for utilization in a FSC-response system. Some are operational presently, while others require a retrofitting effort such as preparing bed space, ensuring utilities and wraparound services, and clearing the facility from other operations. Hotels and sports arenas demand a more extensive retrofitting process to ensure adequate operational facility standards for healthcare provision. Countries such as Sweden have historically had little experience of domestic healthcare provision in nonconventional or standardized facilities. Nonetheless, as part of the response to the COVID-19 pandemic, several areas have been explored to increase the capacity of Swedish healthcare [35,37]. In line with the total defense structure, civilian-military collaboration has also increased, and military field hospitals have been deployed to house additional beds outside of major hospitals. The transportation of critical patients has been performed with military helicopters. However, to avoid misunderstanding and to smooth the pace of collaboration, these efforts should be planned and trained [35].

5.4. System

The responsibility for and management of the proposed FSC-concept must be carefully considered before implementation into a crisis management system. To rapidly deploy and operate ACFs, the logistics and transportation of material, equipment, and patients must be swift and well-coordinated. The efficiency of communication structures and the distribution of resources are of paramount importance. The command and control of the FSC is one of the most critical factors in achieving a successful response. In any context, leadership and decision-making are two critical factors that determine an event's outcome. Besides having a central coordinator, such as a public health agency, the ACF should be operating locally, close to the incident scene, with regional operational guidance and possible material reinforcement distributed from the regional and/or national levels and related agencies [12,19].

The importance of correct and efficient triage during a MID cannot be stressed enough, and selection of the patients for treatment at an ACF is crucial. Over-triage could lead to an unnecessary overflow of patients to hospitals, which could result in the depletion of precious resources, and under-triage may endanger the lives of the victims [30]. Readiness and competence to conduct simple and vital maneuvers, including ventilating a patient until transport to the definitive care, should be presented, and necessary materials must be available. Triage should also give particular concern to vulnerable populations.

Exercises are crucial to create a coherent system that allows for practicing in a FSC and efficient deployment and operation of ACFs. Broad collaborative exercises involving all actors in the crisis management system should be held regularly to streamline efforts from all parties. Appropriate educational initiatives can increase the motivation to help. Educational initiatives should be adapted to the level of care in the assigned task and existing competencies at the facilities of interest [38]. Further studies should determine the content of educational initiatives suitable for professionals and civilians involved in MID management. Findings from a recent study in Sweden indicate a need for new public education initiatives to enable nonprofessionals to become immediate responders [32,36]. There is also the potential to incorporate volunteer resources in some of the ACF operations. All MIDs are likely to affect the mental health of victims, which must be considered and treated alongside their physical injuries and trauma. Mental health preparedness has been deemed insufficient in most countries and must improve [39].

Preserving a network of concurrent material provision and maintenance with education, training, and exercise initiatives continuously running requires significant financial resource allocation, which must be prioritized. Without necessary resources a FSC-response system is toothless. Insufficient program duration has been identified as an essential factor that explains the considerable ineffectiveness of many community-based health and safety programs. Having a long-term program view, active planning against conflicting missions, and mobilizing sufficient resources are necessary to establish, deliver, and sustain the system over time [7].

6. Implications and Recommendations

Integrated participatory and sustainable planning can increase resilience and is closely related to some of the World Health Organization's (WHO) sustainable development goals [40]. If optimally implemented, the FSC-concept can lead to a safer and more resilient society by encouraging increased civil engagement and educational initiatives [12,32]. However, a successful implementation of FSC depends on some essential factors:

1. Mapping capabilities, resources, and networks in the community as part of contingency planning. While decentralizing forces and resources can benefit the independence of communities, they still need support from higher levels. Smaller cities had a higher response rate in this study, which might reflect a higher willingness to engage in their community.

2. Empowering communities, nonprofessionals, and professional individuals to create pools of resources to utilize ACFs, as shown in recent studies and projects.
3. Changing legal and organizational rules and norms necessary to implement the concept into any crisis management system.
4. Financial investment from municipalities, regions, and, ultimately, the state, which might prompt policy and budget changes.
5. Avoiding political interference in public health-related issues to limit crippling the healthcare apparatus more than necessary. The simplicity of disaster plans should be maintained and no excessive changes to the organization, staffing, or supply-chains should occur during a MID.
6. Ethical, safety, and security aspects of using ACFs in response to MIDs should also be considered as the system is implemented.
7. Regulation regarding monitoring and evaluating the initiative is also crucial for the improvement of the response system. Once implemented in policy, the involved parties must exercise and train the FSC-concept in real life for the response system to be efficient and effective.
8. Further research is needed to explore possible use of ACFs and the FSC-concept. FSC can be a reasonable way to increase regional surge capacity, not only within the fields of trauma and surgery but also in other medical emergencies, e.g., CBRNE (Chemical, Biological, Radiological, Nuclear, Explosive)-related events.

7. Limitations and Strengths

The small number of investigated facilities, especially sports facilities, did not allow any statistical analysis of the results. However, the descriptive results confirm that the FSC-concept can be applied in more contexts than the Swedish one and has transferability to other settings in Europe and possibly to other regions as well [41].

The lack of previous studies in this field did not allow any comparison of results with other publications.

8. Conclusions

Management of MID is a multi-professional approach in a chain of reactions. A chain is not stronger than its weakest link. The flexible surge capacity concept is a feasible approach to emergency management that involves all stakeholders within the community. Educational initiatives, drills and exercises, nonprofessionals' empowerment, professional alternatives, organizational and legal changes, and sufficient funding are needed to realize the concept. This response system can also increase societal resilience through community participation and may advance nations' fulfillment of some of the WHO's Sustainable Development Goals. Components that explore possibilities of an attainable increased regional flexible preparedness are novel to the Swedish as well as other contexts. They could lead to a change in the crisis management system. The mobilization of sufficient resources to establish, deliver, and sustain programs over time will be essential to effective implementation of the FSC-concept. This study has found ample will residing in civil society to help the healthcare sector respond to MIDs. It is now up to the crisis management system to channel this will to help in a smart, safe, and efficient way.

Author Contributions: Conceptualization, A.K.-M.; formal analysis, V.G., P.P., E.C., and A.K.-M.; investigation, V.G.; methodology, E.C. and A.K.-M.; project administration, V.K.; resources, A.K.-M.; supervision, A.K.-M.; writing—original draft, V.G.; writing—review and editing, P.P., E.C., and A.K-M. All authors have read and agreed to the published version of the manuscript.

Funding: This research received no external funding.

Acknowledgments: The authors would like to thank Associate Professor Yohan Robinson for his support to this project.

Conflicts of Interest: The authors declare no conflict of interest.

Appendix A

Information Sheet, Questionnaire and interview guide (English Translation for review only)

Flexible Surge Capacity Questionnaire

All resources within a community need to be used to combat a major incident or disaster. This puts high demands on a healthcare system in close collaboration with other partners and authorities. Such collaboration requires both knowledge, planning and practice and must be based on mutual understanding and respect for areas of activity and related responsibilities. In the event of many injured persons needing urgent care, can the need for resources exceed the capacity of the hospitals near your centre/clinic/working place. We would like to investigate how different healthcare players/institutions/organizations can work together in specific events (scenario). Below are several questions that could provide guidance on how such collaboration can be built up in a given scenario. After reading the scenario carefully, please mark the answers that corresponds to the ability of your centre/clinic/working place. It is possible to select several options on the same question.

Participation in this study is voluntary, data would be handled confidentially and the answers will be de-identified. We hope you take the short time needed to answer our questions. This study is part of a PhD program at the University of Gothenburg/Sweden and Mahidol University/Thailand.

On behalf of the research group
Name: xxxxxxxxxxxxxxxxxxxxxxx, Date: xxxxxx

Scenario

After an accident near your centre, there are 120 injured at the site. A sum of 40 severely injured victims require all emergency resources at the major hospital's surgery and intensive care units. Another 40 people are at immediate risk of inhalation injuries and must be under observation with intubation readiness (creating free airways by inserting a tube through the mouth and then into the airway) for the next few hours. Some people also have burn and splinter injuries. The last 40 patients have minor injuries and can be treated either at a hospital or at another unit.

A. Primary care/Health

If your centre is staffed adequately when the event occurs, how can you help?

You can receive the less injured from the incident.

You can receive serious injured from the event for physiological stabilization pending further transport to major hospitals.

You can relieve the hospital emergency departments by receiving other emergency cases, not related to the incident.

Your health care staff can connect to the hospital for reinforcement.

You can can offer resources, e.g., space, instrument, material.

Your centre can handle minor surgical procedures, suture wound injuries, plaster uncomplicated fractures, etc.

Your centre can handle medical patients.

Your centre can offer psychosocial support to patients and staff.

Your centre can coordinate transport for patients to the home.

Your centre cannot help.

Other?

Prerequisites for Healthcare to be able to help.

Equipment/Material:

You have sufficient equipment and materials for the desired ability to assist in special events.

You lack equipment/materials for increased ability. For increased ability, you need _________________.

Other?

Local Supply:

You have adequate facilities for the desired ability to assist in specific events

You do not have adequate facilities for the desired ability to assist in specific events. For increased ability, you need?

Other?

Staffing:

What kind of resource or knowledge your staff need to increase their ability in to take care of injured people?

Other?
Competences:
Do you have the skills required for what you would like to do in the event of a major incident when the needs exceed the available resources?
Yes, absolutely.
Yes, but we need more training/practice.
No, but we can after a directed training/exercise. Suggestion?
Other comments and extensions?

B. Veterinary Clinic
If your centre is staffed adequately when the event occurs, how can you help?
You can receive the less injured from the incident.
You can receive seriously injured from the event for physiological stabilization pending further transport to major hospitals.
You can relieve the hospital emergency departments by receiving other emergency cases not related to the incident.
Your health care staff can connect to the hospital for reinforcement.
You can can offer resources, e.g., space, instrument, material.
Your centre can handle minor surgical procedures, suture wound injuries, plaster uncomplicated fractures, etc.
Your centre can handle medical patients.
Your centre can offer psychosocial support to patients and staff.
Your centre can coordinate transport for patients to the home.
Your centre cannot help.
Other?
Prerequisites for Healthcare to be able to help.
Equipment/Material:
You have sufficient equipment and materials for the desired ability to assist in special events.
You lack equipment/materials for increased ability. For increased ability, you need?
Other?
Local Supply:
You have adequate facilities for the desired ability to assist in specific events
You do not have adequate facilities for the desired ability to assist in specific events. For increased ability, you need?
Other?
Supply of competence:
Do your veterinary clinic have the skills required for what you would like to do in the event of greatly increased care needs?
Yes, absolutely.
Yes, but we need more training/practice.
No, but we can after a directed training/exercise. Suggestions?
Other comments and extensions?

C. Dentistry
If your centre is staffed adequately when the event occurs, how can you help?
You can receive the less injured from the incident.
You can receive seriously injured from the event for physiological stabilization pending further transport to major hospitals.
You can relieve the hospital emergency departments by receiving other emergency cases, not related to the incident.
Your health care staff can connect to the hospital for reinforcement.
You can can offer resources, e.g,. space, instrument, material.
Your centre can handle minor surgical procedures, suture wound injuries, plaster uncomplicated fractures, etc.
Your centre can handle medical patients.
Your centre can offer psychosocial support to patients and staff.
Your centre can coordinate transport for patients to the home.
Your centre cannot help.
Other?

Prerequisites for Healthcare to be able to help.

Equipment/Material:

You have sufficient equipment and materials for the desired ability to assist in special events.

You lack equipment/materials for increased ability. For increased ability, you need?

Other?

Local Supply:

You have adequate facilities for the desired ability to assist in specific events

You do not have adequate facilities for the desired ability to assist in specific events. For increased ability, we need?

Other?

Supply of competence:

Do you have the skills required for what you would like to do in the event of a significant increase care needs?

Yes, absolutely.

Yes, but we need more training/practice. Suggestions?

No, but we can after a directed training/exercise. We suggest?

Other comments and extensions?

D. Schools

How can you help in the urgent care of those affected?

We can stop bleeding, repair wounds, and administer cardiac resuscitation and other emergency procedures.

We can receive the minor injured from the incident.

We can receive shocked people and administer psychosocial support.

We can prepare sleeping accommodation for homeless, evacuated or otherwise afflicted people.

We can prepare food and water for the needy.

We can take care of children so that parents can help elsewhere.

We can send staff to help other authorities.

No, we can't help.

Other?

Do you have the skills for what you would like to do?

Yes, absolutely.

Yes, but we need more education. Suggestions?

No, but we can after a targeted education. Suggestions?

Other?

Prerequisites for your reception to help.

Equipment/Material:

We have enough equipment and materials for the desired ability to help in special cases events.

We lack equipment/materials for increased ability. For increased ability, we need?

Other?

Local Supply:

We have adequate facilities for the desired ability to assist in specific events

We do not have adequate facilities for the desired ability to assist in specific events. For increased ability, we need?

Other?

Supply of competence:

Do you have the skills required for what you would like to do in the event of a significant increase care needs?

Yes, absolutely.

Yes, but we need more training/practice. Suggestions

No, but we can after a directed training/exercise. We suggest?

Other comments and free text?

E. Gym /Sports clubs / Hotel

How can you help in the urgent care of those affected?

We can stop bleeding, repair wounds, and administer cardiac resuscitation and other emergency procedures.

We can receive the minor injured from the incident.

We can receive shocked people and administer psychosocial support.

We can prepare sleeping accommodation for homeless, evacuated or otherwise afflicted people.

We can prepare food and water for the needy.

We can take care of children so that parents can help elsewhere.

We can send staff to help other authorities.

No, we can't help.

Other?

Do you have the skills for what you would like to do?

Yes, absolutely.

Yes, but we need more education. Suggestions?

No, but we can after a targeted education. Suggestions?

Other?

Prerequisites for your reception to help.

Equipment/Material:

We have enough equipment and materials for the desired ability to help in special cases events.

We lack equipment/materials for increased ability. For increased ability, we need?

Other?

Local Supply:

We have adequate facilities for the desired ability to assist in specific events

We do not have adequate facilities for the desired ability to assist in specific events. For increased ability, we need?

Other?

Supply of competence:

Do you have the skills required for what you would like to do in the event of a significant increase care needs?

Yes, absolutely.

Yes, but we need more training/practice. Suggestions

No, but we can after a directed training/exercise. Suggestions

Other comments and free text?

References

1. Skliarov, S.; Kaptan, K.; Khorram-Manesh, A. Definition and General Principles of Disasters. In *Handbook of Disaster and Emergency Management*; Khorram-Manesh, A., Ed.; Kompendiet: Göteborg, Sweden, 2017; Chapter 1; pp. 17–22.
2. Jacobsen, K. *Introduction to Global Health*, 3rd ed.; Jones & Bartlett: Burlington, MA, USA, 2019.
3. Vitalii, S.; Khorram-Manesh, A.; Nyberg, L. Disaster Cycle and Management. In *Handbook of Disaster and Emergency Management*; Khorram-Manesh, A., Ed.; Kompendiet: Göteborg, Sweden, 2017; Chapter 2; pp. 23–29.
4. United Nations International Strategy for Disaster Reduction, (UNISDR). *Terminology on Disaster Risk Reduction*; United Nations: Geneva, Switzerland, May 2009. Available online: https://www.unisdr.org/files/7817_UNISDRTerminologyEnglish.pdf (accessed on 25 June 2020).
5. Stikova, E.; Lazarevski, P.; Gligorov, I. Global public health threats and disaster management. *Health Promot. Dis. Prev.* **2017**, *5*, 746–772.
6. Hick, J.; Christian, M.; Sprung, C. Surge Capacity and Infrastructure considerations for mass critical care. *Intensive Care Med.* **2010**, *36*, 11–20. [CrossRef] [PubMed]
7. Barbich, D.; Koenig, K. Understanding Surge Capacity: Essential Elements. *Acad. Emerg. Med.* **2006**, *6*, 1098–1102. [CrossRef] [PubMed]
8. Kaji, A.; Koenig, K.L.; Bey, T. Surge capacity for healthcare systems: A conceptual framework. *Acad. Emerg. Med.* **2006**, *13*, 1157–1159. [CrossRef]
9. Bonnet, C.; Peery, B.; Cantrill, S.; Pons, P.; Haukoos, J.; McVaney, K.; Colwell, C. Surge capacity: A proposed conceptual framework. *Am. J. Emerg Med.* **2007**, *25*, 297–306. [CrossRef]
10. Runkle, J.D.; Brock-Martin, A.; Karmus, W.; Svendsen, E.R. Secondary Surge Capacity: A framework for understanding long-term access to primary care for medically vulnerable populations in disaster recovery. *Am. J. Public Health.* **2012**, *102*, 24–32. [CrossRef]
11. Adams, L.M. Exploring the concept of surge capacity. *Issues Nurs.* **2009**, *14*, 2. [CrossRef]
12. Khorram-Manesh, A. Flexible Surge Capacity - Public Health, Public Education, and Disaster Management. *Health Promot. Perspect* **2020**, *10*, 175 179. [CrossRef]
13. The Lancet Editorial. Disaster prevention should be equal. *Lancet Glob. Health* **2017**, *5*, 1047. [CrossRef]

14. Krolik, M. Exploring a rights-based approach to disaster management. *Aust. J. Emerg. Manag.* **2013**, *28*, 44–48. Available online: https://knowledge.aidr.org.au/resources/ajem-oct-2013-exploring-a-rights-based-approach-to-disaster-management/ (accessed on 30 June 2020).

15. Rice, K.; Felizzi, M.V.; Hagelgans, D. Human Rights-Based Approach to Disaster Management: Valparaiso, Chile. *J. Hum. Rights Soc. Work* **2017**, *2*, 117–127. [CrossRef]

16. Marston, C.; Hinton, R.; Kean, S.; Baral, S.; Ahuja, A.; Costello, A.; Portela, A. Community participation for transformative action on women's, children's and adolescents' health. *Bull. World Health Org.* **2016**, *94*, 376–382. [CrossRef] [PubMed]

17. Bayram, J.; Zuabi, S.; Subbarao, I. Disaster Metrics: Quantitative Benchmarking of Hospital Surge Capacity in Trauma-Related Multiple Casualty Events. *Disaster Med. Public Health Prep.* **2011**, *5*, 117–124. [CrossRef] [PubMed]

18. Agency for Healthcare Research and Quality (AHRQ). Disaster Alternate Care Facilities. In *Report and Interactive Tools*; Chapter 4; Rockville: Montgomery, MD, USA, 2018. Available online: https://www.ahrq.gov/research/shuttered/acfselection/chapter4.html. (accessed on 25 June 2020).

19. Khorram-Manesh, A.; Hedelin, A.; Örtenwall, P. Regional coordination in medical emergencies and major incidents; plan, execute and teach. *Scand. J. Trauma Resusc. Emerg. Med.* **2009**, *17*, 32. [CrossRef] [PubMed]

20. Szostak, R. Interdiciplinary and Transdiciplinary Multimethod and Mixed Methods Research. In *The Oxford Handbook of Multimethod and Mixed Methods Research Inquiry*; Oxford University Press: Oxford, UK, 2015. [CrossRef]

21. Bowen, P.; Rose, R.; Pilkinton, A. Mixed Methods-Theory and Practice. Sequential, Explanatory Approach. *Int. J. Quant. Qual. Res. Methods* **2017**, *5*, 10–27.

22. Saunders, B.; Sim, J.; Kingstone, T.; Baker, S.; Waterfield, J.; Bartlam, B.; Burroughs, H.; Jinks, C. Saturation in qualitative research: Exploring its conceptualization and operationalization. *Qual. Quant.* **2018**, *52*, 1893–1907. [CrossRef] [PubMed]

23. Sweden, S. Population by Region and Year. 2019. Available online: http://www.statistikdatabasen.scb.se/pxweb/sv/ssd/START__BE__BE0101__BE0101A/BefolkningNy/table/tableViewLayout1/ (accessed on 25 June 2020).

24. Sofaer, S. Qualitative research methods. *Int J. Qual. Health Care* **2002**, *14*, 329–336. [CrossRef]

25. Harvey, N.; Holmes, C.A. Nominal group technique: An effective method for obtaining group consensus. *Int. J. Nurs. Pract.* **2012**, *18*, 188–194. [CrossRef]

26. Brinkmann, S. Unstructured and Semi-Structured Interviewing. In *The Oxford Handbook of Qualitative Research*; Leavy, P., Ed.; Oxford University Press: Oxford, UK, 2014. [CrossRef]

27. Tracy, S. Interview planning and design. In *Qualitative Research Methods–Collecting Evidence, Crafting Analysis, Communicating Impact*; Wiley-Blackwell: Hoboken, NJ, USA, 2013.

28. Tavakol, M.; Dennick, R. Making sense of Cronbach's alpha. *Int. J. Med. Edu.* **2011**, *2*, 53–55. [CrossRef]

29. Ashkenazi, M.; Liebiediev, D. Legal aspects in disasters. In *Handbook of Disaster and Emergency Management*; Khorram-Manesh, A., Ed.; Kompendiet: Göteborg, Sweden, 2017; Chapter 26; pp. 44–47.

30. Khorram-Manesh, A.; Lennquist Montán, K.; Hedelin, A.; Kihlgren, M.; Örtenwall, P. Prehospital triage, discrepancy in priority-setting between emergency medical dispatch centre and ambulance crews. *Eur. J. Trauma Emerg. Surg.* **2011**, *37*, 73–78. [CrossRef]

31. Phattharapornjaroen, P.; Glantz, V.; Dahlén Holmqvist, L.; Carlström, E.; Khorram-Manesh, A. Alternative Leadership in Flexible Surge Capacity—The Perceived Impact of Tabletop Simulation Exercises on Thai Emergency Physicians Capability to Manage a Major Incident. *Sustainability* **2020**, *12*, 6216. [CrossRef]

32. Khorram-Manesh, A.; Plegas, P.; Peyravi, M.; Carlström, E. Immediate Response to Major Incidents: Defining an immediate responder! *Eur. J. Trauma Emerg. Surg.* **2019**. [CrossRef] [PubMed]

33. Khorram-Manesh, A.; Robinsson, Y.; Boffard, K.; Örtenwall, P. The History of Swedish Military Healthcare System and Its Path Toward Civilian-Military Collaboration From a Total Defense Perspective. *Mil. Med.* **2020**, usaa071. [CrossRef] [PubMed]

34. Blimark, M.; Örtenwall, P.; Lönroth, H.; Mattsson, P.; Boffard, K.D.; Robinson, Y. Swedish emergency hospital surgical surge capacity to mass casualty incidents. *Scand. J. Trauma Resusc. Emerg. Med.* **2020**. [CrossRef] [PubMed]

35. Khorram-Manesh, A.; Lönroth, H.; Rotter, P.; Wilhelmsson, M.; Aremyr, J.; Berner, A.; Nero Andersson, A.; Carlström, E. Non-medical aspects of civilian-military collaboration in management of major incidents. *Eur. J. Trauma Emerg. Surg.* **2017**, *43*, 595–603. [CrossRef] [PubMed]

36. Khorram-Manesh, A.; Carlström, E. Civilmilitär samverkan behövs för att Klara masskadelägen. *Lakartidningen* **2019**, *116*. FRZE.
37. Goniexicz, K.; Khorram-Manesh, A.; Hertelendy, A.J.; Goniewicz, M.; Naylor, K.; Burkle, M.B. Current response and management decisions of the European Union to the COVID-19 outbreak: A review. *Sustaianability* **2020**, *12*, 3838. [CrossRef]
38. Khorram-Manesh, A.; Berlin, J.; Carlström, E. Two validated ways of improving the ability of decision-making in emergencies; Results from a literature review. *Bull. Emerg. Trauma* **2016**, *4*, 186–196.
39. Roudini, J.; Khankeh, H.; Witruk, E. Disaster mental health preparedness in the community: A systematic review study. *Health Psychol. Open* **2017**, 1–12. [CrossRef]
40. World Health Organization (WHO). *Sustain. Dev. Goals.* Available online: https://sustainabledevelopment.un.org/?menu=1300 (accessed on 25 June 2020).
41. Franklin, M. Doing Research-Gathering data. In *Understanding Research: Coping with the Quantitative-Qualitative Divide*; Taylor & Francis Group: New York, NY, USA, 2013; Volume 6, pp. 167–210.

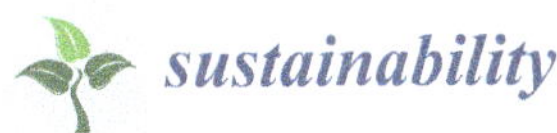 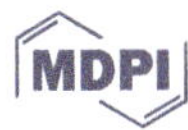

Article

Outcomes of Establishing an Urgent Care Centre in the Same Location as an Emergency Department

Annelie Raidla [1,2], **Katrin Darro** [1,2], **Tobias Carlson** [2,3], **Amir Khorram-Manesh** [2,4], **Johan Berlin** [5] and **Eric Carlström** [2,6,7,*]

[1] Emergency Department at Östra Hospital, Sahlgrenska University Hospital, 413 90 Gothenburg, Sweden; annelie.raidla@vgregion.se (A.R.); katrin.darro@vgregion.se (K.D.)

[2] Gothenburg Emergency Research Group (GEMREG), Sahlgrenska University Hospital, 413 90 Gothenburg, Sweden; tobias.carlson@vgregion.se (T.C.); amir.khorram-manesh@surgery.gu.se (A.K.-M.)

[3] Center of Emergency Department Development, Sahlgrenska University Hospital, 413 90 Gothenburg, Sweden

[4] Institute of Clinical Sciences, Sahlgrenska Academy, Gothenburg University, 405 30 Gothenburg, Sweden

[5] Department of Social and Behavioral Studies, University West, 461 86 Trollhättan, Sweden; johan.berlin@hv.se

[6] Institute of Health and Care Sciences, Sahlgrenska Academy, University of Gothenburg, 405 30 Gothenburg, Sweden

[7] USN School of Business, Campus Vestfold, University of South-Eastern Norway, 3603 Kongsberg, Norway

* Correspondence: eric.carlstrom@gu.se

Received: 2 August 2020; Accepted: 2 October 2020; Published: 4 October 2020

Abstract: The emergency department (ED) is one of the busiest facilities in a hospital, and it is frequently described as a bottleneck that limits space and structures, jeopardising surge capacity during Major Incidents and Disasters (MIDs) and pandemics such as the COVID 19 outbreak. One remedy to facilitate surge capacity is to establish an Urgent Care Centre (UCC), i.e., a secondary ED, co-located and in close collaboration with an ED. This study investigates the outcome of treatment in an ED versus a UCC in terms of length of stay (LOS), time to physician (TTP) and use of medical services. If it was possible to make these parameters equal to or even less than the ED, UCCs could be used as supplementary units to the ED, improving sustainability. The results show reduced waiting times at the UCC, both in terms of TTP and LOS. In conclusion, creating a primary care-like facility in close proximity to the hospitals may not only relieve overcrowding of the hospital's ED in peacetime, but it may also provide an opportunity for use during MIDs and pandemics to facilitate the victims of the incident and society as a whole.

Keywords: urgent care centre; emergency department; length of stay; surge capacity; Sweden

---

1. Introduction

The increasing number of Major Incidents and Disasters (MIDs), either natural or man-made, necessitates preparedness in both human and material resources. This has become evident during the COVID 19 pandemic, which has caused tremendous pressure on Emergency Departments (EDs) in several countries. The concept of surge capacity initiated within the immediate period after an MID or the outbreak of a pandemic has the aim of increasing the number of staff and material, as well as creating spaces and structures based on validated and tested systems and procedures. However, an expanding incident necessitates an additional surge, a so-called secondary surge capacity with the intention of utilizing other possible resources. All these measures are implemented in accordance with the contingency plans for each organization, including healthcare, in order to create a more flexible surge capacity [1].

Most of the hospitals call in their staff and create operational spaces. The first stage entails sending home patients who are already admitted but do not need emergency care, or those who have already been treated and who can continue their recovery at home. This stage creates new beds and spaces for incoming patients. In the second phase, extra space should be created for the admission of emergency cases. Besides the ordinary ED, another admission unit is normally set up to handle either urgent patients or ordinary, non-emergency cases. An outpatient department is usually used. Whilst adequate, this approach needs to be planned as there is a clear need for staff who are familiar with the locales, equipment that has to be adjusted to emergency requirements, and procedures that can be put in place as quickly as possible based on disaster medicine principles [2].

Previous studies have shown that staff who lack such familiarity can cause more harm than save lives, and unfavourable spaces can cause more challenges than facilitating the process. In particular, EDs should have staff qualified in emergency medicine, areas for triage and sorting, and proper devices for the care of the severely injured. The optimum suggestion is actually an existing unit that already handles emergency cases, i.e., a secondary ED [3–6].

The emergency department is one of the hospital's busiest facilities and is frequently described as a bottleneck that limits space and structures, jeopardising surge capacity [7,8]. In recent decades, overcrowding in emergency departments (EDs) has been reported as an increasingly worrying occurrence [9,10]. It has been associated with longer waiting times prior to treatment for severely ill patients, risk of in-hospital mortality and a higher probability of leaving the ED against medical advice or without being seen [11]. During the height of the COVID 19 epidemic in Europe and the US in spring 2020, EDs experienced a tremendous peak in the number of patient presentations. Preparedness for disasters became a significant concern in relation to health-care sustainability, and several city-based hospitals throughout the world were operating at or near to capacity limits [12].

The issue of everyday overcrowding of EDs and the impact on preparedness to handle peaks such as that during COVID 19 appeared to be complex, with several factors including physical distancing, use of personal protective equipment and hygienic measures needing to be considered along with remedies required [13].

In the early 1980s, an increasing number of emergency cases led to the establishment of Urgent Care Centres (UCCs) [14]. They function as a healthcare provider staffed by primary care physicians, registered nurses and nurse practitioners, with the ability to handle emergency conditions that do not need ED amenities. UCCs are often managed by a hosting hospital and share mutual support systems such as laboratory, radiation and medical services. It has been reported that UCCs reduce the overuse of EDs by up to 48% [15]. Doran showed that patients treated by UCCs, sited together with and in close collaboration with an ED, received swift service and better follow-up than the control group in the study [16]. UCCs and EDs have also proven to be horizontally integrated and collaborative and function informally between ED and UCC staff [17].

This paper suggests that UCCs may be suitable units for beneficial use both in peacetime and during an MID. They fulfil the function as a supportive unit in peacetime, and by using the same staff and resources can easily be converted to an extra ED or a pandemic admission unit as evidenced by the current need during the COVID 19 epidemic. With the first UCC having been set up in Sweden, the aim of this study was to investigate the outcome of treatment in the ED versus the UCC in terms of quality, LOS, time to physician (TTP), use of medical services, referrals, revisits, hospitalisation, mortality and costs. If it was the case that these parameters were equal to the ED, the UCC could be used as a complementary unit to the ED, improving sustainability not only in peacetime but also during MIDs.

2. Methods

The ED and UCC studied were situated in a hospital in Gothenburg in western Sweden. The ED was part of a University Hospital, distributed over three main hospital complexes in different districts, with one ED each. Each of the EDs received approximately one-third of the 150,000 presentations annually in the city. The ED included was typical, i.e., treating diseases and injuries from age 16, excluding orthopaedic and psychiatric diseases. It received 53,840 visits during 2018, an increase of 4.8% over the year before (2017). The trend of more visits had been apparent during the last few decades. The ED served the part of the county characterised by the weakest socioeconomic status and highest proportion of immigrants. A UCC was established in spring 2018, staffed with primary care physicians and registered nurses. The UCC shared the triage line with the ED, with attendees being assessed post-triage as either ED or UCC patients. The UCC was expected to optimise shared resources and provide improved services for low-urgency patients. The study was approved by the Regional Ethical Review Board in Gothenburg with approval number: D 374-18.

2.1. Sample

The study was based on 200 patients fulfilling the inclusion criteria for visiting the UCC. The exclusion criteria were patients triaged red, patients with a preliminary diagnosis in most cases referred from the primary care centre to the ED (e.g., potential distal deep vein thrombosis, emergent vertigo etc.) and patients with a preliminary diagnosis potentially developing from non-red triage to a state of emergency (e.g., suspected ectopic pregnancy, dyspnoea, suspected urosepsis, etc.). A list of exclusion criteria based on a literature review was developed and implemented as a selective tool used in the triage at the ED. The STROBE checklist (strengthening the communication of observational studies in epidemiology) was used to guide the study process [18].

The first half ($n = 100$) of the 200 patients were selected retrospectively on a consecutive basis just prior to the UCC being established. Consequently, the first half were treated by the ED. The second half of the patients ($n = 100$) were selected consecutively from patients triaged to the UCC six months after it was established. No other substantial changes in organization or methods occurred at the ED during the study period.

The 200 patients were distributed over 104 men and 96 women, with an average age of 45 (SD = 20.24). The study size was based on a power estimation of a standardized statistical power of 0.80 and medium effect size of 0.3 premeditated the appropriate sample size to 93 participants in each population. The α significance level was 0.05 [19]. The two populations were compared in order to concur in terms of emergency and severity. They were triaged on a five-level scale from red (highest degree of emergency) to blue (non-urgent). The distribution was red = 0, orange = 3, yellow = 107, green = 89 and blue = 13 patients. The patients were all triaged according to the Rapid Emergency Triage Treatment Scale [20]. The most common symptoms were wounds/burns, headache/dizziness, fever/infection and chest pain/vascular symptoms (Table 1).

Table 1. Symptoms distributed over the two samples, before (ED population) and after (UCC population). ($n = 200$).

	Before (ED)	After (UCC)	Total
Headache/Dizziness	20	8	28
Infection/Fever	15	11	26
Wound/Burn	14	16	30
Dyspnoea	8	1	9
Abdominal	7	8	15
Colorectal	7	7	14
Urology	7	8	15
Extremities	7	9	16
Chest pain/Vascular	5	14	19
Unspecific	10	18	28
All	100	100	200

2.2. Analysis

We produced a before (n = 100 ED patients) and after (N = 100 UCC patients) design, i.e., prior and after the UCC being established. Focus was on dimensions concerning the outcome of treatment at the ED in comparison to the UCC. Aspects studied were LOS, TTP, use of medical services (radiology, laboratory analysis), revisits, hospitalisations, mortality and cost. Descriptive statistics included central tendency and dispersion. LOS was defined as the time spent from admission to discharge from the UCC or the ED or admission to a ward. TTP was defined as the time spent from admission to seeing a physician. Paired-sample calculations of LOS, TTP and laboratory analysis showed a statistical difference of means. However, the results of normality measured by the Kolmogorov Smirnov test did indicate LOS, TTP and laboratory analysis to be significantly skewed (LOS sig. 0.00, TTP sig. 0.00, and laboratory analysis sig. 0.00). The samples could consequently not be regarded as normally distributed due to outliers. A complementary non-parametric test was therefore conducted using a Wilcoxon signed-rank test.

3. Results

The results include aspects (mainly LOS, TTP and laboratory analysis) of patients visiting the UCC versus visiting the ED, a Wilcoxon signed-rank test of LOS, TTP and laboratory analysis and the cost in Euros/average attendee at the UCC versus the ED.

Several differences appeared when comparing the first and second half of the sample (treated by the ED versus treated by the UCC). From arrival to discharge, the UCC patients spent an average of 2.11 h less at the hospital than the ED patients. TTP was thus 1.57 h less at the UCC than at the ED. There was also a reduction in terms of laboratory analysis at the UCC compared to the ED. Even though the numbers of radiology, findings, referrals, revisits and hospitalisations were minor (26 and below), the sample visiting the UCC appeared to be almost similar to the one visiting the ED (Table 2).

Table 2. Aspects studied of patients visiting the UCC versus patients visiting the ED (N = 200).

	ED	UCC	All
n	100	100	200
LOS (SD)	3.21 (2.32)	1.10 (0.63)	2.15 (2.00)
TTP (SD)	2.14 (2.28)	0.57 (0.46)	1.36 (1.82)
Laboratory analysis (SD)	449 (5.15)	31 (0.66)	480 (4.22)
Radiology	9	4	13
Radiology findings	1	3	4
Referrals	26	21	47
Revisits 72 Hours	3	1	4
Hospitalisation	1	0	1
5-day Mortality	0	0	0

LOS, TTP and laboratory analyses were selected for the Wilcoxon rank test, confirming both LOS and TTP to be significantly more time consuming at the ED than at the UCC. A similar result emerged with regard to laboratory analysis.

Total cost of attendees at the UCC and the ED differed. The cost of UCC attendees was less than the cost of ED attendees (Table 4). (Table 3).

On average, an UCC attendee was 67–210 Euros cheaper. One reason for the difference was fewer medical services, i.e., radiology and laboratory than at the ED. The total cost of medical services at the UCC for the population studied was an average of 37.28 Euros less than at the ED (radiology = 16.62, laboratory = 20.66) (Table 4).

Table 3. Ranks and statistics of LOS, TTP and laboratory analysis of attendees at UCC versus ED (N = 200).

	Ranks	n	Mean Rank	Sum of Ranks
	Negative Ranks	82 (UCC LOS < ED LOS)	55.23	4474.00
Z based on positive ranks = −7.547	Positive Ranks	16 (UCC LOS > ED LOS)	17.44	279.00
Assympt Sig. (2-tailed) = 0.00	Ties	2 (UCC LOS = ED LOS)		
	Total	100		
	Ranks	**n**	**Mean Rank**	**Sum of Ranks**
	Negative Ranks	80 (UCC TTP < ED TTP)	56.75	4540.00
Z based on positive ranks = −6.928	Positive Ranks	20 (UCC TTP > ED TTP)	25.50	510.00
Assympt Sig. (2-tailed) = 0.00	Ties	0 (UCC TTP = ED TTP)		
	Total	100		
	Ranks	**n**	**Mean Rank**	**Sum of Ranks**
	Negative Ranks	63 (UCC lab. < ED lab.)	36.05	2271.00
Z based on positive ranks = −6.723	Positive Ranks	5 (UCC lab. > ED lab.)	15.00	75.00
Assympt Sig. (2-tailed) = 0.00	Ties	32 (UCC lab. = ED lab.)		
	Total	100		

Table 4. Cost in Euros/average attendee at the UCC and the ED distributed in total cost, radiology cost and laboratory cost.

	Total Cost/Average Attendee	Radiology Cost/Average Attendee in the Population Studied (N = 200)	Laboratory Cost/Average Attendee in the Population Studied (N = 200)
ED (n = 100)	362 E (Physician) 219 E (Nurse)	18.11 E	22.19 E
UCC (n = 100)	152 E (Physician and Nurse)	1.49 E	1.53 E

4. Discussion

This study shows that waiting times for the patients studied who were referred to the UCC were reduced, both in terms of TTP and LOS. There was also a reduction in the number of blood tests performed at the UCC. Accordingly, there was a substantial cost reduction for UCC visits compared to the ED on the studied population. These components contribute to cost-effective and sustainable care. However, the sample was too small to draw any conclusions regarding the outcome in terms of assessment and treatment accuracy, though it was not possible to register any increase in revisits.

The most important effect was probably the reduced LOS. The UCC relieved the ED of low-urgency patients and, in the long run, potential crowding. This might consequently have contributed to fewer complex and diversified assignments at the ED. Extrapolating the results, a consequence of establishing a UCC might contribute to EDs maintaining their focus on emergencies and avoid time-consuming challenges such as maintaining continuity and follow-up routines [21]. The UCC studied cut the LOS by two-thirds in relation to the population studied, which may improve disaster preparedness [22]. An integrated UCC/ED may also be used as a fast track and flexible area of care during pandemic peaks and emergencies [23,24].

It can tentatively be suggested that one more important function of UCC in crisis is its networking capacity as part of the primary care system. Non-urgent and non-MID patients can easily be referred to other primary care centres for follow-up [1]. Patients who have access to continuous primary care are known to have an improved health status and lower rates of unnecessary hospitalisation compared to those which do not have such access [25]. In contrast, crowding in the emergency room not only contributes to patient dissatisfaction, but it also increases the risk of spread of infection, misdiagnosis and delayed administration of drugs and, in the long run, prolongs hospitalisation [22].

The proximity of the UCC used in this study seems to be an advantage, not only for peacetime use but also for a future MID, when immediate staff and material and structures are essential factors in successful MID management. The close distance between the UCC and the ED may not only alleviate the ED's burdens but also improve close interprofessional collaboration between colleagues from both units. A study four months after the establishment of an integrated ED/UCC reported inter-organizational and inter-professional collaboration. The staff, physicians and nurses crossed a stairwell and a corridor to discuss common challenges. Questions about the parties' capacity for diagnosing and treating patients were sorted out, and non-conventional solutions were occasionally invented to handle strenuous situations and tricky cases. Mistakes in assessments and patients whose health conditions rapidly changed could easily be handled by swift re-referrals from the UCC back to the ED [17].

The differences observed in this study regarding the utilization of medical services by UCC and ED on a similar population may simply reflect the ability of UCC to adjust to new conditions, procedures and perspectives when assessing patients. The ED staff may be more focused on recent symptoms and a rapidly emerging illness. The UCC staff, on the other hand, may be focused on long-term medical history [26]. While the ED assesses and reassesses the patient in a broad manner, the UCC may use anamnesis and bedside information to construct a picture of the status of the patient [16]. However, when comparing the strengths of the two units, the UCC has the potential to optimize care for both urgent and non-urgent patients. The difference in working methods can be considered an asset when providing sustainable care to the mix of needs in the population of attendees, and during pandemics and disaster management [27]. Despite fewer blood tests and X-rays at the UCC, the results obtained did not indicate any incorrect assessments or treatments at UCC. However, generalising the results of this study will require studies of larger populations. Placing a UCC close to an ED may, however, become a promising establishment in terms of reduction in costs, LOS, TTP and the use of medical services, which is beneficial in the management of an MID.

The pressure on EDs during COVID 19 underscores the need for further studies on interventions aiming to relieve and facilitate ED capacity. Even though a silver bullet for the issue of ED crowding has not yet been found, different methods may be combined to improve preparedness. UCCs are one promising method when it comes to preparedness, along with cost-reductions and improved continuity.

5. Limitations

As already mentioned, this is a study of a limited population from a single UCC. If the results are to be generalised, a substantial study population from several UCCs will be desirable.

This study did not include a follow-up on patient satisfaction. The next study on the outcome of the UCC established should include such a study. Even though there are reasons to believe that patients perceive the UCC as a favourable alternative to the ED, based on the shorter TTP and LOS, other factors such as treatment, follow-up and expectations may impact on patient satisfaction. Such satisfaction is also important for non-MID patients seeking help during a major emergency. It is important that the public feel secure and that patient safety for non-MID patients can be guaranteed by using ordinary staff, material and structures. Another limitation is the scarcity of research related to hospital-based UCCs, especially in a European context. Hopefully, this limited study might inspire other researchers to conduct new research on UCCs in order to improve the sustainability of healthcare.

6. Conclusions

In conclusion, Major Incidents and Disasters (MIDs) and pandemics such as COVID 19 are inevitable and demand hospital and prehospital preparedness in order to guarantee and enhance the capability of healthcare to save lives. Hospitals need to surge capacity by obtaining the necessary staff, material and structure, as well as valid and tested systems. Professional, trained staffs are an important factor in successful MID management; however, their familiarity with the facility in which they work and the devices they need to use is also essential. In this perspective, creating a primary care-like facility in close proximity to the hospitals may not only relieve overcrowding in hospital EDs in peacetime, but it also provides an opportunity for such units to be used to facilitate care of the victims of MIDs and pandemics.

Author Contributions: Conceptualization, A.R., K.D., T.C., A.K.-M, J.B., E.C.; methodology, E.C., A.R. and K.D.; Writing—original draft, E.C., A.R., K.D., A.K.-M.; Writing—review and editing, A.R., K.D., T.C., A.K.-M., J.B., E.C.; supervision, E.C. All authors have read and agreed to the published version of the manuscript.

Funding: This research was not funded.

Conflicts of Interest: The authors declare no conflict of interest.

References

1. Khorram-Manesh, A. Flexible surge capacity—Public health, public education, and disaster Management. *Health Promot. Perspect.* **2020**, *10*, 175–179. [CrossRef] [PubMed]
2. Khorram-Manesh, A.; Lönroth, H.; Rotter, P.; Wilhelmsson, M.; Aremyr, J.; Berner, A.; Nero Andersson, A.; Carlström, E. Non-medical aspects of civilian–military collaboration in management of major incidents. *Eur. J. Trauma Emerg. Surg.* **2017**, *43*, 595–603. [CrossRef] [PubMed]
3. Khorram-Manesh, A.; Yttermyr, J.; Sörensson, J.; Carlström, E. The impact of disaster and major incidents on vulnerable groups: Risk and medical assessment of patients with advanced care at home. *Home Health Care Manag. Pract.* **2017**, *29*, 183–190. [CrossRef]
4. Ablah, E.; Konda, K.S.; Konda, K.; Melbourne, M.; Ingoglia, J.N.; Gebbie, K.M. Emergency preparedness training and response among community health centers and local health departments: Results from a multi-state survey. *J. Community Health* **2010**, *35*, 285–293. [CrossRef] [PubMed]
5. Jacobs, L.M.; McSwain, N.E.; Rotondo, M.F.; Wade, D.; Fabbri, W.; Eastman, A.L.; Butler, F.K.; Sinclair, J. Improving survival from active shooter events: The Hartford Consensus. *J. Trauma Acute Care Surg.* **2013**, *74*, 1399–1400. [CrossRef] [PubMed]
6. Shoaf, K.I.; Rottman, S.J. The role of public health in disaster preparedness, mitigation, response, and recovery. *Prehospital Disaster Med.* **2000**, *15*, 144–146. [CrossRef]
7. Berlin, J.; Carlström, E. The 20-minutes Team. A critical study from the emergency room. *J. Eval. Clin. Pract.* **2008**, *14*, 569–576. [CrossRef]
8. Berlin, J.; Carlström, E. From Artefact to Effect.—The organising effect of artefacts on teams. *J. Health Organ. Manag.* **2010**, *24*, 412–427. [CrossRef]
9. Carter, E.; Pouch, S.M.; Larson, E.L. The Relationship between Emergency Department Crowding and Patient Outcomes: A Systematic Review. *J. Nurs. Scholarsh.* **2014**, *46*, 106–115. [CrossRef]
10. Kellerman, A.L. Crisis in the emergency department. *N. Engl. J. Med.* **2006**, *355*, 1300–1303. [CrossRef]
11. Bernstein, S.L.; Aronsky, D.; Duseja, R.; Epstein, S.; Handel, D.; Hwang, U.; McCarthy, M.; McConnell, K.J.; Pines, J.M.; Rathlev, N.; et al. The Effect of Emergency Department Crowding on Clinically Oriented Outcomes. *Acad. Emerg. Med.* **2009**, *16*, 1–10. [CrossRef] [PubMed]
12. Rosovski, R.P.; Andonian, J.S.; Hayes, B.D. The impending storm: COVID-19, pandemics and our overwhelmed emergency departments. *Am. J. Emerg. Med.* **2019**, *38*, 1270–1294.
13. Khorram-Manesh, A.; Carlström, E.; Hertelendy, A.J.; Goniewicz, K.; Casady, C.B.; Burkle, F.M. Does the prosperity of a country play a role in COVID 19 outcomes? *Disaster Med. Public Health Prep.* **2020**, *12*, 1–10. [CrossRef] [PubMed]
14. Weinick, R.M.; Bristol, S.J.; DesRoches, C.M. Urgent care centers in the US: Findings from a national survey *BMC Health Serv. Res.* **2009**, *9*, 79. [CrossRef]
15. Yee, T.; Lechner, A.E.; Boukus, E.R. The surge in urgent care centers: Emergency department alternative or costly convenience. *Res. Brief* **2013**, *26*, 1–6.
16. Doran, K.M.; Raven, M.C.; Rosenheck, R.A. What drives frequent emergency department use in an integrated health system? National data from the veterans' health administration. *Annu. Emerg. Med.* **2013**, *62*, 151–159. [CrossRef]

17. Wennman, I.; Wittholt, M.; Carlström, E.; Carlsson, T.; Khorram-Manesh, A. Urgent care centre in Sweden—The integration of teams and perceived effects. *Int. J. Health Plan. Manag.* **2019**, *34*, 1–12. [CrossRef]

18. Vandenbroucke, J.; von Elm, E.; Altman, D.G.; Gøtzsche, P.C.; Mulrow, C.D.; Pocock, S.J. Strengthening the Reporting of Observational Studies in Epidemiology (STROBE): Explanation and Elaboration. *PLoS Med.* **2007**, *4*, 1628–1654. [CrossRef]

19. Cohen, J. *Statistical Power Analysis for the Behavioral Sciences*; Academic Press: Cambridge, MA, USA, 2013.

20. Wircklint, S.C.; Elmqvist, C.; Parenti, N.; Göransson, K.E. A descriptive study of registered nurses' application of the triage scale RETTS©; a Swedish reliability study. *Int. Emerg. Nurs.* **2018**, *38*, 21–28. [CrossRef]

21. Raidla, A.; Dárro, K.; Carlson, T.; Carlström, E. Characterising double frequent users in an emergency department. *J. Hosp. Adm.* **2018**, *7*, 35–39. [CrossRef]

22. Wickman, L.; Svensson, P.; Djärv, T. Effect of crowding on length of stay for common chief complaints in the emergency department: A STROBE cohort study. *Medicine* **2017**, *96*, e8457. [CrossRef] [PubMed]

23. Wennman, I.; Nordling, P.; Herlitz, J.; Lernfelt, B.; Kihlgren, M.; Gustafsson, C.; Hansson, P.-O. The clinical consequences of a prehospital diagnosis of stroke by the emergency medical services. A pilot study. *Scand. J. Trauma Resusc. Emerg. Med.* **2012**, *20*, 48. [CrossRef] [PubMed]

24. Morley, C.; Unwin, M.; Peterson, G.M.; Stankovich, J.; Kinsman, L. Emergency department crowding: A systematic review of causes, consequences and solutions. *PLoS ONE* **2018**, *13*, e0203316. [CrossRef] [PubMed]

25. O'Malley, A.S.; Forrest, C.B.; Politzer, R.M.; Wulu, J.T.; Shi, L. Health center trends, 1994–2001: What do they portend for the federal growth initiative? *Health Aff.* **2005**, *24*, 465–472. [CrossRef]

26. Tricco, A.C.; Antony, J.; Ivers, N.M. Effectiveness of quality improvement strategies for coordination of care to reduce use of healthcare services: A systematic review and meta-analysis. *Can. Med. Assoc. J.* **2014**, *186*, E568–E578. [CrossRef]

27. Wertheimer, B.; Jacobs, R.E.A.; Baily, M. Discharge before noon: An achievable hospital goal. *J. Hosp. Med.* **2014**, *9*, 210–214. [CrossRef]

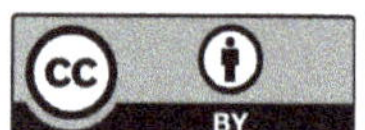

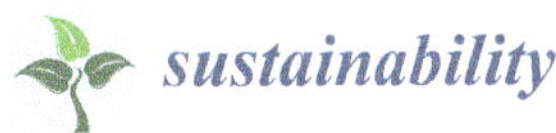 *sustainability*

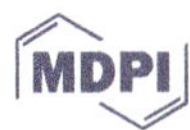

Article

Alternative Leadership in Flexible Surge Capacity—The Perceived Impact of Tabletop Simulation Exercises on Thai Emergency Physicians Capability to Manage a Major Incident

Phatthranit Phattharapornjaroen [1,2], **Viktor Glantz** [1], **Eric Carlström** [3,4], **Lina Dahlén Holmqvist** [5] and **Amir Khorram-Manesh** [1,6,*]

1. Institute of Clinical Sciences, Department of Surgery, Sahlgrenska Academy, Gothenburg University, 40530 Gothenburg, Sweden; phatthranit.pha@mahidol.edu (P.P.); gusglavi@student.gu.se (V.G.)
2. Department of Emergency Medicine, Center of Excellence, Ramathibodi Hospital, Mahidol University, Bangkok 10400, Thailand
3. Institute of Healthcare Sciences, Sahlgrenska Academy, Gothenburg University, 40100 Gothenburg, Sweden; eric.carlstrom@gu.se
4. USN School of Business, University of South-Eastern Norway, P.O. Box 235, 3603 Kongsberg, Norway
5. Institute of Medicine, Department of Molecular and Clinical Medicine, Sahlgrenska University Hospital, 40530 Gothenburg, Sweden; lina.holmqvist@vgregion.se
6. Department of Research and Development, the Swedish Armed Forces Center for Defense Medicine, Västra Frölunda, 42676 Gothenburg, Sweden
* Correspondence: amir.khorram-manesh@surgery.gu.se; Tel.: +46-707-722741

Received: 16 July 2020; Accepted: 1 August 2020; Published: 2 August 2020

Abstract: Flexible surge capacity aims to activate and utilize other resources than normally are surged in a community during the primary and secondary surge capacity. The presence of alternative leadership, skilled and knowledgeable in hospital and prehospital emergency management, is invaluable. Thai emergency physicians work at both levels, emphasizing their important role in emergency management of any source in a disaster-prone country. We aimed to investigate Thai emergency physicians' ability in terms of knowledge and preparedness to manage potential emergencies using tabletop simulation exercises. Using an established method for training collaboration, two training courses were arranged for over 50 Thai emergency physicians, who were divided into three teams of prehospital, hospital, and incident command groups. Three scenarios of a terror attack along with a bomb explosion, riot, and shooting, and high building fire were presented, and the participants' performance was evaluated regarding their preparedness, response and gained knowledge. Two senior observers followed the leadership characteristic in particular. Thai physicians' perceived ability in command and control, communication, collaboration, coordination, and situation assessment improved in all groups systematically. New perspectives and innovative measures were presented by participants, which improved the overall management on the final day. Tabletop simulation exercise increased the perceived ability, knowledge, and attitude of Thai emergency physicians in managing major incidents and disasters. It also enabled them to lead emergency management in a situation when alternative leadership is a necessity as part of the concept of a flexible surge capacity response system.

Keywords: disasters; emergencies; flexible surge capacity; leadership; Thailand; 3LC

---

1. Introduction

Major Incidents and Disasters (MID) affect societies and their inhabitants and result in medical and nonmedical consequences due to the imbalance between the needs and available resources [1].

MID management is a multiprofessional process of organizing and managing the available resources and responsibilities for dealing with all humanitarian aspects of MID, specifically in mitigation, preparedness, response, and recovery phases to lessen the impact of emergencies [2]. Some strategies for MID management include establishing command and control, reliable and efficient ways of communication, information, organization, warning systems, stockpiling of resources, and the development of response plans for the mobilization and management of resources such as personnel, equipment, volunteers, and emergency facilities. The efficiency of the organizational structure in the response is paramount for the outcome of the event [2,3].

The initial approach to proper management of MID is to increase the management system's capacity, i.e., Surge Capacity (SC). Three broad areas of healthcare demand SC in response to a MID [4]. Firstly, Public Health Surge Capacity (the ability of the public health system to increase capacity for patient care, epidemiological investigation, laboratory services, mass fatality management, etc.). Secondly, Healthcare Facility-Based Surge Capacity (augments the response within the healthcare facility structure, e.g., triage-tent on hospital grounds). Finally, Community-based Surge Capacity (the public effort to support and augment the healthcare system). The four essential elements of SC, i.e., Staff, Stuff, Structure, and System (4S), should rapidly and effectively be surged in the affected areas. Staff refers to available/alternative personnel, Stuff refers to available/alternative equipment, Structures refer to Alternate Care Facilities (ACF), and systems are procedures and guidelines that govern the emergency management process [5,6].

The expansion of a MID necessitates a new surge capacity (secondary SC), which underlines the need for extra efforts to obtain additional resources still available within the management system [7–9]. Nevertheless, a further expansion of the incident demands new approaches, policies, and adjustable preparedness within the community to scale up and down resources in a fast, smooth, and productive way, i.e., "flexible surge capacity" (FSC) [10]. The concept of FSC is concordant with the new paradigm of proactivity in disaster management and emphasizes on risk reduction rather than focusing on pure relief operations to reduce vulnerability and increase resilience within communities [11]. Therefore, risk assessment and focus on all four elements of SC is necessary for achieving an FSC. Although the disaster management cycle should incorporate, recognize, and value the participation of affected communities [12], it is necessary that adequate infrastructure is in place to ensure access to emergency services [13]. In this perspective, the readiness of hospitals is essential and among necessary measures, staff pools and new staff categories are needed to replace the regular staffing structure, and to reduce the risk of lacking qualified staff, e.g., leadership.

Although many functions and measures are necessary for proper and successful MID management, the command and control (C2) function remains the most critical function [14,15]. C2 emphasizes the leaderships' characteristics to command, control, communicate, collaborate, and coordinate [2,6,14,15]. Such ability offers an excellent opportunity for the leaders to attain a mutual goal, assess the situation from different perspectives, overview all necessary measures, successfully sort out all injuries, treat them adequately and distribute them equally to designated medical facilities. Most hospitals have an emergency management committee, which consists of predesignated positions and staff. Such a group of professionals needs to be trained to act decisively and quickly during crises. Previous studies have, however, shown that these committees suffer from the rarity of MID, and thus, neither have the experience nor are trained enough to act as needed [15,16]. There is a lack of experience and knowledge about the management process and collaboration with other partners, particularly in hospital and prehospital arenas. One specialty with the ability and knowledge to connect hospitals and prehospital organizations is Emergency Medicine [17].

Thailand is a disaster-prone country with a westernized healthcare system. Emergency Medicine residency training in Thailand started in 2004, during which the first Tsunami hit its southern part and caused mass casualties and structural devastation. One of the outcomes of this deadly event was understanding the needs for organizational and structural changes, and proper knowledge in command and control within the disaster management system. Since then, many educational initiatives such as MIMMS (Major Incident Medical Management and Support), and MRMI (Medical Response to Major Incidents) have been established and yearly conducted to raise the theoretical and practical knowledge of all staff [18–21]. Thai Emergency Physicians (EP), work within and outside the hospitals and are the point of contact and the first line of medical assessment [19,20]. This role requires the right level of structural and organizational knowledge of MID management and merits a more responsible and critical role in response to major emergencies. One way to obtain such knowledge is through tabletop simulations training [21].

The Three-Level Collaboration (3LC) training model is used to train small groups of commanders up to hundreds of participants in the management of MID. The development of the 3LC model was based on hypothesizing that the collaborative elements in a mutual task help reduce the organizational barriers [21]. The method has been compared with traditional exercises in several studies [22–24]. In one of these, the 3LC method improved collaboration as well as learning. At the 3LC exercise, 94.3% of the personnel perceived the exercise to be focused on collaboration. The traditional exercises reported a corresponding figure of 75.6%. The majority of the participants answered that they learned something new during the exercises (78.5%, traditional 64.9%). They also felt that the exercises had an impact on real-life activities during daily work (80.4%, traditional 61.7%) [24]. Organizational capabilities and limitations are enlisted to promote interplay with no hierarchical authority, and to promote the ability to switch between different collaboration strategies as demanded by the specific situation. Collaboration training offers a chance to not only exhibit stability (the quality that one develops through drill and practice), but also to practice transitions, overlaps, fearlessness, improvisation, creative thinking, and the ability to handle unexpected situations. Such education is beyond the repeated learning that comes from the drill in control and command structures and other mechanical structures.

2. Aim

This study aimed to evaluate the progress of knowledge and learning outcomes of a group of Thai EPs before and after 3LC simulation exercise in seven documented and essential areas (CSCATTT): Command and control, Safety, Communication, Triage, Treatment, and Transport, which according to MIMMS concept are essential elements to lead and manage a MID [18].

3. Method

3.1. Population

All EPs voluntarily registered to an Incident Command System course at a major hospital in Bangkok, Thailand. Participants who were present during the entire course session were included. Consequently, those who could not present or left the course for a few hours were excluded. Otherwise, there were no exclusion criteria, and all staff working with MID, including nurses could take part in the course.

3.2. Course Design

Two two-day courses with the same structure consisting of a short introduction and a scenario simulation exercise on the first day, followed by two more scenarios on day two. A round of discussion and comments for the whole course took place at the end of the course. Participants were divided into three groups of (1) a prehospital team (Operational), (2) emergency departments command group (Tactical), and (3) hospital command group (Strategical).

There was a rotation between different groups, which enabled all participants to try different positions to reach consensus in the whole group of participants to achieve similarities rather than differences. No instruction was given about participants' posts in each group, and they had to figure out what they need and how to use all competences, based on the given lectures and earlier knowledge in MIMMS. Three different scenarios (1) fire in a tall building, (2) a terrorist attack and a bomb explosion, and (3) riots, including shooting, were presented to the groups during rotation (Appendix A). After each scenario, the participants in each group had to present their results. Each group received comments from supervisors and other participants. At the end of the presentations, and according to the 3LC model, the participants in each group had to gather again and discuss what they could do better if they had a new opportunity. Each group presented the results of this round, and other participants and supervisors could comment on their findings. Finally, each group gathered to discuss the necessary knowledge and functions and guidelines for each position to be taken home as the quality, which is needed for operational, tactical, and strategic levels. Besides, two supervisors followed each group and evaluated their performance based on MIMMS-CSCATT concept (see below) [18].

3.3. Pre- and Post-Course Test

The pre- and post-course tests were conducted to evaluate the gained knowledge in each participant [25]. The tests were designed using the learning objectives established for the course, i.e., crucial factors for successful management of MID incorporated in CSCATTT (Command and control, Security, Communication, Assessment, Triage, Treatment, Transport), a well-known model used in MIMMS courses internationally [18]. Both tests consist of the same items. The test aimed for each participant's self-assessment in knowledge about the subjects of CSCATTT, displayed as a Likert scale, in which No knowledge was represented by 0%, while 100% was full knowledge. Participants were asked to mark the grade of their understanding in each topic on a five-level Likert Scale. A nonparametric test, Wilcoxon signed rank test, was chosen to compare the means.

3.4. Observational Evaluation

All groups were observed based on a Participant Observation model with a focus on the leadership in all groups [26–28]. Among various signs of good leadership, the following points were mainly observed to evaluate the leadership: Communication and Decision-making ability, Accountability, Delegation, and Empowerment of others. Two observers collected and noted their observations, which were discussed after each scenario to reach a consensus. The observer registered if a commander was identified and appointed during the incident and if the appointed commander possessed the control. The observer did also register if the commander ensured successful medical management, i.e., built a team of multiple staff overcoming a potentially chaotic situation and if the team reached a subtactical, tactical, or operational level [18]. The data were recorded as Event Sampling, which allows focusing on one specific subject. All other types of behavior were ignored [26–28].

3.5. Observational Evaluation

As part of 3LC simulation training, group discussions took place after each scenario. Besides confirming and discussing the results and improvement measures, these discussions also aimed to discuss the observational findings in each occasion. The process aimed to pair data collected by observation to the discussion and interviews to unearth individual motivations or behaviors that were not immediately obvious in a group setting [24–28].

4. Results

There were 56 participants registered, however, only 52 could complete the course. The four physicians excluded (two females and two males) had to go back to work due to emergencies, and were not presented at all levels of simulation training. A sum of 52 EPs took part in the entire course on two occasions. Nurses were also invited to these courses, but none were registered due to hesitance of the spoken language of the course (English). There were 36 females and 16 males. The age of the participants ranged between 26–35 years, with a range of experience between 1–10 years as EP. The majority of participants were from the hospitals in Bangkok. However, 16 physicians were from hospitals in other parts of Thailand. The pre- and post-training tests were conducted before and after the session.

a. Command and control (C2): There was an increasing knowledge of C2 after the course. Around 20% of the EPs ($n = 10$) had little or very little knowledge about C2, and 46% ($n = 24$) had medium knowledge. At the end of the course, there was a shift to the positive end, where the majority of our participants had a good to a very good understanding of C2 function ($n = 49, 94\%$) (Figure 2). The change was statistically significant ($p = 0.00$, z $= -5.436$).

b. Safety: There was an increasing knowledge of safety issues after the course. Around 15% of the EPs ($n = 8$) had no or very little knowledge about safety issues, and 44% ($n = 23$) had medium knowledge. At the end of the course, there was a shift to the positive end, where the majority of our participants had a good to a very good understanding of safety issues ($n = 50, 96\%$) (Figure 3). The change was statistically significant ($p = 0.00$, z $= -6.056$).

c. Communication: There was an increasing knowledge of communication ways and difficulties after the course. Around 21% ($n = 11$) of the EPs had none or very little knowledge about communications issues, and 44% ($n = 23$) had medium knowledge. At the end of the course, there was a shift to the positive end, where the majority of our participants had a good to a very good understanding of safety issues ($n = 48, 92\%$) (Figure 4). The change was statistically significant ($p = 0.00$, z $= -5.872$).

d. Assessment: There was an increasing knowledge about the importance of the assessment during a major incident after the course. Around 17% ($n = 9$) of the EPs had no or very little knowledge about assessment and its association with the incident management, and 48% ($n = 25$) had medium knowledge. At the end of the course, there was a shift to the positive end, where the majority of our participants had a good to a very good understanding of assessment issues ($n = 48, 92\%$) (Figure 5). The change was statistically significant ($p = 0.00$, z $= -5.464$).

e. Triage: There was an increasing knowledge about the importance of triage and associated dilemmas during a major incident after the course. Around 17% ($n = 9$) of the EPs had no or very little knowledge about triage and its role during incident management, and 30% ($n = 16$) had medium knowledge. Although 29 EPs reported a good or very good knowledge, there was still a shift to the positive end at the end of the course, where the majority of our participants had a good to a very good understanding of triage issues ($n = 46, 88\%$) (Figure 6). The change was statistically significant ($p = 0.00$, z $= -4.585$).

f. Treatment: There was an increasing knowledge about the treatment alternatives and options at the right time and right place during a major incident after the course. Around 17% ($n = 9$) of the EPs had none or very little knowledge about the treatment given during incident management, and 28% ($n = 15$) had medium knowledge. Although 28 EPs reported good or very good knowledge, there was still a shift to the positive end at the end of the course, where the majority of the participants had good to a very good understanding of triage issues ($n = 37, 71\%$) (Figure 7). The change was statistically significant ($p = 0.00$, z $= -5.287$).

g. Transport: There was an increasing knowledge about the importance of triage and associated dilemmas during a major incident after the course. Around 21% ($n = 11$) of the EPs had none or very little knowledge about triage and its role during incident management, and 32% ($n = 17$) had medium knowledge. At the end of the course, there was a shift to the positive end, where the majority of our participants had a good to a very good understanding of assessment issues ($n = 38, 73\%$) (Figure 8). The change was statistically significant ($p = 0.00$, z $= -5.634$).

h. Observations: Two critical observations were reported (Figure 1). Both observers collected their documented results in which they had specifically commented on the ability of decision-making, communication, accountability, empowerment of other group member and delegation of tasks. Consensus was made and the groups were exposed to the observers' understanding to unearth individual motivations or behaviors that were not immediately obvious in a group setting [24,25].

    a. During the exercises, each team selected its leader with three leadership styles, without any previous knowledge and spontaneously;

i.   Consensus leadership (G3): The leader tried to reach consensus with other members before any decision. Slower decision-making process.

ii.   Passive leadership (G2): The leader laid back and observed other members and only interrupted if needed. Decisions were made, but sometimes not of the leader.

iii.   Active Leadership (G1): The leader had the last word in every decision and continuously directed the group. Less delegation and empowerment.

b.   Each group developed its communication method consisting of a mobile telephone, paper-based messages, and signs.

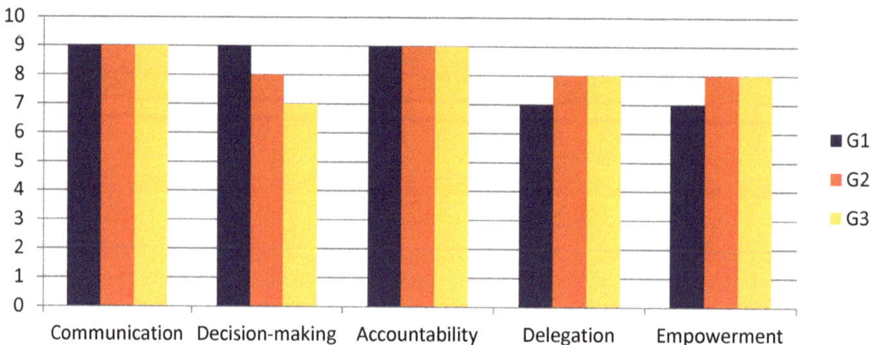

Figure 1. Shows the results of the leadership characteristics during the exercise.

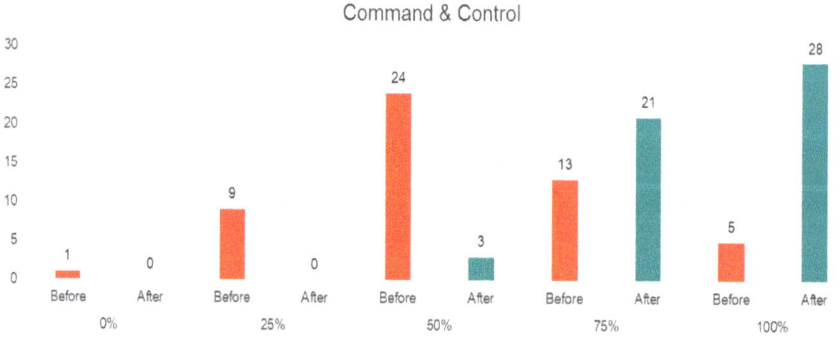

Figure 2. Shows the results of the pre-, and post-test in Command and Control.

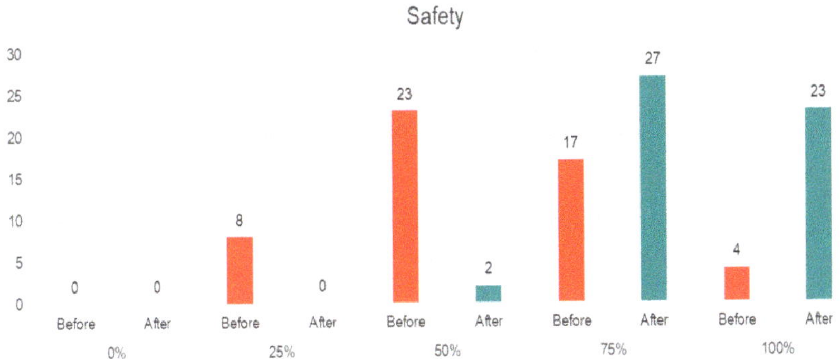

Figure 3. Shows the results of the pre-, and post-test in Safety issues.

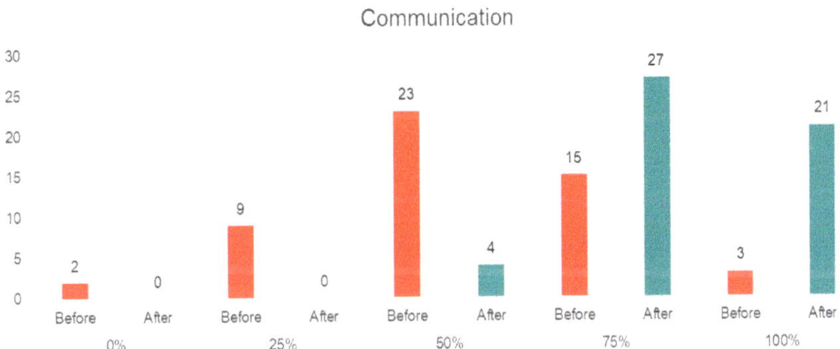

Figure 4. Shows the results of the pre-, and post-test in Communication.

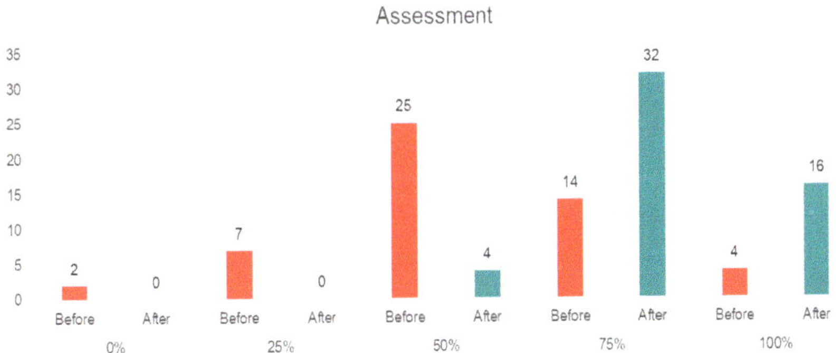

Figure 5. Shows the results of the pre-, and post-test in situation Assessment.

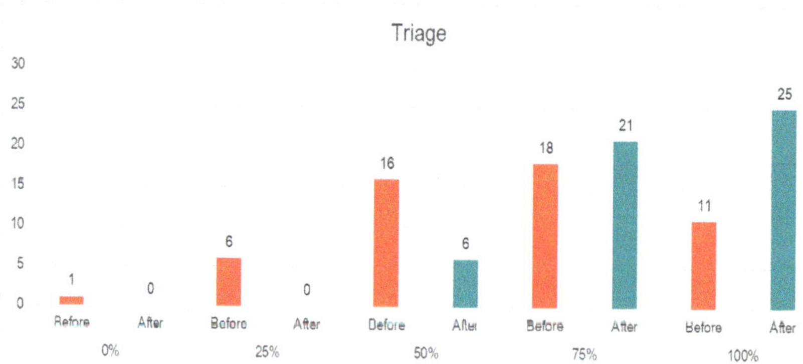

Figure 6. Shows the results of the pre-, and post-test in Triage.

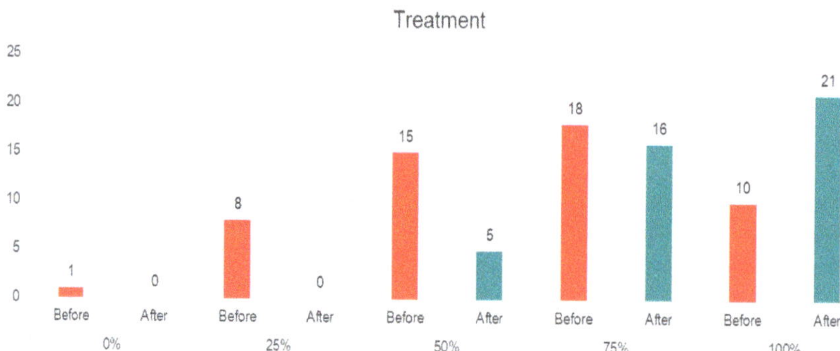

Figure 7. Shows the results of the pre-, and post-test Treatment issues.

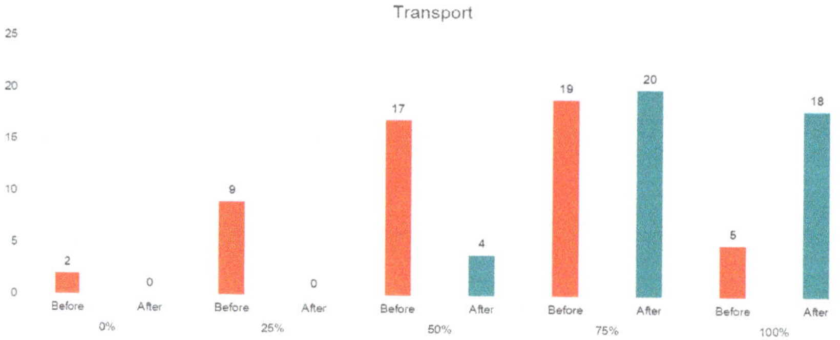

Figure 8. Shows the results of the pre-, and post-test Transport issues.

5. Discussion

The essential raise of knowledge among Thai EPs was registered in Command and control, Safety, Communication, and situation Assessment. At the same time, the understanding of the subject areas, Triage, Treatment, and Transport did not develop to the same extent. All changes were statistically significant. Since these physicians are working at both hospital and prehospital levels, it is not surprising that the grade of their knowledge in strict medical areas, e.g., Triage, Treatment, and Transport, is higher than other subjects within CSCATTT, which specifically deal with leadership characteristics.

Earlier studies have discussed the medical and nonmedical aspects of MID management, showing critical shortcomings in the latter [15]. Disaster and major incidents are rare, but they need to be mitigated and managed if they occur. In successful management, collaboration is one crucial factor that demands skilled leadership and reliable communication. In this group of EPs with no earlier experience of MID, the collaborative elements in a mutual task helped to reduce the organizational barriers, enlisted their abilities and limitations, and promoted interplay with no hierarchical authority, as well as the ability to switch between different collaboration strategies as demanded by the specific situation and leadership styles. The groups grew up to be more stable, practiced transitions, overlaps, fearlessness, and improvised to create new ways of handling the unexpected situation by discovering different communication alternatives. During training, their ability to try out the situation developed their confidence, increased their trust to each other, and reduced the internal fear of doing wrong. They could test a model, evaluate its effect in the next stage, create a new approach, test it, and develop their approach continuously [21,23,24,29]. All these elements are necessary for successful teamwork at the time of emergency. The ultimate requirement is to act in a flexible surge capacity (FSC) when hospitals and communities must activate their resources, respectively [10].

Choosing EPs as one of the major players in MID management is a natural selection [17,19,20]. In countries such as Thailand, they work at both hospital and prehospital levels and thus have a logical connection to both entities [19,20]. In a changing world, when resources may not be enough to match the needs, there must be more material and personal options than what is offered by standard disaster plans. FSC aims to provide new innovative solutions to these shortcomings [10]. Other reports have high lightened the need for FSC and discussed the need for ACF [30]. This paper tried to examine the possibility of using a simulation model to increase the knowledge and understanding of a new set of professionals to lead MID management. Training EPs for the next MID will strengthen the whole chain of disaster management and partly accommodate the WHO´s policy of proactivity and increase the strength and ability of communities to handle the first waves of MID impacts since EPs are one group, who will face upcoming incidents [17,19]. Other measures within the community, such as civilians' empowerment as immediate responders, and the necessity of creating new guidelines and systems have been reported elsewhere [31–33]. Altogether, they facilitate the concept of FSC (Flexible Surge Capacity). Using the elements of CSCATTT as a model enables a direct assessment of critical features that need to be in place during MID management [18]. These elements are part of educational initiatives given to all healthcare staff, and are not only perceived abilities and knowledge but also what they practice in every-day missions, and emphasize the importance of medical and nonmedical aspects of MID management. In a future with limited resources and expanding needs, civilian help can be decisive in creating Resilience in each society [31–33]. The same method and elements can be used to educate other groups of people to act at different levels of management or maybe increase their awareness about any given event to mitigate the adverse outcomes of any incidents [15,30–34].

Moynihan [29] emphasizes the value of trying it out, i.e., to test a model to cope with an event, evaluate the effect of the model in the next stage, create a new approach, test it, and develop the method continuously. Through the 3LC-exercise, the EPs practiced their ability to make a concerted and coherent assessment of which collaboration form is applicable at a given time. The collaboration is not a static activity but subject to construction, deconstruction, and reconstruction, depending on what is appropriate for a specific time, place, or event. The 3LC exercise illustrates the primary goal of practicing the different forms of collaboration and switching between them by including asymmetries in the scenarios [21–24]. For instance, the police can arrive first at the scene and begin caring for victims with serious injuries, or understaffed emergency rescue services have to get help from the police and paramedics at a fire incident. The exercise also reveals the need for a joint assessment and the importance of knowing both prehospital and hospital fields. The latter offers a valuable opportunity to increase the collaborative segment of MID management. At the same time, decisions can be made based on knowledge about the different organizations' limitations and capabilities [15,16].

6. Limitations

This study did not compare the 3LC and traditional types of exercises. In earlier studies, 3LC had a significant impact on perceived collaboration, learning as well as performance. Based on these findings, before and after design control was chosen (pre- and post-test) [22–25]. Measuring the perceived effects of exercises, using a self-assessment tool, may be considered as a limitation. The possibility of over- or underreporting cannot be ignored. However, there are some advantages with the tool too, such as it encourages the participants to reflect over their own learning progress and performance, to be more responsible for their own learning, to develop their judgment skills while they have no pressure of peer evaluation, make participants more autonomous learners and finally make them aware of their weaknesses and strength. To verify the causality and generalizability of the results, a study that is not just based on a written test would give additional insightful and important information.

As an alternative, a comparative design, including a control group, should be considered in future studies. However, pre- and post-test scores provide information on whether or not participants have learned from the training. Besides, a well-designed pre- and post-test can help trainers understand which concepts or competencies were well taught during the training and which ones need additional time, or need to be covered using alternative methods [25,33]. Pre- and post-tests may not be the best tools to use for every type of training but still offer a good overview of the tested group's advancement. Wishing to understand what knowledge can be credited to the training itself, using a pre- and post-test methodology is essential. As shown statistically in this study, the knowledge of EPs in all areas of CSCATT increased significantly. Another limitation was that the data collection occurred immediately after the exercises and not supplemented with data collected weeks or months after the exercises [27,28].

An alternative method of evaluating learning, such as the observation of skills demonstrated in a role-play, might be more appropriate in some situations. In this study, we combined the Participant observation method as a complement to the pre- and post-course tests [26–29]. It is a variant of the natural observations model. Still, the researcher joins in and becomes part of the group they are studying to get a more in-depth insight into their activities. In this overt observation model, the researchers revealed their identity and purpose to the group and asked permission to observe. There are some limitations to this model. It can be challenging to get time/privacy for recording, which means observers have to wait until they are alone and rely on their memory, which is a problem as they may forget details and are unlikely to remember direct quotations. Furthermore, if the researcher becomes too involved, they may lose objectivity and become bias, and thus reduce the validity of the data.

The participants in this study were all physicians, while other staff such as nurses, paramedics, administrators, etc. are also important parts of a hospitals' MID management. This study was the first step in a series of studies that are planned to evaluate the concept of FSC, and physicians were simply chosen due to their actual position within the Thai healthcare and their knowledge in English. It is clear that other knowledgeable staff could also possess the leadership position [34].

Finally, although statistically significant results were obtained in this study, the number of included EPs can be challenged. However, for everyone working within healthcare, it is clear that a larger number of physicians cannot be gathered at the same time for any kind of exercise or training. This is a challenging fact that affects all types of education and training within all healthcare systems [21,35]. Similar argument is true concerning the provision of a control group. It is hard to get enough healthcare workers in a training session, and still harder to have one third of them as a control group. Simulation exercises emerged as a solution to this issue since reality-based exercises demand not only a large number of participants but also cost a lot and often evaluate just one part of the disaster management chain [21,35].

7. Conclusions

In conclusion, the findings in this report indicate that the ability in all elements of CSCATTT, particularly expertise in command and control, communication, collaboration and coordination, and situation assessment, improved in all groups of EPs systematically and after each scenario. The 3LC method also enabled all participants to create new perspectives and innovative measures, which improved the overall management of scenarios on the final day. The 3LC increases the ability, knowledge, and attitude of Thai emergency physicians in managing MID. It also enables them to lead emergency management in an unexpected situation, as alternative leaders in a flexible surge capacity-response system [10,30].

Author Contributions: Conceptualization, A.K.-M.; data curation, P.P.; formal analysis, P.P., V.G., E.C. and A.K.-M.; investigation, P.P. and A.K.-M.; methodology, E.C. and A.K.-M.; project administration, P.P.; resources, P.P., A.K.-M.; supervision, A.K.-M.; validation, L.D.H.; writing—original draft, P.P.; writing—review & editing, V.G., E.C., L.D.H. and A.K.-M. All authors have read and agreed to the published version of the manuscript.

Funding: This research received no external funding.

Acknowledgments: The authors would like to thank Yohan Robinson for his support to this project.

Conflicts of Interest: The authors declare no conflict of interest.

Appendix A

Appendix A.1. Scenarios, 3LC Exercises, Bangkok, Thailand

Scenario 1: A bomb

On 15 September 2017, the dispatch center contacted and informed you about a Bomb found 5 km from your hospital. There was another hospital 200 m next to the scene. More than 100 people were injured. Mange situation based on CSCATTT.

Around 30 min after the first contact, a second bomb is found at the middle of the scene. How would you manage the scene now?

Scenario 2: A Fire in a Tall Building

On 15 December 2017, the dispatch center contacted and informed you that there was a fire on the fifth floor of an 11 floors apartment 5 km away from your hospital. More than 50 people were injured. How do you manage the situation based on CSCATTT?

Around 30 min after the fire incident and when there is a crowd and gathering of people, a truck drives into the treatment zones inside the area, and hit many people.

Scenario 3: Riot and Active Shooter

On 15 May 2015, you were on a night shift at the hospital and saw Riots on the news; the place of the incident was 5 km from your hospital. Some people starts shooting and ambulances started and kept bringing injured people to your hospital. How would you manage your emergency department based on CSCATTT?

One of the injured victim had a bomb strapped on his chest. How would you manage the situation? Would you evacuate your emergency department?

References

1. WHO. Hospital Emergency Response Checklist. An All-Hazards Tool for Hospital Administrators and Emergency Managers. 2011. Available online: http://www.euro.who.int/__data/assets/pdf_file/0008/268766/Hospital-emergency-response-checklist-Eng.pdf (accessed on 25 June 2020).
2. Vitalii, S.; Khorram-Manesh, A.; Nyberg, L. Disaster cycle and management. In *Handbook of Disaster and Emergency Management*; Khorram-Manesh, A., Ed.; Kompendiet: Göteborg, Sweden, 2017; Chapter 2; pp. 23–29.
3. United Nations International Strategy for Disaster Reduction (UNISDR). *Terminology on Disaster Risk Reduction*; United Nations: Geneva, Switzerland, 2009. Available online: https://www.unisdr.org/files/7817_UNISDRTerminologyEnglish.pdf (accessed on 25 June 2020).
4. Hick, J.; Christian, M.; Sprung, C. Surge Capacity and Infrastructure considerations for mass critical care. *Intensive Care Med.* **2010**, *36*, 11–20. [CrossRef]
5. Barbich, D.; Koenig, K. Understanding Surge Capacity: Essential Elements. *Acad. Emerg. Med.* **2006**, *6*, 1098–1102. [CrossRef] [PubMed]
6. Kaji, A.; Koenig, K.L.; Bey, T. Surge capacity for healthcare systems: A conceptual framework. *Acad. Emerg. Med.* **2006**, *13*, 1157–1159. [CrossRef] [PubMed]
7. Bonnet, C.; Peery, B.; Cantrill, S.; Pons, P.; Haukoos, J.; McVaney, K.; Colwell, C. Surge capacity: A proposed conceptual framework. *Am. J. Emerg. Med.* **2007**, *25*, 297–306. [CrossRef] [PubMed]
8. Runkle, J.D.; Brock-Martin, A.; Karmus, W.; Svendsen, E.R. Secondary Surge Capacity: A framework for understanding long-term access to primary care for medically vulnerable populations in disaster recovery. *Am. J. Public Health* **2012**, *102*, 24–32. [CrossRef] [PubMed]
9. Adams, L.M. Exploring the concept of surge capacity. *Issues Nurs.* **2009**, *14*, 2. [CrossRef]
10. Khorram-Manesh, A. Flexible Surge Capacity—Public Health, Public Education, and Disaster Management. *Health Promot. Perspect* **2020**, *10*, 175–179. [CrossRef]
11. The Lancet Editorial. Disaster prevention should be equal. *Lancet Glob. Health* **2017**, *5*, 1047. [CrossRef]
12. Krolik, M. Exploring a rights-based approach to disaster management. *Aust. J. Emerg. Manag.* **2013**, *28*, 44–48. Available online: https://knowledge.aidr.org.au/resources/ajem-oct-2013-exploring-a-rights-based-approach-to-disaster-management/ (accessed on 14 July 2020).
13. Rice, K.; Felizzi, M.V.; Hagelgans, D. Human Rights-Based Approach to Disaster Management: Valparaiso, Chile. *J. Hum. Rights Soc. Work* **2017**, *2*, 117–127. [CrossRef]
14. Prytz, E.G.; Rybing, J.; Carlström, E.; Khorram-Manesh, A.; Jonson, C.O. Exploring prehospital C2-work during a mass gathering event. *Int. J. Emerg. Serv.* **2015**, *4*, 227–241. [CrossRef]
15. Khorram-Manesh, A.; Lönroth, H.; Rotter, P.; Wilhelmsson, M.; Aremyr, J.; Berner, A.; Nero Andersson, A.; Carlström, E. Non-medical aspects of civilian-military collaboration in management of major incidents. *Eur. J. Trauma Emerg. Surg.* **2017**, *43*, 595–603. [CrossRef]
16. Khorram-Manesh, A.; Hedelin, A.; Örtenwall, P. Regional coordination in medical emergencies and major incidents; plan, execute and teach. *Scand. J. Trauma Resusc. Emerg. Med.* **2009**, *17*, 32. [CrossRef]
17. Kahn, C.A.; Koenig, K.L.; Schultz, C.H. Emergency physician disaster deployment: Issues to consider and model policy. *Prehosp. Disaster Med.* **2017**, *32*, 462–464. [CrossRef]
18. Sammut, J.; Cato, D.; Homer, T. Major Incident Medical Management and Support (MIMMS): A practical multiple casualty, disaster-site training course for all Australian healthcare personnel. *Emerg. Med.* **2001**, *13*, 174–180. [CrossRef]
19. Sittichanbuncha, Y.; Prachanukool, T.; Sarathep, P.; Sawanyawisuth, K. An emergency medical service in Thailand—Providers perspectives. *J. Med. Assoc. Thai* **2014**, *97*, 1016–1021.
20. Khorram-Manesh, A.; Angthong, C.; Pangma, A.; Sulannakarn, S.; Burivong, R.; Jarayabhand, R.; Örtenwall, P. Hospital Evacuation; Learning from the Past? Flooding of Bangkok 2011. *BJMMR* **2014**, *4*, 395–415. [CrossRef]
21. Khorram-Manesh, A.; Berlin, J.; Carlström, E. Two validated ways of the ability of decision-making in emergencies, Results from a literature review. *Bull. Emerg. Trauma* **2016**, *4*, 186–196.
22. Sorensen, J.; Magnussen, L.I.; Torgersen, G.E.; Christiansen, A.M.; Carlstrom, E. Percieved Usefulness of Maritime Cross-Border Collaboration Exercises. *Arts Soc. Sci. J.* **2018**, *9*, 1–5. [CrossRef]

23. Magnussen, L.I.; Carlström, E.; Sörensen, J.L.; Torgersen, G.E.; Hagenes, E.F.; Kristiansen, E. Learning and Usefulness stemming from collaboration in a maritime crisis management exercise in Northern Norway. *Disaster Prev. Manag.* **2018**, *27*, 129–140. [CrossRef]

24. Berlin, J.; Carlström, E. The three level collaboration exercise—Impact of learning and usefulness. *J. Conting. Crisis Manag. (JCCM)* **2015**, *23*, 257–265. [CrossRef]

25. Aykal, G.; Kespali, M.; Aydin, Ö.; Esen, H.; Yegin, A.; Gungör, F.; Yilmaz, N. Pre-Test and Post-Test Applications to Shape the Education of Phlebotomists in a Quality Management Program: An Experience in a Training Hospital. *J. Med. Biochem.* **2016**, *35*, 347–353. [PubMed]

26. Takala, E.P.; Pehkonen, I.; Forsman, M.; Hansson, G.Å.; Mathiassen, S.E.; Neumann, W.P.; Sjögaard, G.; Veiersted, K.B.; Westgaard, R.H.; Winkel, J. Systematic evaluation of observational methods assessing biomechanical exposures at work. *Scand. J. Work Environ. Health* **2010**, *36*, 3–24. [CrossRef] [PubMed]

27. Luna-Reyes, L.F.; Lines Andersen, D. Collecting and analyzing qualitative data for system dynamics: Methods and models. *Syst. Dyn. Rev.* **2004**. [CrossRef]

28. Lofland, J.; Lofland, L.H. *Analyzing Social Setting: A Guide to Qualitative Observation and Analysis*, 2nd ed.; Wadsworth: Belmont, CA, USA, 1984.

29. Moynihan, D.P. Learning under uncertainty: Networks in crisis management. *Public Admin. Rev.* **2008**, *68*, 350–365. [CrossRef]

30. Glantz, V.; Phattharapornjaroen, P.; Carlström, E.; Khorram-Manesh, A. Regional Flexible Surge Capacity—A flexible response system. *Sustainability* **2020**, *12*, 5984. [CrossRef]

31. World Health Organization (WHO). Sustainable Development Goals (SDGs). Available online: https://www.who.int/sdg/en/ (accessed on 25 June 2020).

32. Khorram-Manesh, A.; Plegas, P.; Peyravi, M.; Carlström, E. Immediate Response to Major Incidents: Defining an immediate responder! *Eur. J. Trauma Emerg. Surg.* **2019**. [CrossRef]

33. Khorram-Manesh, A.; Berlin, J.; Ljung Roseke, L.; Aremyr, J.; Sörensson, J.; Carlström, E. Emergency Management and Preparedness Training for Youth (EMPTY): The Results of the First Swedish pilot Study. *Disaster Med. Public Health Prep.* **2018**, *12*, 685–688. [CrossRef]

34. Khorram-Manesh, A. *Learning to Respect Diversity, Gender Equality, and Collaboration: A childhood Agenda or the Content of a Leadership Development Program*; Magnussen, L.I., Ed.; Disaster, Diversity, and Emergency Preparation; IOS Press: Amsterdam, The Netherlands, 2019; pp. 11–18. [CrossRef]

35. Jahangirian, M.; Naseer, A.; Stergioulas, L.; Young, T.; Eldabi, T.; Brailsford, S.; Patel, B.; Harper, P. Simulation in health-care: Lessons from other sectors. *Oper. Res. Int. J.* **2012**, *12*, 45–55. [CrossRef]

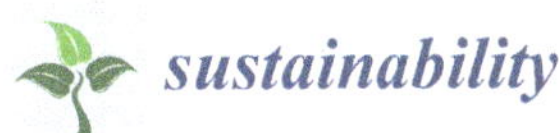 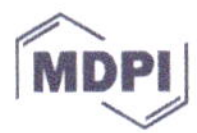

Article

A Coronavirus (COVID-19) Triage Framework for (Sub)National Public–Private Partnership (PPP) Programs

David Baxter [1] and Carter B. Casady [2,*]

[1] Infrastructure Development/PPP Consultant and Steering Committee Member for the World Association of PPP Units & Professionals (WAPPP), Washington, DC 22312, USA; dbaxter@wappp.org
[2] Bartlett School of Construction and Project Management, University College London, London WC1E 7HB, UK
* Correspondence: c.casady@ucl.ac.uk

Received: 3 June 2020; Accepted: 24 June 2020; Published: 29 June 2020

Abstract: Around the world, countries are struggling to address the immediate and long-term impacts of the novel coronavirus (COVID-19) pandemic on their (sub)national public–private partnership (PPP) programs. Burdened with the real possibility of widespread project failures and constrained budgets, governments are searching for ways to prioritize projects in need of relief and bolster post-pandemic recovery plans. To meet this need, this article conceptualizes a triage system for PPP programs based on five categories: (1) projects without a need for economic stimulus (blue); (2) projects experiencing minor economic/financial losses (green); (3) projects needing temporary/stop-gap support or restructuring (yellow); (4) projects unable to survive without significant economic relief (red); and (5) projects that cannot survive, even with government intervention (black). This research also stresses the importance of launching and sustaining a crisis command center to support PPP triage decisions and encourages PPP stakeholders to collectively craft win–win solutions for post-pandemic recovery efforts.

Keywords: coronavirus (COVID-19); public–private partnerships (PPPs) triage; crisis management; resilience

---

1. An Unprecedented Battle

The novel coronavirus (COVID-19) pandemic caught most public agencies at all levels of government off-guard, leaving them ill-equipped to address the immediate and long-term impacts on their (sub)national public–private partnership (PPP) programs. In the United States alone, procurements for several infrastructure PPP projects have already been delayed, put on hold, or cancelled altogether [1]. With uncertainty increasing around demand–risk transit and toll road projects, more project failures are anticipated. States are also projected to face a 30 percent drop in transportation-related revenues (e.g., gas tax) over the next 12–18 months. Combined with sharp declines in sales tax revenue, the fiscal position of state and local governments will continue to deteriorate through at least fiscal year (FY) 2021 [2] and "catch-up" funding mechanisms may be needed for state and local infrastructure development and recovery efforts [3].

Without flexible surge capacity "to scale up and down resources in a fast, smooth, and productive way" [4] (p. 1), many governments, banking organizations, and development institutions still do not fully understand the current strengths and weaknesses of their existing PPP programs. They are, therefore, looking for ways to assess the massive, sudden, and unprecedented impacts of the COVID-19 pandemic on PPP projects and (sub)national programs. More specifically, "a new model to exercise or simulate all phases of multiagency disaster management" is needed, "based on real scenarios, to find out strengths and weaknesses of [their PPP] organizations and to improve … access to all resources" [4] (p. 4). This article thus offers a conceptual triage framework for PPP programs. Borrowing from medical and business triage procedures, we outline several triage heuristics for PPP practitioners. We begin by briefly describing the concept of medical triage. Next, we discuss how medical triage models have been adapted by the private sector into decision-making frameworks. Then, we use both medical and business triage approaches as a template for conceptualizing a PPP triage framework. After reflecting on additional considerations for PPP triage actions, we ultimately conclude by encouraging PPP stakeholders to collectively craft win–win solutions for post-pandemic recovery efforts.

2. Medical Triage

Medical triage involves identifying and sorting people most urgently in need of care. Adopted from battlefield medicine, triage procedures assess a patient's health status to determine their relative priority for treatment. In practice, triage is reserved for situations (e.g., wars, natural disasters, pandemics, etc.) when both supplies and staff are limited and care must be rationed [5]. In medical settings, injured or ill patients are typically categorized into various treatment groups based on need and urgency. These groupings generally use the following color scheme to identify priority levels:

1. Blue: patients not in need of urgent medical attention or hospitalization;
2. Green: patients with minor injuries or illnesses (i.e., "walking wounded");
3. Yellow: more serious cases whose lives are not yet threatened;
4. Red: those who will die without immediate treatment, and
5. Black: a fifth category reserved for the deceased, or those with no chance of survival [5,6].

With so many patients becoming critical ill simultaneously, many countries have found it impossible to meet the unprecedented healthcare demands of the COVID-19 pandemic [7]. This has forced doctors to make excruciating triage decisions on who to treat [8]. Although some scholars, such as Ouyang, Argon, and Ziya [9], have recently developed mathematical modeling and analysis techniques to improve intensive care unit (ICU) allocation decisions during periods of high patient demand, many of these triage decisions are often based on heuristics (e.g., age, comorbidities, etc.), which value "saving people with the greatest chance of short-term survival, followed by saving those who, thanks to a relative lack of coexisting conditions, have the greatest chance of long-term survival" [7] (p. 1875); see also [10]. When faced with such ethical dilemmas, many scenarios "will still feel morally untenable, particularly in the face of heightened prognostic uncertainty" and resource scarcity [7] (p. 1875). Nevertheless, rationing is often required in the direst circumstances. The COVID-19 pandemic is no exception. King and Kissoon [11] (p. 1794) stress that, "while research during pandemics is fraught with many obstacles, we must be courageous" and test triage models when the opportunity presents.

3. Business Triage

Over time, medical triage approaches have been adapted by the private sector into decision-making frameworks. These frameworks help businesses prioritize organizational goals and resource allocation. In global disasters like the COVID-19 pandemic, business enterprises must face "difficult decisions with regard to allocating limited resources between multiple 'mission-critical' functions" [12] (p. 21). In such times of crisis, business triage methodologies offer a simplified means of decision making based on objective, evidence-based criteria. Using similar categories employed by military and disaster–medical services—i.e., red (essential/critical), yellow (important/urgent), and green (optional/supportive)—these models identify tiers of service/operational criticality for the long-term health of a company. Crises force businesses to prioritize their essential/critical (red) expenses and relieve obvious "pain points" plaguing the organization. Once these "urgent care" needs are stabilized, other important (yellow) functions can be addressed, followed by auxiliary/supportive capabilities [13]. To determine relative organizational priorities, triage determinations will typically involve:

1. centralized decision making for consistency, speed, and decisiveness;
2. cataloging sources of funds (e.g., cash, lines of credit, equity infusions, etc.);
3. rapidly identifying economic scenarios;
4. modeling projected impacts;
5. defining non-negotiables (i.e., essential/critical functions);
6. drawing on available levers of leadership (expense reductions; hiring freezes, etc.);
7. determining immediate actions to take [14].

Accepted and understood throughout the organization, these triage procedures ultimately promote business continuity during rapidly evolving and unpredictable events. By identifying the sickest "patients" (i.e., processes) first and quickly stabilizing them, businesses can then prioritize other urgent operations that will need more planning and resources to fix [15].

4. Public–Private Partnership (PPP) Triage: A Conceptual Framework

Taken together, both medical and business triage processes offer a useful template for conceptualizing a PPP triage framework in the COVID-19 epoch. Because the likelihood of widespread PPP project failures is all but inevitable, governments will soon face the difficult and unenviable task of triaging PPP projects in their (sub)national programs so they can maximize project survival and kickstart national recovery efforts. Such a "mass-casualty event" will require rapid assessment of the "current health" of PPP projects to determine if they are in a terminal downward trajectory or show signs of resuscitation and recovery.

In this assessment process, government institutions (i.e., PPP units, ministries of finance, treasury units, and other line ministries) may find themselves in almost the same situation as hospital ICUs, facing critical shortages of funding, financing, and material resources to keep their projects functioning. Governments facing such constraints should thus develop "several triage heuristics policies that can potentially be used in practice" [9] (p. 592). For instance, a sophisticated and objective PPP triage system might begin by separating current PPP projects (and candidate projects) into the following categories (see Table 1).

Table 1. Public–Private Partnership (PPP) Triage Framework.

Triage Code	Criteria	Action or Priority
Blue	Project without a need for economic stimulus	Periodically (re)assess project key performance indicators (KPIs)
Green	Project experiencing minor financial/economic losses	Closely monitor project KPIs for early signs of project distress/default
Yellow	Project needs temporary/stop-gap support or restructuring	Explore contractual renegotiation procedures and other conciliation mechanisms
Red	Project will not survive without significant economic relief	Evaluate existing government guarantees and other opportunities for economic resuscitation
Black	Project cannot survive, even with government intervention	Prepare for contract termination and/or buyout procedures

To illustrate, take, for example, the LBJ-managed lanes in Texas. This PPP recorded a 20 percent traffic drop in March due to the COVID-19 pandemic. However, Ferrovial (the private concessionaire) still recorded growth in both revenues and EBITDA across its toll road division. This stronger-than-expected performance led Moody's to revise its outlook on the LBJ PPP from positive to stable and reaffirm its Baa3 rating despite uncertainty about the project's traffic and revenue recovery [16]. Because the liquidity of the PPP is also expected to remain strong, this project would likely be coded in the triage framework as "blue" and only need to be periodically (re)assessed.

A similar performance assessment could also be applied to airport PPPs affected by the COVID-19 pandemic. For instance, passenger numbers at Heathrow Airport have declined by 18.3 percent, and both revenues and EBITDA have fallen 12.7 percent and 22.4 percent, respectively. However, since Heathrow "has the necessary resources to continue operating for at least the next 12 months even in the absence of passengers[,] this PPP would be initially coded as "green" (i.e., experiencing minor financial/economic losses) but potentially reclassified as "yellow" if signs of project distress and/or potential default persist [16].

Finally, the COVID-19 pandemic is exacerbating problems plaguing transit projects like the $2 billion Purple Line light-rail PPP in Maryland. Already 976 days—more than $2\frac{1}{2}$ years—behind schedule and $755 million (i.e., 37 percent) over budget, Purple Line Transit Constructors (i.e., the joint-venture between Fluor, Lane Construction Corp. and Traylor Bros) is now threatening to walk away from the 36-year PPP. Efforts are currently underway to save this code "red" project, but a failed settlement could add up to a year to the project's schedule, cost millions more, and end in a protracted legal battle. If the parties are going to find a resolution, all will likely need to share in the sacrifice. However, this prospect comes at a particularly bad time for government budgets suffering from tax revenue losses due to the pandemic [17]. Without any relief or new significant funding from Maryland's Department of Transportation, this PPP may ultimately have to be re-triaged as "black" and prepared for contract termination.

Overall, governments (in conjunction with private sector counterparties, consultants, etc.) could begin using this conceptual PPP triage framework to label each "patient" (i.e., project) by sector or specific service offered, develop preliminary damage assessment records (see, e.g., FEMA [18]), identify project triage priorities for economic mitigation, track triage statuses, and identify additional risks associated with context-specific political, economic, and social factors. Categorizing desired outcomes/goals using such a PPP triage model would ultimately ensure limited resource allocation support and maintain national recovery goals.

5. Additional Considerations for PPP Triage Actions

Naturally, the utility of any PPP triage framework for decision making, goal prioritization, and resource allocation will depend on a country's institutional capacity and surrounding PPP-enabling environment [19,20]. Governments should thus consider launching and sustaining a crisis command center to effectively triage PPP projects [14]. Within this center, one of the first and most important tasks is to separate PPP specialists providing "care" for projects from those making triage decisions. A "triage officer", backed by a team with expertise in PPP preparation, procurement, and management, would make resource allocation decisions and communicate them within their PPP unit, ministry of finance, treasury unit, or other line ministry overseeing a country's (sub)national PPP program. Using revised and recalibrated Value for Money (VfM) assessments, Public Sector Comparators (PSCs), and other PPP screening tools, this triage team would provide economic and commercial rationales for triage decisions rather than quick fixes based on political headwinds. These decisions would then be reviewed regularly by a centralized (sub)national-level monitoring committee to ensure other factors, such as "People First PPP" considerations, project sustainability, and resilience, are given weight in decisions to rescue current PPP projects and reprioritize procurements for future PPPs [21]. Such oversight and governance will ensure countries do not mortgage their futures for ill-conceived, short-term recovery actions.

Finally, the triage framework should be reviewed regularly, as knowledge about the impacts of the pandemic evolves [7]. In this phase, governments may revisit commitments to Sustainable Development Goals (SDGs), see how the pandemic has affected them, and recalibrate national development strategies accordingly. Governments may also wish to (re)consider unsolicited proposals for stalled PPP program initiatives, (re)evaluate the resilience of PPPs to force majeure events, and develop short-, medium- and long-term solutions that strike a balance between investing in the future and reducing costs to survive [22,23]. Overall, post-pandemic recovery efforts should produce new PPP policy guidance and sector-specific models "that may respond, in a logical, consistent, and consultative way, to inevitable changes in policy and the market" [24] (p. 19).

6. Conclusions

Although the "point at which preparedness dissolves into panic will always be context-dependent … the best outcome of this pandemic would be being accused of having overprepared" [7] (p. 1875). Governments will thus need to begin carrying out extensive and systematic triage assessments of their (sub)national PPPs in order to mitigate the impacts of the COVID-19 pandemic. This article offers an initial conceptualization of PPP triage processes, but hard and decisive decisions still need to be made on both current and planned PPP projects. If PPPs are going to be a central tool for national economic recovery efforts, "trust, shared vision and long-term commitments" are needed so "contracting parties [can] change their adversarial relationships to a more cooperative, team-based approach" [25] (p. 441); see also [26]. Through cooperation, openness, and innovation, PPP stakeholders can collectively craft win–win incentives that maximize opportunities in the face of shared risks [27].

Overall, "[d]ue to the complexity, intensity, and frequency of complex disasters, global leaders in healthcare, government, and business will need to pivot from siloed approaches of decision-making to embrace multidisciplinary and transdisciplinary levels of cooperation" [28] (p. 3838). Doing so will fundamentally change the way transportation, transit, school, and hospital PPPs are designed and operated. Although "a lot of projects have been able to continue, and some, such as hospitals and schools, have even been accelerated[,]" governments still need to provide relief to struggling projects to get them through this tough time [29]. After all, "[p]erfect is the enemy of good, especially during crises when prompt action is required" [14]. Moving forward, much more work still needs to be done to combat COVID-19 and prepare for the next pandemic. Let us not repeat the same mistakes. Instead, let us challenge the complacency of construction management research, "engage in more robust critique and analysis of construction systems, as they are realised in practice[,]" and develop sustainable, resilient, and future-proofed PPPs [30] (p. 1).

Author Contributions: The authors confirm contribution to the paper as follows: conceptualization (D.B. and C.B.C.); writing—original draft preparation (D.B.); writing—review and editing (C.B.C). All authors have read and agreed to the published version of the manuscript.

Funding: Article processing charges (APCs) for open access publication were covered by UCL's Open Access Team. No other external funding was received for this research.

Conflicts of Interest: The authors declare no conflict of interest.

References

1. Inframation. *US P3 Market Summary|May 2020*; Inframation—An Acuris Company: New York, NY, USA, 2020.
2. American Association of State Highway and Transportation Officials (AASHTO). State DOTs Feeling the Budgetary Impact of COVID-19. 2020. Available online: https://aashtojournal.org/2020/04/24/state-dots-feeling-the-budgetary-impact-of-covid-19/ (accessed on 25 May 2020).
3. Casady, C.B.; Geddes, R.R. Asset Recycling for Social Infrastructure in the United States. *Public Works Manag. Policy* **2020**, *25*, 281–297. [CrossRef]
4. Khorram-Manesh, A. Flexible surge capacity–public health, public education, and disaster management. *Health Promot. Perspect.* **2020**, *10*, 1–5.
5. Harbaugh, K. The Next, Terrible Phase of This Crisis|After Cancellation Comes Triage. 2020. Available online: https://www.theatlantic.com/ideas/archive/2020/03/after-cancellation-comes-triage/608146/ (accessed on 25 May 2020).
6. Barfod, C.; Danker, J.; Forberg, J.; Lauritzen, M.M. The distribution of triage categories and the impact of emergency symptoms and signs on the triage level. *Scand. J. Trauma Resusc. Emerg. Med.* **2010**, *18*, 34. [CrossRef]
7. Rosenbaum, L. Facing Covid-19 in Italy—Ethics, logistics, and therapeutics on the epidemic's front line. *N. Engl. J. Med.* **2020**, *382*, 1873–1875. [CrossRef]
8. Romeo, N. The Grim Ethical Dilemma of Rationing Medical Care, Explained|How Hospitals Decide Which Covid-19 Patients to Prioritize When Resources Are Scarce. 2020. Available online: https://www.vox.com/coronavirus-covid19/2020/3/31/21199721/coronavirus-covid-19-hospitals-triage-rationing-italy-new-york (accessed on 25 May 2020).

9.   Ouyang, H.; Argon, N.T.; Ziya, S. Allocation of intensive care unit beds in periods of high demand. *Oper. Res.* **2020**, *68*, 591–608. [CrossRef]

10. Farrohknia, N.; Castrén, M.; Ehrenberg, A.; Lind, L.; Oredsson, S.; Jonsson, H.; Asplund, K.; Göransson, K.E. Emergency department triage scales and their components: A systematic review of the scientific evidence. *Scand. J. Trauma Resusc. Emerg. Med.* **2011**, *19*, 42. [CrossRef] [PubMed]

11. King, M.A.; Kissoon, N. Triage during pandemics: Difficult choices when business as usual is not an ethically defensible option. *Crit. Care Med.* **2016**, *44*, 1793–1795. [CrossRef] [PubMed]

12. Moore, B.; Bone, E.A. Decision-making in crisis: Applying a healthcare triage methodology to business continuity management. *J. Bus. Contin. Emerg. Plan.* **2017**, *11*, 21–26.

13. Small Business Network (SBN). A Triage Approach to Operational Efficiency. 2017. Available online: https://www.sbnonline.com/article/triage-approach-operational-efficiency/ (accessed on 23 May 2020).

14. Renjen, P. The Heart of Resilient Leadership: Responding to COVID-19. 2020. Available online: https://www2.deloitte.com/us/en/insights/economy/covid-19/heart of resilient-leadership-responding-to-covid-19.html (accessed on 28 May 2020).

15. Cerocke, S. How to Conduct a Business Process Triage. 2015. Available online: https://ncet.org/how-to-conduct-a-business-process-triage/ (accessed on 26 May 2020).

16. Fabrizio, A. *Ferrovial 1Q20 Toll Road Revenue Up Despite COVID-19*; Inframation—An Acuris Company: New York, NY, USA, 2020.

17. Shaver, K. Maryland Likely to Be on the Hook for Millions If It Wants to Save the Purple Line Project, Analysts Say. 2020. Available online: https://www-washingtonpost-com.cdn.ampproject.org/c/s/www.washingtonpost.com/local/trafficandcommuting/maryland-likely-to-be-on-the-hook-for-millions-if-it-wants-to-save-the-purple-line-project-analysts-say/2020/06/12/29b40dda-ab39-11ea-a9d9-a81c1a491c52_story.html?outputType=amp (accessed on 14 June 2020).

18. Federal Emergency Management Agency (FEMA). *PDA Pocket Guide*; FEMA: Washington, DC, USA, 2020.

19. Casady, C.B.; Eriksson, K.; Levitt, R.E.; Scott, W.R. (Re) defining public-private partnerships (PPPs) in the new public governance (NPG) paradigm: An institutional maturity perspective. *Public Manag. Rev.* **2020**, *22*, 161–183. [CrossRef]

20. Casady, C.B. Examining the institutional drivers of Public-Private Partnership (PPP) market performance: A fuzzy set Qualitative Comparative Analysis (fsQCA). *Public Manag. Rev.* **2020**, 1–25. [CrossRef]

21. United Nations Economic Commission for Europe (UNECE). *"What are People-First PPPs?"*; UNECE International Center of Excellence: Geneva, Switzerland, 2019.

22. Baxter, D.; Casady, C.B. Proactive and Strategic Healthcare Public-Private Partnerships (PPPs) in the Coronavirus (Covid-19) Epoch. *Sustainability* **2020**, *12*, 5097. [CrossRef]

23. Gulati, R.; Nohria, N.; Wohlgezogen, F. Roaring out of Recession. 2010. Available online: https://hbr.org/2010/03/roaring-out-of-recession (accessed on 28 May 2020).

24. Farquharson, E.; Torres de Mastle, C.; Yescombe, E.R.; Encinas, J. *How to Engage with the Private Sector in Public-Private Partnerships in Emerging Markets*; World Bank: Washington, DC, USA, 2011.

25. Weston, D.C.; Gibson, G.E., Jr. Partnering-project performance in US Army Corps of Engineers. *J. Manag. Eng.* **1993**, *9*, 410–425. [CrossRef]

26. Henisz, W.J.; Levitt, R.E.; Scott, W.R. Toward a unified theory of project governance: Economic, sociological and psychological supports for relational contracting. *Eng. Project Organ. J.* **2012**, *2*, 37–55. [CrossRef]

27. Crowley, L.G.; Karim, M.A. Conceptual model of partnering. *J. Manag. Eng.* **1995**, *11*, 33–39. [CrossRef]

28. Goniewicz, K.; Khorram-Manesh, A.; Hertelendy, A.J.; Goniewicz, M.; Naylor, K.; Burkle, F.M. Current Response and Management Decisions of the European Union to the COVID-19 Outbreak: A Review. *Sustainability* **2020**, *12*, 3838. [CrossRef]

29. Gismondi, A. P3 Projects Moving Ahead Despite Pandemic, Some Accelerated. 2020. Available online: https://canada.constructconnect.com/dcn/news/projects/2020/05/p3-projects-moving-ahead-despite-pandemic-some-accelerated (accessed on 1 June 2020).

30. Sherratt, F.; Sherratt, S.; Ivory, C. Challenging complacency in construction management research: The case of PPPs. *Constr. Manag. Econ.* **2020**, 1–15. [CrossRef]

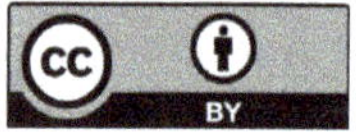

MDPI

St. Alban-Anlage 66

4052 Basel

Switzerland

Tel. +41 61 683 77 34

Fax +41 61 302 89 18

www.mdpi.com

Sustainability Editorial Office

E-mail: sustainability@mdpi.com

www.mdpi.com/journal/sustainability